Discipline of Nursing

Series Editor
Bruno Salgues

Discipline of Nursing

Three-time Knowledge

Michel Nadot

iSTE

WILEY

First published 2020 in Great Britain and the United States by ISTE Ltd and John Wiley & Sons, Inc.

ISTE Ltd
27-37 St George's Road
London SW19 4EU
UK

www.iste.co.uk

John Wiley & Sons, Inc.
111 River Street
Hoboken, NJ 07030
USA

www.wiley.com

Library of Congress Control Number: 2020942263

British Library Cataloguing-in-Publication Data
A CIP record for this book is available from the British Library
ISBN 978-1-78630-429-2

MIX
Paper from responsible sources
FSC® C013604

Contents

Foreword

Nurses are searching for what characterizes the nursing discipline or the nursing sciences. Publications as well as conferences have been held around the world with the aim of specifying the purpose of the discipline. However, there is no consensus on the subject. What is nursing knowledge made of? What are the foundations of the discipline, what is its purpose and what is its scientific identity?

This book by Michel Nadot provides concrete answers to the questions raised. Nadot proposes an epistemological analysis of the three phases of nursing knowledge in a unique way by following a historical chronology. Drawing on his long experience as a writer, he is keen to present the traditions of our languages and their influences on knowledge and, consequently, on the nursing discipline. Through his research as a philosopher and nurse, he proposes an innovative schematization of nursing knowledge and takes up his conceptual model in nursing sciences (health mediology) conceived through his empirical research as an alternative to the name "nursing sciences".

This book entitled *The Discipline of Nursing – Three-time Knowledge* is Michel Nadot's masterpiece, which is composed of three main parts. This volume focuses on the foundations of the discipline, a subject little discussed in Europe and the Middle East. His style of writing, the structure of the text and the illustrations provided, followed by proposals for the development of the discipline, add to the maturity of this book, which is reflected in the pleasure of an enjoyable reading, reinforced by the "image feedback" and a summary of the key ideas at the end of each part.

Nadot's involvement in his work is that of a nurse who is both a historian and a philosopher at the same time, who tries to demonstrate in his book that the nursing discipline was built up chronologically in three stages: lay knowledge, which was documented as early as the 14th Century, protodisciplinary knowledge as early as the middle of the 19th Century, and finally scientific knowledge as early as the last third of the 20th Century.

In the first chapter of his book, Nadot argues that caring or caregiving is a three-dimensional field that gives rise to the first languages from traditions and by extracting experience and nursing practice. The basic triptych of the nursing discipline has its origins in lay knowledge: *Domus* (care environment)–*Familia* (family)–*Hominem* (person), and is at the center of a three-dimensional field of competences "*Domus–Familia–Hominem*", which, according to Nadot, constitutes the foundation of the nursing discipline on which new knowledge and new roles will be superimposed.

Then, in the second part of his work, appears *protodisciplinary knowledge*. During this period, two distinct training models proposed by two great women marked the formalization of nursing knowledge. The first model was developed in Switzerland thanks to Valérie de Gasparin, discovered by Michel Nadot, who created the "school-hospital[1]" training model, and the second in England with Florence Nightingale, known throughout the world and who in turn created the "hospital-school[2]" training model. These two training models have influenced many schools around the world.

In the third chapter of his book, Nadot shows through his multiple publications that the nursing discipline was born implicitly with reference to the medical sciences; however, it is, in fact, situated in the humanities. He insists by saying that in the game of science, scientists are the only people to produce knowledge in order to obtain recognition, including recognition of the discipline in question. In this scientific part of knowledge, Nadot situates himself as an epistemologist, who aims to understand the origin of nursing sciences and the world in which the knowledge of the nursing discipline and its problematic identity develops.

According to Nadot, it seems that clinical research is more developed at the expense of basic nursing research. This is due, according to him, to the valorization of the practical side of the profession at the expense of nursing theory and research.

However, Nadot adds that nurses' access to university has provided access to scientific language and methods, as well as to research and epistemological thinking, which constitute a pillar of recognition for the nursing discipline. It is therefore incumbent on nurses, researchers and university professors to take responsibility for

1 Where the hospital depends on the school on a geographical, administrative and financial basis.

2 An opposing model to the previous, where the school depends on the hospital on a geographical, administrative and financial basis.

the direction of our discipline, because the profession is in crisis and does not seem to be able to rely on legislation or its theorists to get out of it. According to Nadot, only basic research, which has long been absent from nursing faculties, will be able to do a conceptual and historical clean-up, revise our linguistic codes and produce knowledge specific to our discipline. This will create a paradigm shift that will allow disciplinary identity to be enhanced.

Several factors will contribute to this conceptual clean-up. According to Nadot, the fact of being part of a reflexive science, or rather I would say a "reflexive practitioner" attitude, of taking a distance, having a critical look to examine the existing knowledge, not only at the individual level but also at the collective level, from experience, from the historical roots of our profession, as well as through the destructuring and restructuring of our traditions, allows us to better propagate and value nursing knowledge. Hence, the role of universities to train nursing students who are not only called upon to acquire specific knowledge and know-how, but also who must prepare themselves to have a reflexive attitude and research, analysis and questioning skills in order to bring about the emergence of a disciplinary "green knowledge". This "green knowledge" is demonstrated in this book.

Nadot's book proposes a very original schematization of the aggregation of knowledge where disciplinary "green knowledge" forms the core of practical knowledge and is immersed in a cultural environment represented by institutional culture, healthcare culture and medical culture. According to Nadot, it should not be denied that the knowledge emanating from these three cultures is developing in such a way that it gradually comes to the moor, and masks the "green ball" at the origin of fundamental knowledge. Hence, the problem of disciplinary visibility that only basic research on the elements of the discipline, namely the environment (*Domus*), care, health and the individual/family (*Familia/Hominem*), enriches nursing knowledge. It is a matter of proving that nursing is not only a collection of knowledge borrowed from other disciplines, particularly medicine and humanities, but also that it has a distinct identity. Thus, the schematization would be more harmonious by constructing a knowledge that places the human being at the center and in continuous interaction with a changing healthcare environment.

In this book, Nadot sheds light on several factors, highlighting that our nursing science has not reached the same level compared to other existing sciences. According to him, it is a question of the female status of the profession, and the evolution of this status in our societies at different rates of development of scientific research. However, for a discipline to develop, it must be neutral, exclusive of gender, consistent and must reflect the world it came from. For Karl Popper [POP 85], for example, a discipline can only claim the status of a scientific discipline if it produces falsifiable statements, that is, statements that are capable, in the form of testable hypotheses, of being subjected to the test of experimentation.

Nadot's book is one of the European reference works that calls on the reflexivity of nursing researchers, teachers, managers and theorists from North America, Europe, Africa and the Middle East to formulate, based on their theories and scientific statements, hypotheses that are supposed to be subjected to experimentation with the aim of attaining a consensual construction of a scientific status for the nursing discipline in the 21st Century. Let us thus take advantage of the globalization of nursing knowledge to develop a disciplinary identity that takes into account the influence of the demographic, political, economic, scientific, social, regulatory, cultural and technological environment of a constantly changing healthcare environment.

This is what makes this book innovative, a true disciplinary revolution, a call for a major paradigmatic change or better, a real conceptual clean-up to come. It calls for the construction of a clear status for the discipline, a distinct professional identity and a scientific discipline that only increases the credibility of the nursing profession, as well as the confidence of other healthcare professionals and, above all, of all the beneficiaries of the services provided by nurses in response to ever-increasing healthcare needs.

Finally, I conclude with Bachelard [BAC 83] who said that nothing is self-evident. Nothing is given, everything is built. This is the case with this book. So let us demystify and overcome the nursing myth that we currently know and build together the nursing sciences of the 21st Century!

Rima SASSINE KAZAN
Dean of the Faculty of Nursing
Saint-Joseph University of Beirut, Lebanon
August 2020

Preface

Female caregivers[1], and with them their knowledge or their own discipline, are still epistemologically subject to a historical cultural domination imposed at the end of the 18th Century. Nurses have few historians. Others took it upon themselves to write their own history. As the narrator of the Howard Zinn film about American popular history would say, "Until the rabbits have a historian, the story will be told by the hunters". Can we get rid of the cliché? Of course, it is up to the discipline and its members (the rabbits) to appropriate their history and define its object. However, as Gélis pointed out, "historians of health practices were for a long time doctors anxious to write the past of their profession; the helpers, the guards, the caretakers, were in their eyes only auxiliaries. The humble, everyday life; this was not… history!" [GÉL 88]. This may partly explain why nursing professors did not take ownership of the history of their knowledge from the very beginning. As a nurse, health executive or researcher, it is not common to study history. Who would fund such studies? Why not, however, try to expose the knowledge of the past, notably by publishing this book, in order to identify what our spaces of speech and language traditions are made of? "After all, why should we deny the right of the members of a profession to take up their past for themselves, as long as they meet the requirements of historical research?" [GÉL 88].

The role and conditions favoring the emergence of the history of knowledge within the nursing profession are not always well perceived and understood, as they are difficult to access. It did not all start with Florence Nightingale! Retrieving traces of daily care presents many difficulties for the nurse historian engaged in

1 Women have always been predominantly represented in the care world. Today, they still represent the majority of professionals in practice. On average, between 7% and 11% of the profession's members are men, depending on the source or country.

research. These traces, too ordinary to constitute scholarly heritage, have eluded health historians until recently. Before being able to describe and interpret the world that was theirs, women caregivers were linguistically colonized by dominant cultures. In order: church, medicine and the military (Red Cross). As Gérard Noiriel rightly points out, "one of the essential forms of domination in history was between those who had the power to describe and interpret the world through writing and those who had only oral language" [NOI 18].

Writing has status, and to write about nursing requires access to the legitimate places of knowledge production (e.g. university) and a cultural understanding of professional practices and the environment in which they are practiced. According to Marrou, "in order to know its purpose, the historian must have in his personal culture, in the very structure of his mind, the psychological affinities that will allow him to imagine, feel and understand the feelings of the past that he will find in the documents" [MAR 54].

Precisely in terms of personal culture, it may be relevant to describe the main stages, given the rather atypical profile of my educational and professional background. I was born under the bombing of the town of Montbéliard (France) in preparation for its liberation during the offensive of Marshal de Lattre de Tassigny between November 14 and 17, 1944. After technical training at the Peugeot Automobiles Apprenticeship School and several months of practice in this national company, I left my home region for a complete change of air and orientation. I couldn't breathe! Being subservient to machines and workshop managers was not really meant to please.

It was then the restart of a training cycle. After training as a psychiatric nurse in French-speaking Switzerland and several years of care practice as a nurse in various hospital institutions, followed by two to three years of management practice as a nursing executive, followed by more than 30 years of teaching practice and 10 years of scientific research practice at the *Haute école de santé de Fribourg* (Freiburg's Higher School of Health), my experience seems to be well diversified to be able to talk about it. After having climbed one by one up the ladder from primary school to post-doctorate, it is as a professor of nursing that my interest in studying the history and epistemology of this as yet little-known discipline developed.

These lived experiences allow this somewhat naive explorer to open paths. Without having really programmed it, I find myself in new avenues with the feeling of being the "first" under different horizons. Being the "first" male nurse, a lay graduate in a Catholic hospital in the Swiss Jura region run by the Sisters of Saint Martha of Beaune, the "first" lay director of care in a small hospital on the Neuchâtel coast run by Protestant deaconess sisters, the "first" professor of history[2] and epistemology in nursing sciences in French-speaking Switzerland, the "first" teacher with a doctorate in a nursing school that was not yet a university level school at the time, the "first" professor at the *Haute école de santé de Fribourg* to have the status of associate professor in foreign nursing faculties (Canada, Lebanon), the "first" historian to bring the founder of the world's first school of nursing out of the shadows (Valérie de Gasparin) and, finally, the "first" man to appear alongside major theorists of the nursing discipline on the websites of some North American nursing faculties, it is easy to understand why I keep traces in my memory that will help me grasp history. Without forgetting the fact that I am the first author of a conceptual model in nursing that is the "first" in French-speaking Europe. This model identified by researchers in the discipline in North America aroused a few curiosities. Since 2005, I have also been in charge of a network of researchers in the field of health and social work at the regional level, and with a post-doctorate in "Higher education and research policies" (*Ecole polytechnique fédérale de Lausanne* – EPFL), I can now take on the challenges of scientific research. Add, on a more personal level, two marriages, four children and twenty-six moves, and you can understand why I sometimes feel dizzy on this atypical, completely unexpected and yet well-filled career path. This "first" part, which goes off the beaten track and which seeks not only to escape from its main starting determinisms, but, above all, to understand where this incessant desire to know comes from, is really not to displease in the end.

I also discovered that it is not through the history of language traditions that nursing research began. Aside from a few cleverly maintained myths, the results of research say little about the historical foundations of the knowledge that constitutes the discipline today. The nursing discipline, situated in the human order in terms of science, is struggling to go beyond its ordinary social representations and its own myths to construct its specific knowledge and give it a name.

Focusing on what is now known as "nursing knowledge", "nursing discipline" or "nursing sciences", this book deals with a subject little discussed in the literature, particularly in Europe. Each of the three parts ends with a short critical analysis of the knowledge presented (image feedback). This image feedback is a kind of self-reflexivity on the content and context of knowledge emergence.

Several excerpts from this book are based on the author's doctoral thesis [NAD 93], especially the unpublished passages. Also included are the results and reports of scientific research financed by the Swiss National Science Foundation (SNF) and developed since 1999 by the Health Mediology Laboratory of the Fribourg University

2 At a time when the first word-processing typewriters heralded the arrival of the first computers.

of Applied Sciences (HES-SO)[3]. First-hand documents from partially published empirical research [NAD 12b, NAD 13] are also used, supplemented by a series of reflections published since 1982 and numerous scientific conferences held on several continents between 2000 and 2016.

Drawing inspiration from a diagram of the development of fundamental knowledge with reference to the philosophy of science (Figures 11.2 and 11.7), I believe that I can verify, through a succession of questions, whether the increase in knowledge reveals a thought process that has "as a starting point and as a term, the formulation of problems that are ever more fundamental and whose fruitfulness continues to increase, giving rise to other problems that are as yet unpublished" [POP 85]. Not only is an understanding of the language tradition a necessary condition for innovation, but also the knowledge carried by several concepts worked on as needs and questions arise makes it possible to envisage a reality that goes from the macroscopic to the microscopic. These concepts serve to delimit the object of the study carried out within the researcher's specific discipline and practice, and drive the dynamics of the research. They have analytical value while delimiting both the object of the research and the disciplinary field concerned. They allow the object of the study to be treated from authoritative sources of knowledge found in what Popper calls the "third world" or what he calls "objective knowledge" [POP 91].

This book is primarily intended for nursing students, their professors and researchers involved in the development of the discipline. Although indirectly concerned, nurses in healthcare settings are also likely to be interested in this book, if only out of curiosity. It is also intended to contribute to the nascent academic debate on nursing knowledge, its origins, the discipline, nursing science, its existence, its orientations, its identity or the reasons for the indifference it arouses. How is the term "discipline" represented in the healthcare environment and why do the advancement of nursing science and its theories remain inaudible in the scientific community, the media, politics and the economy despite the efforts invested in this endeavor?

Michel NADOT
August 2020

3 This will exist for about 10 years (1999–2009), directed by the author.

Introduction

At present, there are very few books on the foundations of the nursing discipline[1] and the progressive construction of its knowledge. Most of those that do exist start from the nursing reform carried out by Florence Nightingale, who, presented at the time as a pioneer (the English aristocratic heroine), found herself projected onto the nursing scene as the one who brought about the knowledge of care through spontaneous generation of knowledge. Yet care has been provided for a long time and long before Florence Nightingale's entry into the hospital scene. Nursing practices and their knowledge did not wait until the middle of the 19th Century to exist. However, there is not much in common between Florence Nightingale's social status and that of the hospital maids and governesses of the 19th Century. A good example of this is the prominent image of the English heroine Florence Nightingale or a confessional past of "nuns" among the caretakers. The emergence and foundations of the discipline of care are much more complex than this, and the role

1 There are a multitude of ways to approach the notion of discipline. The place of language traditions in the constitution of a discipline must be taken into account and allows us to see the discipline as "a historically rooted articulation of composite elements that can make sense in a sustainable way and constitute a rational instance of knowledge" [BER 04]. However, the notion of discipline "is irremediably associated with the development of the university, of which it is an organizing principle" [FAB 13]. Today, it is known that the "epistemological analysis of the theoretical bases of nursing science shows the anchoring points around which the body of scientific knowledge belonging to the discipline is organized and defines its object according to four concepts: environment, person, care and health" [DAL 08a]. For Pépin *et al.*, a discipline is also "a field of investigation and practice with a unique perspective or a distinct way of examining phenomena" [PÉP 10]. But we also know "that it is impossible to deal with the disciplinary question today without associating it with the political dimension of scientific activity. Discipline is an operation of domination before being a structure of knowledge production" [FAB 13].

played by French-speaking Switzerland in the emergence of the first schools for care workers should not be overlooked. Florence Nightingale did indeed exist, but we cannot understand her involvement in care if we do not place her thinking in the context of the time, and this in relation to Valérie de Gasparin-Boissier, the Swiss woman who founded the first school for care workers in the world and who, in terms of values, was both her forerunner and her rival. Just as it is difficult to understand the role of nuns and the Church in hospitals if we do not know why at one time the Catholic Church began to send its nuns to civilian hospitals to replace the lay personnel already in place or, as in Quebec, to develop healthcare institutions that were to be established in the wake of French colonization, so too is it difficult to understand the role of the sisters and the Church in hospitals.

Contrary to existing beliefs, the nursing profession does not have good nuns as forebearers and has no medical paternity from the outset. With practices sometimes almost similar to those of today, but in different contexts, the knowledge at work in lay hospitals in secular times cannot be called "nursing". The term nurse, moreover, is an exclusively religious term, as will be seen later, and belongs to the Catholic Church according to values proper to the ancient Scriptures. Why do the lay people still use it today?

NOTE.– The terms "*infirmière*" (i.e. "nurse" in French) and "*garde-malade*" (i.e. sick nurse in French) are neither synonymous, nor interchangeable and are rather historically in competition to qualify (the real!) professional care. Each term has its own history, and the latter does not tolerate mix-ups. It is not by chance, as Canadian nursing researchers point out, that the name to be given to future faculties of care poses a problem for rectors to gallicize the term *nursing* and illustrates "the difficulty of adequately translating the word *nursing*" [COH 02]. The difficulty is of the same order when it is necessary to explain the nature of the nursing discipline and to find a name for it.

Some nursing students, who are traditionally familiar with biomedical books or manuals and data sheets during their studies, are rarely required to obtain books that address the fundamentals of their discipline as is often the case in other academic disciplines. Moreover, there are very few critical works on the development of the discipline and its early theories. As Debout points out, "the English-language preponderance for scientific activities makes English the primary language of dissemination of the discipline's work. Nursing research often does not take into consideration existing disciplinary knowledge and theories, but prefers to borrow those of related disciplines". This, of course, has paradoxical consequences. "The professional group claims to be recognized in its singularity, but rejects a disciplinary content that seeks to establish this specific nursing perspective" [DEB 08].

Books on the history of nursing, women caregivers and the history of the profession are also available in bookstores. This history is sometimes local, with a short periodical time, rarely long term, as is the case with medicine, for example. Indeed, as Canadian historians note [BAT 05], "while medical historians trace the origin of their profession to Greek and Roman antiquity, nurses present a historical perspective with *nursing* dating back to Florence Nightingale" [BAT 05]. Before referring to Anglo-Protestant care models, we might wonder how care was provided in the ancient nations, for example, before the French colonists imposed a Franco-Catholic model on the Aboriginal or Métis populations, as well as on themselves. The Outaouais, Stadaconeans and other Hochelaguians were never asked about their pre-colonial conceptions of "caregiving". The questioning of the status of the nursing discipline was not on the agenda. "Little is known about the nature or extent of healthcare practices in the Amerindian nations" [COH 02]. This shortcut around Florence Nightingale and the values of the English aristocracy does not really help in understanding the foundations of the discipline of care and the construction of its identity. Care practices and their knowledge existed long before Florence Nightingale. With contemporary North American researchers systematically referring to the English heroine Florence Nightingale to mark the beginnings of the discipline of *nursing*, and a discipline that bears the name *nursing science*, we are still far from identifying the real foundations of the knowledge that underlies the discipline in question.

Why present a book that focuses on the history of knowledge within the nursing discipline rather than on its actors? Because this knowledge, like the discipline itself for that matter, continues to be inaudible. The actors are known, symbolically at least. What they know or what they experience is still sometimes a form of angelism. We certainly talk about nurses, but little about their discipline. Even in the era of nursing faculties, universities and doctorates in nursing, the discipline is still seen as something that allows nurses to do, in a general way, "a little bit of everything, anything and nothing special", as one Canadian nursing professor famously put it [ADA 79]. Admittedly, this formula does not really help the professional or scientist to build a unique identity through successive socializations, and does not really tell society what nurses bring to it in terms of skills and costs. The nurse is not an interchangeable pawn on the health chessboard. What is her own discipline made up of, what is the locus of discourse, what are its foundations, what is its purpose, what is its scientific identity and what is it used for?

The different types of knowledge produced within the discipline are fragmented knowledge, just like the places where knowledge is produced, without links between them, without an epistemological foundation that would be in continuity with the traditions of language. Without links between them, knowledge struggles to ensure its visibility. However, these fragmented parts of knowledge can still be linked to each other in a fragile way over the long term. The knowledge that guides practices is arranged in different layers of sedimentation. The separation between the layers is blurred and varies in time and space depending on the region of the globe. It should also be noted that the discipline is still orphaned in terms of identity. The research methodologies are multiple and the scientific frames of reference are also used. Knowledge is scattered and volatile, applied research, sometimes called "clinical" research, proliferates and basic research is at a standstill.

Should nursing research be exclusively at the service of the profession's four fields[2,3] of practice, or is it possible to envisage, for example, basic or free research for the nursing discipline? In the absence of basic research, we often have a partial picture of the nursing discipline. An overview and a homogeneous synthesis of knowledge built up over the long term is sorely lacking. Moreover, the vocabulary used has often been so mixed up in meaning that the origin, values and profile of the care professional (nurse) are not recognized today. This knowledge, produced and instrumented over the long term by groups with different value systems, as can be seen in Figure 13.1, does not always reveal its origins. A distinction must be made in terms of values between religious knowledge (French-Catholic or Anglo-Protestant) and lay knowledge. The activity at the Hôtel-Dieu differs from that of the civil hospital. The foundations of the discipline lie not in the natural sciences such as medicine, but within the human and social sciences. In the long term, the medical profession, since it has been authorized for practice in the hospital, often delegates new knowledge to nurses in order for them to develop advanced practices. However, each time advancement presupposes a higher requirement in terms of knowledge and not specialized knowledge specific to the discipline in order to clarify ordinary practice.

2 In order of appearance: 1) care practice, 2) teaching practice, 3) management practice, 4) research practice.

3 Practice is a human action that is controlled and guided by symbolic elements included in a cultural system (knowledge, values, ideologies). Practice, even if it is only healthcare practice, "is then a consequence of the translation and understanding of values into norms of action" [NAD 93].

PART 1

Lay Knowledge

1

Role of History

1.1. Lay knowledge

Lay knowledge is that which goes back to periods when a group of people used knowledge when that group did not yet exist as a corporation. It is knowledge that is not necessarily shared collectively and not yet standardized. People who needed this lay knowledge to carry out their occupations were not aware that they had common knowledge and shared it with others. They only did their work in conditions that were sometimes close to hospital slavery. There were still no schools and structured training in the age of lay knowledge. However, and this is an important discovery, those who performed their duties needed to pass on their knowledge to those who would replace them. Everyone was alone with the hospital managers of the time. The hospital governesses, maids and servants took an oath to perform their duties in exchange for a salary in kind and in cash. They mobilized tacit knowledge in action, domestic knowledge, knowledge necessary to run a household, take care of a family, mobilize knowledge related to the characteristics of gender, the woman, the mother, the governess and her servant or mistress of the house. In any case, there was a household to organize!

There were no new roles, new knowledge or modern nursing without reference to previous knowledge. Just as it is difficult to talk about advanced practice without knowing what ordinary practice consists of, we cannot value the role of Florence Nightingale without understanding why she suddenly appeared and was talked about in the mid-19th Century. There is always a before. There were treatments before her. The evolution of knowledge is always an improvement of previous knowledge. And this, even when the latter does not give rise to extraordinary words, to writing and its visibility. Ancient knowledge can even prove to be timeless. It is still part of the care practice. For example, practices of moving around in the hospital or collective hygiene practices have survived for centuries. They still prevail, and we can prove it. What has changed is the environment and the characteristics of the space in which we move. Lay knowledge is not to be contrasted with professional or scientific knowledge. It has simply not yet reached this stage of standardization and recognition. This was much earlier.

The knowledge of the age of lay knowledge was heterogeneous, disparate, vulgar, tacit and implicit. This knowledge had little to do with medicine. But it was in line with local knowledge of experience related to the exploitation of a domain, efforts to ensure survival and representations about health. We do not recognize them because we do not talk about them. Those who used this knowledge did not even exist. They had no status other than that of a servant conferred by the patricians of a city or the hospital's Board of Directors. An existence to be enjoyed in some way. Women had no existence in the medieval hospital. Yet there was no lack of work! Women were still excluded from collective identities in the age of lay knowledge. The most literate even found it difficult to publish under their real names. In fact, "the lay knowledge of healthcare was structured according to the history and culture of the group from which it originates" [DAL 08b]. It is modestly and with difficulty found in the category of women, domestic servants, housekeepers and hospital maids. However, it must be recognized that this is the group from which nursing originated. As you can see, we come from very far away!

Even at the level of hospital archives, it happens that the traces of domestic work were those of the working classes and maids, and no effort was made to list, classify and identify them. What was the point? Thus, we can sometimes find whole bundles of forgotten hospital parchments or books of accounts which concern precisely care in the secular period.

The sources of knowledge on aid to daily and institutional life are sometimes found abandoned under the stairs of a museum or in the civil defense shelters of a town hall, because there has not yet been time to inventory them. This is how, for example, the history of medicine comes before the history of knowledge about care.

However, let us recognize that there are certainly more medical historians than there are nursing historians. The research budget in nursing faculties on this topic is probably lower than the budget that has long been spent in history faculties for medicine.

1.2. A difficult history for an ordinary experience

The daily care routine can be both a lure and a necessary detour. You have to learn to navigate between the two. The lure lies in the fact that the perceptions, sensations and emotions of caregivers cannot be reached by today's historian. Servants who were both wives and servants did not write! Therefore, any projection into the past is to be forgotten. However, it is still interesting by this necessary detour to try to reconstruct their working world from the traces of their activity in the daily life of hospital care. The geographical space, the job descriptions and rules, the relationship with the powers in place, their living conditions, the capacities demanded in the use of care equipment, the relationship with things and people and the use of their work spaces at least allow us to question their living conditions, the knowledge required for their occupations and the reality of their careers.

During 1970–1980 or so, work on the history of the nursing profession gained momentum within the French-speaking community with the work of historians and/or anthropologists intrigued by traditions relating to the body, health, the dimensions of care and the practical and identity-related conditions of those who provided it. Marie-Françoise Collière, then professor at the *École internationale d'enseignement infirmier supérieur de Lyon*[1] (EIEIS), paved the way for reflection in 1982 by publishing a historical–anthropological work on care, a work that was noticed by the profession at the international level [COL 82]. Ten years later, she identified with great foresight the difficulties encountered by researchers in nursing sciences when they were interested in the history of their profession.

Restoring the professional group's memory is not a matter of course. The writings of women caregivers are indeed quite rare. They have an oral tradition and have not left many traces of their activity. "Either they are not introduced to writing or they are denied access to it so as not to write their own writings" [COL 92]. Not very initiated to writing, this is the case of those who were presented as governesses, servants, hospital maids under the *Ancien Régime*[2] and graduate nurses until the end of the 20th Century. We also know that historical sources relevant to the nursing profession and the history of women are not always kept in an official archive department. The public archives "were constituted by men on the actions of men; women only appear in the background, when they appear" [DIÉ 88]. Some hospital archives are rather difficult to access due to the lack of awareness of places of memory.

After the difficulties related to the sources of care practice, Collière also mentions the difficulties related to the subject itself. "Care belongs first and foremost to the history of daily life, of which it is one of the major components. Now, this daily experience is not spectacular; it is part of the mundane, the obvious, what is repeated, but which we cannot do without" [COL 92]. Any elucidation of the history of care practices risks threatening the status quo established within the

1 The school was closed in 1995.

2 The Ancien Régime in France was its political and social system from the Late Middle Ages until the French Revolution of 1789, which led to the abolition of hereditary monarchy and the feudal system of nobility.

discipline, because it is representative of the place and role assigned to women caregivers by institutional authorities. If the nurse thinks that she is working in the natural sciences (medicine), discovering that this is not the case and that her discipline is more in the humanities can destabilize the constructed identity. Moreover, for Collière, historical works do not reach "the deculturated mass of midwives, nurses who – with a few exceptions – are unaware of their publication, do not see the interest, do not feel concerned[3]. Moreover, this is not the concern of professional leaders who, for the most part, are unaware of history or fear its questions" [COL 92]. Nearly 30 years later, we can generally see that this statement still applies!

We can agree with some of the students' concerns. History does not really help to heal. But it has never displayed that purpose! Nor does it help to apply an ordinary healing technique. It does not help to master the knowledge and daily gestures necessary to take care of people who expect service from nurses. This disillusionment among some students taking a history course when they are impatient to discover their future place of work so that they can finally "be able to give injections or treatments", to use a cliché, means that the history resulting from fundamental research on the discipline does not provide them with any means of establishing their know-how. This is a fact. The impact of history has no relevance if the motivation to know the traditions of language and where one comes from is met with indifference or incomprehension.

On the contrary, history helps students to build an identity in order to position themselves among the many health professions. It allows them to emancipate themselves from the role attributed to them in the 18th Century by medicine and the ruling classes. "From the nurse's aide, whose subordinate tasks are defined with industrial precision, to the 'professional' nurse, who translates the doctor's prescriptions into tasks for nurses' aides, the status of nurses is that of uniformed servants in the service of dominant male professionals" [EHR 15]. We may agree with this view, but the word "domestic" perhaps deserves some attention. It had some value at the time it was introduced. It is then beneficial if the so-called domestic activity is seen as one that makes it possible, in the noble sense of the term, to take care of the life of the estate, the *Domus*, the house, the hospital, that is, of the living environment of care, of the languages required and of the first spaces of speech. Apart from this kind of representative alienation of women from domestic and free work, which is very present at the beginning of institutional *care*, it already

3 Collière seems to be speaking here more to history teachers in nursing schools than to the nurses themselves. In fact, most of the instructors of yesteryear (now educators) who taught the history of the profession in nursing schools and institutes in France, for example, were not, in general, researchers in history.

requires some spatio-temporal skills to understand the organization required for a collective household to function.

History is the mother of all human sciences, Michel Foucault told us [FOU 66]. This is an important statement for the nursing discipline. Nursing is concerned with the human being, and therefore belongs to the human sciences. Are today's doctors of the nursing sciences aware of this? Now, the history of our language traditions is part of the first research to be carried out in order to imagine an identity for our discipline. "It is indeed more important for a discipline to determine the identity of its knowledge than to question the identity of the people who refer to it" [NAD 12a]. One does not become a nurse before using knowledge of the same nature as the proclaimed identity. History clearly shows that the title "nurse" is a myth for lay people [NAD 12b]. It came into being before the conceptualization of knowledge took shape or before the "nursing metaparadigm" and its theories became known. At a time when charitable and welfare institutions are growing and common sense is mixing their values or ideologies at the end of the 18th Century, it is important to rediscover according to which values and in which space of origin the activity of those who today are seeking a scientific identity to give to their own discipline began. In the French-speaking tradition, in the first half of the 20th Century, people began to call themselves "nurses" after having been given an identity imposed by doctors. This was in reference to a Franco-Catholic model of care (nuns), but before having been able to give a name to the discipline and conceptualize theoretical conceptual models in nursing or care theories.

It is the weight of the past that makes the invention of the future possible, it is said. This statement by the French historian Fernand Braudel highlights the fact that history brings to individuals the substance of their consciousness. Without history, individuals are condemned to follow the system of the moment. Not always giving the right place to historical knowledge in a training program, especially for nurses, or not evaluating the knowledge acquired in the field, also allows leaders (in our case, in the health field) or other disciplines to better instrument the values and ideologies of a field. When nurses seen as cheaply trained labor are sometimes manipulated, for example solely on the basis of health costs or socio-economic needs, they cannot fail to assert themselves in the name of their language traditions, convince politicians of their actions, form a scientific identity or participate in the critique of reason. If we are not careful, one day, for economic reasons, we will end up replacing nurses with their assistants. "The concept of identity thus refers both to the permanence of the social means of recognition and to the capacity of the subject to give lasting meaning to his or her experience" [SAI 85].

History also avoids the alienation of future generations and avoids the production of "efficient consumer workers and beings without memory, without identity, without roots" [BUG 04]. History participates in the construction of professional identity.

But since we have been talking about it, what can it be used for? As Rocher points out, "professional identity is this essential condition for the maturity of the personality, it allows the harmonious social functioning of a person in his environment, as well as the cohesion of groups" [ROC 68]. It is nevertheless preferable for the harmonious social functioning of interdisciplinary work[4], for example, to know the origins, contents and logic of action of the discipline we represent!

"The teaching of history also gives, whether premeditated or not, nourishment to what is and will be the work of the memory of those who follow us" [MON 93]. The function of memory represented by the saying to know where we are going, is to know (and accept) where we come from "is not to celebrate the office of the past, but to help us imagine the future" [MON 93]. It is therefore incumbent on nursing educators to update the collective memory of their own discipline. It is also the role of universities, particularly nursing faculties, to promote basic nursing research. While it is interesting to discover what the language traditions of caring are made of ethnographically, we must also accept a past that was not necessarily glorious or spectacular in the secular era or in the *Ancien Régime* according to the representations in use.

Initial nursing training today is increasingly being given in academic settings, particularly in English-speaking countries. This is why the term "discipline" appears. In the French-speaking community, there are also nursing faculties (Canada, Lebanon) and high schools (Switzerland, Belgium). As SIDIIEF (*Secrétariat international des infirmières et infirmiers de l'espace francophone*) stated in 2011: "The pursuit of graduate studies in nursing is fundamental to ensure the training of competent teachers capable of guaranteeing quality initial training as well as the training of clinical nurse specialists and the training of researchers. The development of nursing research remains an essential condition for the renewal of care practices and the evolution of knowledge" [SID 11]. But how can nursing faculty researchers produce new knowledge to develop their discipline if they ignore the language traditions inherited from the past and the ancient knowledge on which it is based?

NOTE.– Nursing researchers rarely refer to their language traditions, which, according to the philosophy, "represent the most important source of knowledge, both qualitative and quantitative" [POP 85]. New knowledge is often knowledge that modifies or enriches previous knowledge.

While language traditions thus play a primordial role in the constitution of knowledge, it is normal that this tradition be rediscovered (history of knowledge),

4 We sometimes speak of inter-trade or inter-professionality.

maintained and updated to serve as a basis for subsequent knowledge produced by scientific research. These language traditions, whose importance Popper emphasized, are precisely those statements and those units of discourse that allow specific phenomena related to the action of caregiving in the field of discourse to emerge in the long term. These traditions, which, as we have seen [NAD 12a], are passed on by caregivers from generation to generation, are also mainly units that should be considered:

> By what right they can claim a domain that specifies them in space and a continuity that individualizes them in time; according to what laws they are formed; on the basis of what discursive events they are divided; and if finally they are not, in their accepted and quasi-institutional indivisibility of duality, the surface effect of more consistent units. [FOU 69]

It is from this questioning that the history of the discipline known as "nursing" can access its statements. It is in fact a matter of finding the original statements:

> How far and how often they are repeated, through what channels they are disseminated, in what groups they circulate; what general horizon they draw for men's thinking, what limits they impose on it; and how, in characterizing an epoch, they make it possible to distinguish it from others. [FOU 69]

Certainly, historical research for the nursing discipline has little influence on day-to-day nursing practice, as noted above. However, it remains a necessity if only to teach students about the history of their own discipline. This has long been a seemingly normal procedure at university where, depending on the discipline taught, we can find the history of psychology, the history of medicine, the history of sociology or the history of education sciences, to name but a few. This logic is much less obvious within the nursing discipline where history when taught (!) often takes on hybrid, redundant, stereotyped, laudatory and even hagiographic aspects. But why should we be surprised? Moreover, what place do history courses have in the training programs? On a purely informative basis and without claiming to draw any comparison whatsoever, we find that between 1980 and 2009, for example, "the history of nursing" represented between 6 and 16 hours of teaching in the nursing course at the Fribourg University of Health (Switzerland). It also represented about 24 hours of teaching (foundations of the nursing discipline) and 4 credits in the master's degree program in nursing research in 2016 at the Faculty of Nursing of the Saint-Joseph University in Beirut (Lebanon). It is also 15 hours of "history of the profession" courses that were registered in the curriculum of the schools of nursing run by Quebec hospitals in 1960 [COH 00] and between 2 hours (!) and 8 hours of "history courses" for five French nursing institutes (IFSI) in 2009 [HOM 12]. In contrast, we do not find the word "history" in the 1996 Bachelor of Science in Nursing program of the Faculty of Nursing at the Université de Montréal. It is assumed here that the course title "Introduction to the Discipline of Nursing" plays this role [COH 02].

In the history of the nursing profession, we know Florence Nightingale, but we often ignore the name of the woman who inspired Florence Nightingale to found a nursing school in Great Britain. It is around a religious problem resulting from a conflict of values between Valérie de Gasparin-Boissier and Florence Nightingale that training began in Europe. Why does one of these women take center stage and not the other? And of course, the history of the nursing discipline has nothing to do with the history of medicine or religion. There is often a tendency, not only in the media, for example, but also within the profession, to confuse disciplines and the places where knowledge is produced.

Why always position oneself as an "auxiliary profession" or present oneself as "para something"? Legislation on the profession does not explain everything. Just because women care workers from the servant and working classes were unable to access education in the 18th Century does not mean that the specificity and complexity of their task should be ignored today, especially if we interpret it from a biomedical paradigm that only very partially reflects actual practice.

Caring in ancient societies and in popular circles also means taking into account the environmental conditions and those of the habitat or domestic uses of the time. But, as Ehrenreich and English point out in connection with the witch hunt (empirical healers at the service of the peasant population), "domestic work is much more than cleaning the house. It is about physically, emotionally, sexually serving those who bring in the wages, keeping them ready for work day in and day out". In the devaluation of women's social role, "witch hunts have served the sexual division of labor and the control of men over women, their bodies and their labor" [EHR 15]. To understand also how care was instituted in pre-industrial society, it must be kept in mind that most secular healthcare professionals in institutional settings at the end of the 18th Century came from rural or domestic settings and school was not yet compulsory. There has to be a start to everything!

The history of nursing knowledge has little to do with the history of religion or the history of medicine. Rather, it would be the history of the organization of collective households, of the way they are run and how they function that is at issue. This history is simply concomitant with the history of hospitals (that of the house, the household, the *Domus*, the hospital). These hospital establishments are then the first spaces of speech devoted to hospitality. They are the first spaces for "discursive events" [FOU 69] to take institutional care of it or for the specialization of hospital domestic work.

2

The Hospital as a Place to Talk

It is at the time when the hospital was built and organized that the traditions of language of the care discipline began to emerge and thus find their singularity. Symbols of the central power of the urban bourgeoisie in the legal sense, some of these hospital buildings underwent successive major architectural changes or were rebuilt (more beautiful and larger than before)[1]. In this particular space and time, of prime importance in determining the place of emergence of what would later become the nursing discipline and its knowledge, stood a language of a welcoming nature, a form of life support and protection of human beings similar to that held by an ordinary housewife or mother looking after the home, her spouse, children, parents and other relatives.

NOTE.– Here, it is important to distinguish between the different places of care and not to mix everything together. We can have a space in which a religious language is shaped by the values of the hierarchy of the Church, sacred or doctrinal texts (practical charity of the Church, alms, hospitality, works of mercy, etc.). These religious spaces were first created in Catholic regions and then in Protestant regions. There are also public secular spaces whose organization and functioning sometimes differ from those of the Hôtel-Dieu (the French municipal or communal hospital, often dependent on the bourgeois fiefdom) built by the patricians of a city.

---

1 For example, in the city of Freiburg (Switzerland), four public hospitals followed in the wake of the first: the *hôpital Notre-Dame* (Notre-Dame hospital), the *hôpital des Bourgeois* (the Bourgeois hospital), the *hôpital cantonal I* (Cantonal I hospital) and the *hôpital cantonal II* (Cantonal II hospital). The latter, which is still in operation, is today called the "*Hôpital Fribourgeois*", on the Bertigny site in Freiburg. With each transformation, the existing staff is transferred to the new building and their knowledge also evolves with the characteristics of the new place.

2.1. The origin of the hospital

Rather, the public hospital was an institution of reception and assistance to life that provided a practical economic and material benefit to those who worked there. At the same time, by offering hospitality to the poor, the hospital could in return expect from them work in the service of the prosperity of the hospital's land holdings. The era of feudalism based on land ownership and serfdom was not far off the mark: the bourgeoisie made its appearance. Thus, at the *hôpital de Fribourg* (Freiburg hospital), founded between 1248 and 1252, the hospital keeper "was assisted in his task by his wife (*Magistra*), who took care of the housekeeping and directed the female staff of the establishment. The hospital, governed by a layman, was also served by servants and not by religious men or women. This secular and bourgeois character allows us to classify the hospital as a communal or municipal hospital" [NIQ 21]. In comparison, the *hôpital de Genève* (Geneva hospital) welcomed 135 patients in 1600 [LES 85]. It was establishments of this kind, small (4–12 beds) or large (100–150 beds) that were favored to evoke the emergence of lay nursing knowledge. However, even though only one category of institutions was chosen, it is clear that these institutions could sometimes differ in their management, organization and staffing. "The differences between institutions, even within the same city, are as great as their commonalities. Within the major trends that are shaping the overall hospital landscape in French-speaking Switzerland, for example, each establishment also adopts its own rhythm, depending on local determinations" [DON 03]. We can extend this observation to all the countries concerned by the founding of hospitals. Hospitals therefore present different characteristics in terms of the quality of their services.

The adventure of the so-called "nursing" care began in a fairly limited field of hospital action. At the beginning, the story was mundane and there was nothing medicalized[2]. We owned land or bought a piece of land, if possible close to a river and along communication routes, we began by building, buying or receiving an ordinary house devoted to hospitality in order to welcome passers-by, the poor[3] who were often isolated or without social ties, orphans, the elderly or any wandering person in need of help to live their daily life and we regulated the collective life. A hospital was born! There were "*maisons*" (houses) or "ménages" (households) according to ancient texts.

---

2 Nothing new, but we tend to forget this when we talk today about nursing knowledge or "advanced practices". "From the outset, one fact is clear: the general hospital is not a medical institution. In its functioning or in its purpose, the general hospital is not similar to any medical idea" [FOU 72].

3 For Teysseire, who was inspired by the abbot of St. Peter, "in the 18th century, a person was called poor if he had only his work to survive" [TEY 93].

The terms "*maison*" or "*ménage*" often appeared in the documents (status, job descriptions, accounts, reports) that were created once the house was in operation. There was a need to hire (household) staff to operate it and to offer hospitality. The term "*ménage*" had a special status. The word was often used "as a separate entity with a defined position within the communal structures that were being established and becoming more complex" [ROD 05].

2.2. The care environment

The hospital is an institution that, as a care environment, shapes practices and connects the people who reside there. While this environment transforms its mission, expands or benefits from new equipment, then new knowledge emerges and will be acquired by those who work or live in the hospital. In fact, the hospital environment in a way describes the nature of the background in which care is given. This environment becomes central when the foundations of the discipline and the space and time in which knowledge is created must be rediscovered. "The institution thus shapes the interpretative procedures of situations. Institutions are shaped by models of rationality that they develop reflexively" [DEM 99].

The foundations of the nursing discipline are rooted in hospital space and time. The lay era of the discipline, by linking language to "the only truly scientific concepts that were those related to the geometry of space and time" for Thom, gave meaning to the knowledge in use. The nursing discipline did not grow "above ground". Hospital spaces allowed the knowledge of care and assistance to life to exist. This knowledge could then be transformed into deeds and words. "Only concepts that can be geometrized and related to space and time are susceptible to universalization and therefore scientificity (…). We know and act only locally" [THO 83]. Hospital space and time as an environment thus determined the first scientific element of the discipline still to be born. With the birth of the hospital, these traditions of language became important for the quality of knowledge and the background of discursive events dear to Foucault in which the nursing discipline could appear. The framework was set. These are the reasons why we place the care environment (the hospital) as the first and central concept that conditions the unique perspective of the so-called "nursing" sciences. For many theorists today, the care environment is also a central concept that characterizes the substance of the nursing discipline [DAL 08a]. Space refers to place, time is what escapes and reminds us of our condition as mortals. These two elements allow us to perceive movement.

Without these two particular dimensions, space and time, language first, discipline second, as signs of human activity, cannot exist. For he or she who could hold this language would have had no place to speak or to make speak, to write or to make write, and consequently, no discursive activity to carry out either. For Auffray "space and time are the familiar benchmarks within which we interpret what we perceive of the world around us, especially movement. This has been the case since the beginning of humanity" [AUF 96]. Therefore, identifying the space in which knowledge of action begins is fundamental to account for the transformation of tacit knowledge into scientific knowledge and to recover the knowledge of care that inhabits the discipline. The first words pertaining to lay care thus constituted "a set of anonymous, historical rules, always determined in time and space, which have defined at a given time and for a given social, economic, geographical or linguistic area, the conditions for exercising the enunciative function" [FOU 69].

From the Middle Ages to the end of the 18th Century in Europe, particularly in French-speaking Switzerland, cities had their lay hospital institutions to "take care" of people who were often marginalized or lonely and bear the miseries of life. These institutions, financed by the bourgeoisies of the time, began to organize themselves in many ways, but were very often inspired by the ordinary family dynamic associated with models from old-style communities, inns, farms or various collective households. For example, the Geneva hospital in 1744 (a Protestant canton), which could accommodate about 136 people for a population of 14,400 inhabitants around 1590, already represented a veritable spatial mosaic through its multiple work and speech spaces, among which was the "general hospital", more often referred to as "the house", the cellar, the bakery, the butcher's shop, the stables, the factories, the house of correction, the shoemaker's shop, the school for the children housed in the hospital, the tailor's room, the mills, the granary of the seed collector, the hospital funds (the countryside with farms, vineyards, meadows and gardens, the forests of Jussy, des frères, de Bay, of La Petite Grave and Céligny)[4], the hospital shop, the houses belonging to the hospital (staff accommodation), the temple of the house, the refectory, the shops and pyres, the large kitchen, the room "of the bourgeois women and girls", the room "of the poor of the house", the room "of the working class", the room "of the able-bodied women and girls", the room of the sick "both men and boys and women and girls received in the house", the room of passers-by and beggars, the room of "those bleeding, epileptic and others" who had unfortunate illnesses, the room of "those who suffered from venereal diseases, shameful illnesses or of a particular character" [NAD 93].

These talking spaces of course had their occupants with their lifestyles and languages. As early as 1759, the Freiburg Hospital (Catholic canton) could accommodate between 80 and 110 people for a town with a population of about 6,100. The distribution of the premises in Freiburg in 1759 demonstrated some differences with those of the Geneva hospital in 1744. It is rather classes (from the

4 At the end of the 18th Century, the Geneva hospital owned 180 hectares of forest, which represented about "18% of the forest heritage of the territory of the Seigneury of Geneva" [ZUM 85].

first to the eighth) and statuses that we are talking about. Thus, we can distinguish the apartments of the hospital staff, their family and servants, the men's dormitory, the women's dormitory (the *dormiaudes*), the servants' room, which were often, as the texts say, "fed, housed, heated, lit, whitewashed and medicated", the room or *stove* for the sick or *krankenstube*, the children's room (*kinderstube*), a space (often in the basement) for the inpatients, foolish, chained, dumb[5] and a space for the "poor passers-by" who were often "foreign beggars, French deserters, prowlers" [NAD 93, NAD 12b].

There was also an investment in stone[6]. "In the 15th century, the hospital became a large landowner with a high income" [ROD 05] and made the institution a source of liquidity for the municipal authorities. This situation was not unusual in many medieval hospitals. Sometimes it worked, sometimes it did not, because of wars, bad management, spoliations or difficulties in maintaining the constructed heritage. The Freiburg Hospital was managed to function as usual between the 14th and early 19th Centuries (over five centuries), despite the invasion, economic and disciplinary problems caused by Napoleonic troops as early as March 2, 1798. The hospitals of the Franche-Comté region near the Franco-Swiss border were also destroyed, particularly in the 15th Century. This remark shows the difference that could sometimes exist between hospitals with regard to the integrity of the places and structures. Out of 33 establishments listed by Nicole Brocart, "three were reported destroyed between 1363 and 1376, twelve were destroyed in 1435 and 1459, and eleven again between 1479 and 1484". The 15th Century proved to be particularly disastrous for the Franc-Comté hospitals, "whose temporality was turning into a time of ruin and lesser value". The difficult economic situation also contributed to compromising their management and reducing their revenues [BRO 98].

The urban or rural space where there were hospitals, some of which have now disappeared, was "a highly compartmentalized world, a mosaic of territories with extremely diverse statuses. We can speak of an atomized urban fabric" [WAL 94]. The size of the regions was often a function of the accessibility threshold. In the 18th Century, this threshold was defined as 2 hours of walking, or 8 km or 10 to 20 km by stagecoach. Cities were then used as staging posts in the era of slow transport. "Nomadism was also a fundamental feature of the population structure in the 18th century" [WAL 94]. Under these conditions, small, medium or large towns at the same time welcomed travelers who could not afford an inn and made their properties and the products of hospital work bear fruit. This may also explain the

5 Mental patients were also received in hospitals, but they were not considered as patients to be treated; they were locked up and, if necessary, chained up [NIQ 21].

6 "Already in the 16th century, hospitals were extremely rich institutions, with a large amount of capital and a vast, though very heterogeneous, land heritage (fields, meadows, forests, vineyards, houses, mills, etc.)" [DON 03].

presence of small hospitals as well as hospitality houses along the communication routes.

Around the hospital, in buildings sometimes adjoining it, it was not uncommon to find, depending on the size of the town, functional buildings such as barns, stables, attics, sheds, stores, an oven, a butcher's shop or slaughterhouses, as well as buildings that could be used as functional housing for employees. In comparison with the urban Geneva hospital, the rural lay Bulle hospital in 1738, had only one floor, a kitchen, the "*poile des pauvres*" (6–12 places in "two poorly constructed bedframes"[7]), the "*poile du gardien de l'hôpital*" (functional housing), a room with a bunk, toilets, a barn and an enclosure with a garden and goat's field. Also in the same area of the hospital in 1722 and on either side of it, the "*Fleur-de-lys*" and "*De la Mort vivante*" arrangements. It was thus a very "hospitable" district, which was on the outskirts of the town of Bulle. In 1763, it was noted by the public prosecutors of the Geneva hospital "that the wooden beds were subject to bedbugs and ringworms". They were then replaced by iron beds between 1765 and 1808 [LOU 00].

Located on the outskirts of the town or village, the hospital, since the Middle Ages, has been a community that requires a minimum of organization. It is close to a spring, a river or the ditches of the town[8]. From a cadastral and architectural point of view, the main "built volumes" (the largest buildings) of a small town in the Middle Ages, particularly in Freiburg (see Figure 2.1), Bulle and Romont, up to the end of the 18th Century, were the castle, the church, the hospital and the "*fief bourgeois*" (town house or town hall).

The lay hospitals under the *Ancien Régime*, particularly in French-speaking Switzerland, then bore a name whose very term, "*l'hospital*", *lospitaul* or *l'épetau* or *l'épetô* in 1749[9], recalled a mission of welcoming, providing hospitality and protection to human beings. These terms were confused with the terms "*maison*" or "*ménage*" mentioned above. In other regions or countries, we found similar characteristics to this space and time that we have just presented. For example, a bourgeois hospital was founded in Porrentruy in 1406, and a bourgeois hospital also

7 Gruerian hospital furniture, old wooden bed comprising three levels with a width of 1.20 m. On the other side of the border, the *hôpital de Montbéliard* (Montbéliard hospital) (eastern France) also had "twelve beds with mattresses, eiderdowns, pillows and crossbars" [CUS 86]. This bedframe was thus the predecessor of today's electric bed.

8 This may initially have been a comprehensive benefit for daily hygiene (for the toilet or kitchen, for example) or for the need to dispose of daily waste. But it also proved a difficulty in ensuring hygiene, when insalubrity, dilapidated facilities or lack of ventilation in buildings promoted dampness.

9 Gruyère patois is a Franco-Provençal dialect spoken in the Gruyère district (south of the canton of Freiburg, Switzerland).

existed in Neuchâtel in 1539 [DON 00]. Also in 1377, the *hôpital de Lausanne* (the Lausanne hospital) bought a pair of shoes and a few lengths of cloth to make a garment for a hospital employee (Jaqueta Botlery) [MOS 05].

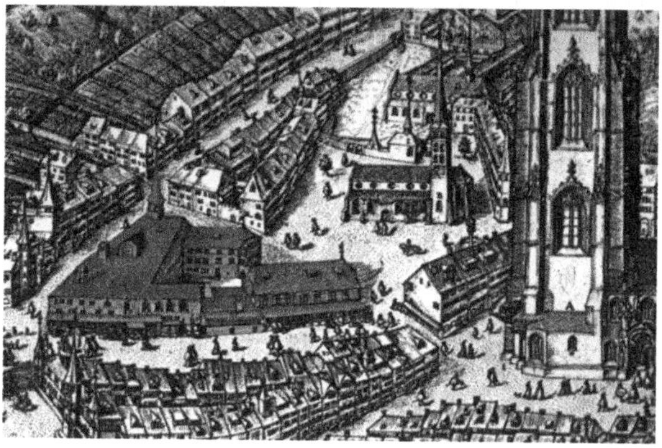

Figure 2.1. *A lay hospital on Catholic soil in 1606 (source: Musée d'art et d'histoire de Fribourg. Plan of Freiburg by Martin Martini – Copperplate engraving published in 1606. Photo B. Rochat 2006, retouched to highlight the hospital building). For a color version of the figure, see www.iste.co.uk/nadot/nursing.zip*

This practice of providing shoes and work clothes was common for hospital servants, as very often their meager salary was paid in cash and in kind. There were also establishments in France similar to those in French-speaking Switzerland. In 1745, for example, the governess of the *hôpital français d'Avranches* (French hospital of Avranches) was paid an annual salary of 100 pounds and employed six servants to help her, who were given 30 pounds a year in addition to food and lodging [NAD 93]. Finally, in Montbéliard (France), for example, in the 15th Century, when the town had 1,500 inhabitants, the establishment with its outbuildings, kitchens, barns, stables and cowsheds had a capacity of 12 beds and a 13.77-meter-long façade on the street [CUS 86, BRO 98]. With its kitchen, cellar, equipment, barn, stables, garden, meadows and vineyard, this establishment was very similar to other establishments in Switzerland (Bulle, Romont, Yverdon, for example). With its 12 hectares of cultivable land, "the hospital at the end of the 15th century was a notable agricultural owner in the Montbéliard area" [CUS 86]. Near Montbéliard, the city of Belfort also (600 inhabitants in 1442) had its lay hospital with 10 beds [BRO 98]. Similarly in Canada, we know of Jeanne Mance who had a first hospital built in Ville-Marie (Montreal) in 1642 with a capacity of 8 beds (six for men and two for women). In this new work space thus created, "it seems that Jeanne Mance was, from 1642 to 1653, the only resource person in the colony in matters of health, assisted by servants, between one and four, and at least two other women of the colony: the wife of Louis d'Ailleboust and Madame de la Bardillière" [YOU 05].

These "*maisons*", this "*ménage*", this "*hôpital*" and ultimately this institution, needed to function. Only, "institutions don't think, they don't have goals or motivation. Only the flesh and blood participants in institutional life think, have goals and reasons to act" [DEM 99]. A hospital institution is therefore not just a set of rules or functions, but "a set of normative schemes that allow both situational and discourse settings of practical interactions between people and with the world. As schemas, norms are reflexive procedures, linking knowledge and capacities" [DEM 99]. So, which participants can we rely on to make a healthcare institution work?

Generally speaking, the activity of the staff and their know-how are close to the traditional occupations of women on large farms or in collective households. Women (governesses or servants) may serve the hospital (caring for residents) according to a maternalistic ideology. "When the rector was married, his wife was, as it were, a partner in the hospital management" [ROD 05]. The men (servants), if any, were more likely to have outside activities on the estate (maintenance, leaf removal, harvesting, livestock supervision, etc.). A sort of handyman, they were also in charge of the heavy work. The Romont hospital (Switzerland) in 1733, for example, had a "master of low works" to help the *gardienne* (caretaker). He was housed in the hospital [NAD 12b].

Once the care environment had been constructed, the first written statements served as prescriptions. They focused on how to carry out the activities of daily living in a community. If we want to find the first knowledge of the care discipline, we need to find the first walls framing the word and the first texts indicating what needed to be done to make everything work. In general, as Louis-Courvoisier points out, "the importance of those involved in healthcare is inversely proportional to the information disclosed by the sources" [LOU 00]. This is also what we have seen repeatedly. Within the hospital in the lay age of knowledge, "the nursing staff was the real hub and representative of the influences of the various healthcare protagonists" [LOU 00]. This still seems to be true today, even though the hospital has changed a great deal. That is why in our conceptual model of nursing published in 2013, we sometimes refer to "cultural intermediaries"[10] and "health mediators" to describe the professional role of nurses as intermediaries between the various health stakeholders [NAD 13]. In fact, as we also specify in this conceptual model, "any intermediary is a mediator, even if often it is not recognized as such" [DES 19].

10 Daniel Teysseire, in his presentation of Tissot's work (*Avis au Peuple sur sa santé*), points out the works written for the people, but by doctors and which are "intended to be read and used by social groups serving as a relay between doctors and the people" [TEY 93]. He calls these social groups "cultural intermediaries". For the anthropologist Françoise Loux too, the notion of intermediaries is present in her reflections. Nurses are then "perceived by the patients as real intermediaries to whom it is possible to entrust more things than to the doctor". Nurses "play a central role as informers and discreet intermediaries between doctors and healers" [LOU 83].

3

Care Before 1850

Reading carefully the texts and job descriptions of the hospital staff of the 18th Century in both Catholic and Protestant regions, we get a strange feeling. It is as if, in turn, those who provided care, appeared at times as depraved, devoid of any morals, infamous, ignorant, without culture and at the same time, full of common sense, intelligent, committed, resistant, sensitive and courageous. In fact, both present and absent. It is as if contemporary works on hospitals of the *Ancien Régime* denounced an evil to be fought. That the written representations resulting from our historical discoveries fed by more recent works on the history of everyday hospital life revealed "a hidden treasure" of qualities stifled by the history we have made of them and which we perceive with a different sensitivity.

The image is moving. By moving this convex and magnifying lens (what we can read), but magnifying too much for it to be sharp (our perception), we are taken by a form of vertigo where, in turn, evil replaces the good, the right is superimposed on the wrong and the doubt that emerges from it (our intuition), accompanied by our astonishment, then transforming the image into a moving image.

Even though the qualities required of hospital governesses and hospital servants by the hospital authorities seemed to refer to noble moral values, the working and material conditions of the time were no less degrading. There was no running water; it was necessary to ensure the production of hot water, the use of firewood, fats, fabrics; lighting with tallow candles sometimes made of brick on the spot, conveniences exposed to draughts; sound and heat insulation almost non-existent, rudimentary sewage disposal, difficult food preservation, etc. Under these conditions, work in the hospital was more akin to serfdom or domestic slavery than to a vocation. However, the daily life of female nursing staff in the lay era brought little satisfaction. In any case, one had to try to earn a living without being sure of succeeding!

3.1. *Maison* staff

Let us perhaps return to the activity of the governesses and servants to understand it well. The lay hospital was the mirror of the popular class (the ordinary people) and the servants (the common people). The wealthy and cultured class (clergy and quality people) had their own care structure and did not share the same hospital living quarters, at least not before 1860.

Municipal and public governments had staff to run their care institutions. Of course, the number of staff hired by the hospital and their status depended on the size of the institution, the resources available and the location. Generally speaking, the larger the institution, the more structured and hierarchical it was. The hospital was generally larger in urban areas than in rural areas. At the municipal hospital in Yverdon (Switzerland), founded shortly before 1308, the domestic staff[1] in 1450 included, for example, *dietates, famuli*[2] and *ancilles.* This was a Protestant region and we could find staff approximately identical to that of the Catholic regions which also had their lay hospitals (Romont, Freiburg or Bulle). Thus, in the lay hospital of the city of Freiburg in 1262, the term "hospital mistress" (*Magistra hospitalis*) was used to describe the one who played the role of "house mistress" and who was responsible for care. In the same hospital, but in 1759 (about 110 beds), we would find a *hospitalier* (hospital master) and his wife in the capacity of *hospitalières* (literally, hospital mistresses). The texts reveal some aspects of their status:

> In addition to the above-mentioned benefits, the hospital master will receive an annual salary of one hundred pounds (twenty écus), as above, the same as the hospital master, and twelve ells of ritual cloth[3]. If the hospital master has no wife, he may take a widow or a daughter of good morals, good reputation and of a certain age. [REG 59]
>
> The hospital master's food will be bourgeois. It will be served in fat at the expense of the hospital only in common meats; for neither poultry nor game will be passed on to him in his expenditure or in his accounts, still less sweets, tea, coffee, chocolates or similar things; however, he may take poultry[4] from direct means, but in moderation. [REG 59]

1 Someone who took care of the estate (*domus*, household, house), who organized it, who ensured its functioning.

2 The hospital rector, his family and the servants, together with the residents, formed the hospital's *familia* [ROD 05].

3 Six ells each. One ell = about 1.18–1.20 m. At the Freiburg hospital in 1759 the *hospitalièrs* had had equal pay for men and women, starting from 1657.

4 A fixed royalty that the owner of a land paid to the Lord of the fief.

The staff assigned to daily care was often in the presence of other employees necessary for the operation of the collective household. Sometimes they were referred to as the "big" servant and the "small" servant. The big servant had more responsibilities. The small one was their helper. The Bulle hospital had a *gardienne* or a *gardienne* (male and female forms of caretakers) of the hospital. Still in the Freiburg Hospital, in the 17th Century, the general service of the house and the sick was provided by four or five servants. One of them (the "*dignan*" or "*dignain*") took care of the children (called "*gittons*"). In 1694, there were 34 children in the hospital, divided into three categories: foundlings, illegitimate children and orphans. Two servants were especially dedicated to the service of the sick. One of them named "*musshafera*" or governess of the sick distributed soup to the passers-by every day. Indeed, called by the ringing of a small bell, the people of the town in need came to the hospital for the distribution of leftover hospital food. The care of the hospital cellar was the responsibility of the "*cellerière*" [NAD 12b]. The hospital in the small town of Romont (Switzerland) on Catholic soil did not always have a hospital master at the head of the hospital. It was a woman who ran the hospital in 1733. In the "bourgeois statutes of the noble town of Romont", one found the duties of the hospital[5] caretaker, next to the duties and the organization of all the city authorities, including those of the "scindic" or "city governor" (*sic*). In 1733, we learn in particular:

> That a caretaker be placed there and appointed in the place of Antoine Badoud[6] from now on, who will conform to what is decreed and ordered by the Council to receive the poor and to care, as well as cloths, furniture and other things from the said hospital for the use of the hospital and the poor alone, as well as for small change, why she will go and take marks from the Banneret in charge, which she will give to the poor to go and receive their money as usual (Original of the 1733 statutes of the town of Romont) [NAD 12b].

The caretaker of the hospital therefore had the capacity to economically manage the daily lives of the poor and their care. In 1700, the cook at the Freiburg hospital received an annual salary of 50 pounds, the children's maid 30 pounds; the baker 30 pounds as well; the maid for the sick 32.5 pounds, but was lodged in the house. On certain occasions, these servants were helped by auxiliaries (day laborers or

5 The term "*gardienne de l'hôpital*" was the term that preceded the term "*garde-malade*" in time. "Custody also means a woman who serves the sick, and lives from that work" [ACA 94]. "To look after a sick person is to be with him or her assiduously to assist him or her in his or her needs" [ACA 62]. This is what those who care for others have probably known how to do since the dawn of time with more or less benevolence.

6 Former hospital master at the *hôpital de Romont* (Romont Hospital).

"small" servants[7]). The salaries of the staff in money and in kind already occupying an important place in the economy of the house. For example, in a very detailed accounting study of the lay hospital in Lausanne, we find that personnel expenses represented 51.76% of the overall expenses in the 14th Century. As a result, "the expenses for the upkeep of the guests were small in comparison with the expenses for the staff" [MOS 05]. It was also customary for the expenses incurred by the hospital caretaker for the upkeep of guests, as can be seen in the case of the Romont Hospital, for example, to be reimbursed by the hospital authorities on the basis of supporting documents. The same was true for the Yverdon hospital in the Canton of Vaud (Switzerland), where the largest accounting item concerned the salaries of permanent and temporary staff. As Yann Rod very rightly mentions: "Permanent staff mentioned in the sources mainly under the heading of *salaria,* which included all the salaries in cash and in kind paid to them. An analysis of the data reveals a division into two groups: first of all, the rector, his family circle and the servants who, together with the residents, formed the hospital's *familia.* In the second group were the paid personnel who did not live in the hospital, such as shepherds, nannies and notaries" [ROD 05].

Geneva also had its lay employees. An important figure in the running of the hospital was the hospital master and his wife, the hospital mistress. In 1535 in Geneva, for example, the hospital master was seen as being "simultaneously a nurse, staff supervisor, bursar, emissary and gardener" [LOU 85]. As we have said, the complexity of the functions varied with the size of the institution, its status and the scope of the field. This function, which may seem heterogeneous, was already representative of the complexity of the functioning of state hospitals. The hospital was part of a complex system of obligations and services rendered by free men similar to slaves. Thus, the income from care work often brought an added value to hospital capital (donations, legacies, alms from priests and nuns in the Christian faith, etc.). The hospital master managed the day-to-day running of the hospital. Helped by his wife and sometimes by his children, he had administrative and economic activities and supervised the daily care given in the hospital. "As head of staff, he was in charge of all the governors, governesses, cooks, gardeners, washers, valets and other employees, which represented a small number of 100 people to be supervised. And finally, he knew, welcomed and visited all the residents, both able-bodied and sick" [LOU 00]. "The hospital master or his wife needed to visit the sick every day in order to provide for their needs and have them served both for food and

7 The titular servant (the one with the most experience), who took an oath at the beginning of each year to carry out her trade faithfully, had one or more "small maids" to assist her. One can therefore already distinguish a division of care work in the medieval hospital. Whether some sociologists like it or not, this was not yet a division of medical work or "dirty work" since the hospital was not yet medicalized.

for the cleanliness of their bodies" [LOU 00]. At the Montbéliard hospital, in neighboring France in 1758, the hospital master also had bursar, receiver and cashier duties. He was housed in the hospital as was customary and "benefited from the service of the second *chambellière*". A recipient hired the staff and registered the admissions of the poor. A "lady of the hospital" or "mistress" played the role of supervisor, second bursar and controlled certain transactions as a housewife would do in the private sector. In France, there was also a maid, the "*chambellière*", who was a sort of maid for all purposes and who was doubled up with a servant, stable hand, farm laborer and carpenter. Thus, in 1540 at the Montbéliard hospital, "with 400 francs a year, 16 people were fed, housed, heated, enlightened and exonerated" [CUS 86]. Here we find conditions approximately identical to those of the Freiburg hospitals [NAD 12b].

Generally speaking, in the 18th Century and on both sides of the border, those hired to provide care came from the servant or working class. While some could read, write or count and sometimes speak two languages, as in Freiburg, others lacked these abilities and had only experience of "running a household". They were "mature" in age 8 and had experience of community work "at the farmer's house" or sometimes even of domestic service in a "bourgeois boarding house". They worked as nurses in medium-sized lay hospitals (80–110 beds).

The first caregivers were known by local French names such as "*gardienne de l'hôpital*", "*gouvernante des malades*", "*grande ou petite servante de la gouvernante*", "*servante des malades*", "*servante des pauvres*", "*gardienne ou gardien de l'hôpital*", "*garde-malade*", *musshafera*[9], *kindermutter*[10] or mother of the children. They were already engaged in a trade that took the shape of a human activity as well as a domestic activity. This activity was vital for institutional functioning and for the protection and survival of the human species.

With a culture and customary practices of life support, household activities or the traditional role of women, caregivers are confronted daily with multiple languages that must necessarily be coordinated and will evolve in the midst of people with very different statuses depending on the size of the institution. The person in a relationship with the caregiver is not "just a patient" or a care receiver. Above all, he or she is an everyday "sociological" person with a different status, culture and powers. Even in a hospital in the *Ancien Régime*, these people were already

8 An age in which "one has knowledge, reflection, without being disturbed" [ACA 94].

9 Legitimate title requiring the taking of an oath, in use in the secular hospital of the city of Freiburg (Switzerland) from the 13th to the 18th Centuries.

10 Freiburg being a bilingual city, German-speaking designations are sometimes found in documents.

numerous in the work place. It was impossible for the caregivers not to come across one day or another one of the many interlocutors with whom they needed to exchange information that was later transformed into action or words. These people, these different interlocutors circulating in the hospital, were on the move and sometimes forced caregivers to process information that varied in intensity, quantity and quality. Depending on the size of the hospital, this information could come from, among others, the hospital master and his wife, the hospital mistress, the hospital secretary, the *sautier*[11], the public prosecutors, the head of the offices, tailors, bakers, butchers, cooks, grooms, porters, apprentices, winemakers, doctors, (city physicists[12], apothecaries, masters or boys surgeons, servants, burials, servants (large and small) and governesses of the sick, chambermaids, foresters, carters, hunters or rogue hunters (security), farmers, sommeliers, bursars, school teachers, visitors (anatomo-pathologist), singers, chaplains, etc. [NAD 12b].

In general, staff who assisted living and cared for "those in the hospital" were guided by job descriptions. These various job descriptions, sometimes brief, were supplemented on several occasions by specific written regulations and injunctions from the hospital authorities. In fact, the institution delegated in these texts knowledge about what was to be done. It was a first cultural system (values, knowledge, ideologies), which was imposed by delegation on the carers. This staff was sometimes sworn in and needed to deposit a so-called "bourgeois" guarantee at the beginning of their employment. In addition, each expense incurred by the hospital caretaker to meet the activities of daily life (candles or oil for lighting, butter, tobacco, teas, laundry, firewood, brooms, starch for ironing, etc.) was, as already mentioned, reimbursed on presentation of vouchers and supporting documents kept in a memorandum. Having an apartment, food, shoes, clothing, heating, candles for lighting, knowing how to keep busy, having a vegetable garden or a garden, a goat farm, chickens, a cow or a horse[13], was already almost "a luxury" in the 18th Century compared to the living conditions of domesticity, working class and servants living in the surrounding cities or countryside.

11 A sort of bailiff who would collect income and interest of little importance or sometimes accompanied the hospital or rector on his travels and could also "help everyone a little" [NAD 93].

12 Some doctors and surgeons subordinate to doctors were sometimes found in large institutions (Geneva in 1744), but rural hospitals or small towns only called upon their services on an ad-hoc basis.

13 Owning a domestic animal was sometimes a requirement to hold the office as stated in the regulations and statutes of the caretaker of the Bulle hospital in Switzerland, in 1749 [NAD 12b].

The hospital was a space occupied by a living community that resembled a farm, of a particular type and produced everyday[14] consumer goods. It had a large and heterogeneous land base. It had its own land, forests, vineyards, mills, herds and all the logistics, as well as craftsmen useful to the functioning of the whole. For example, the lay hospital in Lausanne would employ up to 88 reapers per year [MOS 05].

In addition to the general house service, the hospital's outbuildings also needed to be taken care of. There were farmers, servants and farm handmaids, shepherds, cowherds and carters. Let's not lose sight of the fact that the hospital was at the same time a collective household, a property, an agricultural enterprise, in short, an estate that needed to be managed. It was in fact a domestic economy of the state and monetary type to help live and take care of the most destitute or those who had lost everything. This is also what Cusenier remarks about the Montbéliard hospital in France. "In short, the hospital presents itself as a community where about sixteen people work, subsisting on a farm based on a fairly comfortable capital base" [CUS 86].

This situation was not unique to French-speaking Switzerland. In France, Canada and Belgium, there were also care institutions. This care was not yet qualified as "nursing": lay personnel did not use the word nurse. We will see further on why. What changed, from one country to another, in the arrival of the term "nurse", were the dates or periods when lay care institutions were taken over by the private charity of the churches. And even when religious and lay people worked together, "the former most often served as supervisory personnel for the latter". Let us recall that, still at the beginning of the 20th Century, the French administration used the terms "*domestiques*" (domestic personnel), "*personnel de service*" (service personnel) and "*personnel subalterne*" (secondary personnel) [DIÉ 90] to designate lay personnel in the hospital environment. In Canada, another example, the only health resource in the French colony of New France was Jeanne Mance, assisted by a few maids from 1642 to 1653. As early as the 19th Century, English-speaking Canada also saw a nursing profession practiced by women (and a few men) "undoubtedly part of the working class, characterized by a diversity of skills and character traits, ranging from the highly respectable and intelligent practitioner to the ignorant and unsavory". As in Switzerland, early Canadian hospitals considered life support, hospital care or nursing to be "the vilest domestic work" [YOU 05]. It was this domestic work that would continue to be operational in the "time dimension" of the nursing

14 As an example, in the 17th Century, the Freiburg Hospital was allowed to sell the numerous hens that the hospital had received from its censor farmers. In addition to the goods in kind, this is what ensured its income. As early as 1650, the sale of hens was abolished and the hospital masters received an annual salary of 100 pounds [NIQ 21].

communities that arrived in Quebec in the 17th Century in a colonial situation, insofar as hospital nurses[15] and officers (head of offices) provided what Brigitte Violette called general care: reception of the sick, washing, beds, meals, general order, assistance to the dying, etc. [VIO 05]. Unfortunately, the cliché of "Sairey Gamp, the drunken and filthy night watchwoman from Charles Dickens' novel" [MCP 05] is used as an emblem to disqualify the nursing staff in order to allow the aristocracy to occupy the grounds. It is from Anna Hamilton's thesis at the Faculty of Medicine in Montpellier in 1900, which also saw in ordinary nurses "mercenaries of the lowest extraction" [KRE 32], that prejudice was reinforced. The point deserves to be nuanced! In the jungle of the *Ancien Régime* hospital personnel, as in the individuals who made up the population, there were both perfectly respectable practitioners and unsavory servants.

It was not because female nursing staff in the class of servants and governesses sometimes lived in the painful conditions of hospital domesticity and without the right to benefit from the necessary instruction enabling them, for example, to write about what they did, that the singularity, complexity and arduousness of their roles, as well as the knowledge enabling them to carry them out, should be ignored, downgraded or rejected. People always knew more than they could say! But also, one may wonder: how were the representations about the demands of care and the working conditions they required from the working class, the maids and the poor perceived by the ruling classes? Perhaps the educated class or the local bourgeoisie, who also had experience of the work done by their own maids and servants in their homes, had not yet realized "that cultures different from our own are always considered inferior, especially when such an attitude proves both useful and profitable" [ZIN 14].

NOTE.– There were no "nurses" at work in the public hospitals of the *Ancien Régime* in French-speaking Switzerland. This meant that from about the 11th Century to the last third of the 18th Century (a period of 600 years, after all!), the activity of taking care of the life of the estate (*Domus*), taking care of the life of the group or community (*familia*) and taking care of the human being (*homo, ad-hominem*) was mainly the business of governesses and lay maids who belonged to hospital domesticity.

But the status should not make us forget the language and the knowledge of experience that went with the role and that were called to be transmitted. Female

15 Note here the use of the term "*hospitalière*" in female form which, like the *hospitalier* and *hospitalière* of Swiss lay hospitals in lay times, "was the de facto superintendent of the hospital; she was responsible for the management, organization and general administration of the institution in all matters concerning the hospitalization of the sick. She formed the center of the care structure" [VIO 05].

nursing staff and sometimes a few men, "*hospitaliers*", "*gouverneurs*" and "*gardien de l'hôpital*" (Bulle in 1749), took care of the people housed in the hospitals. In the hospitals of Geneva, Neuchâtel, Lausanne, Yverdon, (Protestant regions) as well as in Freiburg, Bulle, Romont, Porrentruy (Catholic regions), there was a service staff to take care of the domain, the human being and the group as a whole (collective relations). This personnel, especially the governesses and their servants, was already the object of a division of labor. The "*gardes-malades*" with their "small servants" who were different from the "big ones", that is, the ones who were responsible for care and who took an oath to do their job well, were the emblematic figures of the personnel entrusted with the task of "caregiving" [NAD 12b].

From 1759 onwards, the authorities of the Freiburg hospital were concerned about how to continue recruiting staff useful to the running of the hospital. As a reminder, their desire was "always to take for the service of the sick everything that was best in these respects". But, "as people endowed with these advantages of mind and body are not common, and therefore difficult to find, thought was given to the introduction of hospital nuns called the Gray Nuns[16], who would be no less suitable for the sick than for other jobs, for the economy of the house, which in time could be introduced into the hospital" [REG 59].

Therefore, a religious congregation was being considered to address the shortage of competent lay personnel. The hospital authorities had heard positively of the Catholic hospital congregations of Sion, Pontarlier and Besançon, close to the border, who call themselves "*infirmières*" (literally "nurses", but with a religious meaning or connotation in French, which is absent when "nurse" is used to refer to lay caregivers). The latter "turned professional to serve the hospitals and were called the Gray Nuns" [REG 59].

We will then follow in detail how, through cultural colonization, settlement and occupation of space, a lay hospital was transformed into a religious community and, at the same time, how we passed from a tradition of secular care to the instilling of religious knowledge about care.

16 Named so because they were often dressed in gray serge; hence the name which the people gave them. For example, the nuns of the Hôtel-Dieu de Beaune had to do a six-month internship in secular dress to evaluate their competence (time of probation) before putting on a black novice's robe, then finally, a gray robe as a sign of profession [NAD 12b]. The nuns of St. Joseph who arrived in a colonial situation at the Montreal hospital in 1639 from La Flèche in France were also "commonly known as the Gray Nuns" [COH 00].

3.2. Sacred values in the period of lay knowledge

The introduction of sacred knowledge from the language traditions of the Catholic Church into the space of lay knowledge considerably influenced hospital care practices from the last third of the 18th Century to the middle of the 19th Century. From 1759 onwards, the term "*infirmière*", a religious term meaning "nurse" in French, gradually became fashionable in the lay hospital of the city of Freiburg. A religious term made its appearance in the lay world and of course brought with it a different system of values from those in place. Bringing to the hospital a group as different as the one already occupying the field was in fact shaping a major cultural change in the organization of the knowledge and gestures that accompanied care.

Even though there were no nurses at the Freiburg hospital, the word nurse was circulating in society and was making a name for itself. Thus, the lay term still in use at the Freiburg hospital (Switzerland) on April 13, 1760 "*musshafera* or governess of the sick" was suddenly replaced on September 28, 1762 by a religious one: "the hospital nurse". The governess of the patients became "the nurse" in the language! It is important to note that there were still no working nurses in the hospital. Language therefore preceded the desired figure.

> The nurse of the hospital having taken the resolution to leave her office, Babelon Wicht of Praroman, presently a servant at the farmer's, presented herself to want to replace her under the same footing; the hospital master presents the conditions under which she could be engaged under the good will of my honorable Lords; among other things, it is indicated to this Babelon, that if she does her duty well, and that she remains in this role for 15 years, that she will have her bread there for the rest of her days. And said that he promised her 10 pounds of pledge and allowed the hospital master to hire her, on condition that the former stays for a while to give her the necessary instructions, which the hospital master had asked the Honorable Lords for his consolation and what more of those men! (*sic*) [FON 61]

Based on this proposal, but without rushing too much[17], the Board of Directors tried to find a reliable religious congregation, willing to take care of the space and time both temporally and spiritually. Slowly, insidiously, change was coming. First words, an expected language, then finally, an official and sacred text accompanied by a modification and occupation of the space in which the new language would be used,

---

17 It is assumed here that the hospital management did not want to rush things too much and that entrusting the lay hospital to a religious community required careful planning for change on all levels (political, economic, architectural, personnel status, etc.).

announced the change that took place in the lay Freiburg hospital between 1762 and July 12, 1784 (date of the adoption of the Rules of the Religious Hospital Community by the Bishop of the diocese). Twenty-two years of waiting all the same!

As was often the case, existing caregivers were not part of the change. It was imposed on them! But the former governess was still being asked to stay on for some time beyond the term of her contract to give the necessary instructions to this future "hospital nurse". This practice at the time was common and remunerated. There was so much tacit knowledge to be passed on in the lay age, and no school yet, that the hospital management was not prepared to see one person in possession of experienced knowledge go away and leave the other to fend for himself for his learning. Before it was seen as a "female vocation", caring was an activity with knowledge from experiences passed on by peers. This specific knowledge for caring could be analogous to what is sometimes referred to today as "primary nursing" and represents the basic knowledge of the discipline. The length of time required to transmit knowledge and lay knowledge useful to the service was generally "a few months" without further details [NAD 93]. Based on the texts reviewed, we estimate it to be between three and seven months depending on the institution.

Towards the end of the 18th Century, the canton of Freiburg was experiencing serious economic difficulties. Freedoms, food shortages and a famine of the most notable kind caused people in need of care to flock to the hospital. The governess could no longer cope with the difficulties caused by the influx of people in hospital. "The nurse was so busy with the number of sick people that it was necessary to give her help. Since she could not receive this help in time and could no longer cope with her workload, the *musshafera* or governess of the sick requested her discharge on May 12, 1771" [FON 61-74]. The departure of an "expert" in the tacit knowledge of care caused a serious crisis in the hospital and forced the Board of Directors to become seriously concerned about the shortage of personnel and its consequences.

A certain Mademoiselle Dufour was hired on August 4, 1771 to replace her. "The hospital master was authorized to issue her with up to two coins of new gold to make her all the more attached to the service of the poor. The Most Honored Lords approved and reviewed the said Demoiselle Dufour as a 'superior nurse' under the conditions set forth" [NAD 93]. The appearance in 1771 of this new term "super nurse" was still a sudden event in the language of the hospital and marked a probable hierarchy of roles which was beginning to be envisaged. There was some hesitation among the "Most Honored Lords" as to the appropriate term to use to describe the professionals in place. Mademoiselle Dufour replaced the hospital's lay governess (*musshafera*). She was given the status of "a super nurse" and the "small servant" of the governess found herself in the position of "sub-nurse". The hesitation over the term to be used in recruiting staff shows that the hospital's governing authorities were not too clear about the status, mission and skills required for the caring profession.

These new terms (superior-nurse, sub-nurse) appeared in hospital language as early as August 4, 1771, while the "real" nurses (the nuns) were still not active. Announcing major changes within the hospital, this suggests that the hospital management was unsure how to go about both introducing religious personnel and maintaining the roles and privileges of the lay people who remained in place. It also raised the question of whether, through this expected change (which was taking place without the knowledge of the existing caregivers), there was not a connivance of views between the clergy and the doctors who would have perhaps liked to have more power within the hospital to develop or apply clinical knowledge. Another hypothesis to explain the sudden appearance of a new vocabulary (nurse, super nurse, sub-nurse) to qualify the caregivers: in 1771, it was Schueler Laurent-Bernard, who was both a doctor (trained in Montpellier) and a hospital master at the *Hôpital des Bourgois de Fribourg* between 1764 and 1772. Could he be a relative of Ignace Schueler (Schüler)? The latter was in fact director of the Sion Hospital in 1763 and it was he who collaborated with the Freiburg authorities to introduce the nurses from Sainte-Marthe de Beaune, whom he himself had brought to Sion in 1771 (coincidence of name? Place? Role?).

On September 13, 1771, a supplement to the hospital regulations of 1759 institutionalized and officialized the functions of "super nurse" and "sub-nurse", even though there were still no nurses in the hospital. In this new regulation for the "direction of nurses", a distinction was made between what was expected in terms of the knowledge required to perform this function. Of course, we were still in the age of lay knowledge! Reading this document, it is as if we discover, as it were, a work plan for the day. This document seemed to us to be of primary importance in order to speak of the foundations of care knowledge, because written knowledge about ordinary care in a hospital of the Ancien Régime, still of a lay nature in 1771, was rare. Hospital prescriptive writing thus shaped ordinary practices and could advantageously enrich the representations that were usually made about the care to be given and the knowledge that went with it.

The reason why we extend so much detail and attention to the arrival of nurses at the lay bourgeois hospital in Freiburg is because the procedure put forward was almost the same from one religious community to another. It describes well how a community of Catholic nuns took possession of a hospital. Moreover, the documents that reported on this process were relatively rare, mentioned at least once. Certainly, there was often competition between the different religious orders in charge of hospitals. But whether the nuns came from Beaune, Bourg-en-Bresse, La Flèche,

Dieppe, Lyon, Sion, Pontarlier, Besançon, etc., was only secondary to the establishment process, which was almost the same in different parts of the world, including the reference to the rule which then became the written standard that guided the logic of action among religious communities.

When a nurse entered training, it was to access the knowledge that would make her a nun. Imbert rightly reminds us that in the Middle Ages, the vast majority of hospital congregations had one thing in common:

> This was taken from a letter that St. Augustine[18] had sent to nuns to guide them on the path to perfection. This text simply contains some general advice that can be applied to any religious community: it forbids the possession of nothing of one's own, the wearing of clothes other than those provided by the community, orders obedience to the superior, the practice of fasting, encourages religious to purity, humility and charity. Each hospital will add particular prescriptions which will deal more specifically with the care of the sick. [IMB 47]

As mentioned, the traces of healthcare activity and of the knowledge required are rare enough that we allow ourselves to present them to the reader in their entirety. The important passages in the text on "the direction of nurses" will then be framed. What is in fact a description of the role, bears knowledge which is added to the knowledge already exercised and set out from the regulations and texts of the hospitals of Geneva, Freiburg, Bulle, Romont, Yverdon, Lausanne, and from Carrère's 1786 care manual. The body of knowledge that this presupposed was already part of the heterogeneous heritage and multiple legacies of the care discipline (which did not yet have this status at the end of the 18th Century) and this, long before Florence Nightingale was born (1820) and at a time when there were no professional schools. Let us recall that there were no schools, but there was knowledge.

The service asked of the nursing sisters was to provide the care required by the estate (*Domus*) and its inhabitants (*familia*, *ad-hominem* regrouped) in exchange for remuneration for the service rendered, not paid directly to the nuns, but paid to the mother house of the congregation as was often the case at the time. Taking care of the estate concerned "the temporal" aspect.

18 The feminine version of the letter of St. Augustine is the letter 211 or *Objurgatio or regularis informatio*.

Direction for nurses[19] ratified in the Chamber on September 13, 1771 (*sic*)

The sub-nurse will make soup in the morning as usual. When the super nurse is established at the hospital, she will let the sub-nurse make the soups and she will insist that they are made properly and hygienically.

The super nurse will distribute the patients' soup, while the sub-nurse will distribute it to the hospital honorary positions and to the passers-by room, observing not to put bread in the bowls of those, whom the doctor or surgeons will order to be kept on a diet, and of those who will be purged the same day.

The chamber pots are then emptied and taken to the latrine where they are rinsed with hot water, which is boiled in the small boiler for this purpose.

Remedies will be administered as prescribed.

The beds will be made, and after those in one room have been made, it will be swept while those in the other room are made, and then the room in which the beds were made last will be swept.

If a few patients have taken to vomiting or purgation, both the super nurse and the sub-nurse will not only provide them with butter broths or hot water, but will also assist them as needed.

When meal times arrive, they will prepare the dishes and bowls for the patients and arrange them on the boards for transporting soups and portions, following the order of the bed numbers. They will then go down to the kitchen where the soups or broths will first be served according to the prescription; they will distribute them and come back to collect the portions while the patients eat their soup, to be distributed to them afterwards.

During the distribution in the kitchen the superior-nurse will have before her the list that the doctors and surgeons have made, so that each patient will be fed according to their prescription, and while the patients take their meals, they will stay one in one room and the other in the other to see if the patients eat their portions and if no one comes to their house to remove their leftovers, and if one of them should arrive, they will come to warn one or the other of the attendants. They will also have to take the patients' leftovers back to the kitchen. The same order will be observed for the distribution of snacking soup and the distribution of the supper.

19 Book of sentences: Urteil Buch, August 12, 1740–October 10, 1796, 403 pages, only the front is numbered, Archives de l'État de Fribourg (AEF), Fonds de l'hôpital des Bourgeois, unclassified work, bilingual French/German, 336 × 213 mm, 2,100 kg, p. 180–181. Transcribed January 28, 1991 [NAD 93, NAD 12b]. Difficult to find. We had to describe (weigh and measure) the documents found.

The bowls should be washed thoroughly after each soup made and the dishes after each meal.

Following a visit from the doctors and surgeons, the nurse will present them with the list of the plan so that any changes they want to make can be inserted.

During the day, the super nurse will stay in the patients' room to make sure that there is no disorder: that the patients do not assault each other and that no one enters the wards without first having permission from one of the attendants. If during this time she has intervals or is not busy around the patients, she may complete works for herself, for her own need only, or darn the patients' linen.

If the sub-nurse during all this time has something to do around the patients, she will do it especially with regard to the passers-by, and the super nurse will see to it that all these articles are punctually carried out; of all which she will make her report each evening to one of the attendants.

Neither the super nurse nor the sub-nurse shall give to any person, sick or otherwise, anything of any kind whatsoever, other than what the doctors or attendants order or permit, and if anyone in the hospital asks them for anything, they shall return it to the attendants.

The twelve articles above were approved and ratified in the Chamber on September 13, 1771.

Box 3.1. *Planned job description for nurses in 1771 in the Freiburg hospital (Switzerland)*

Caring for people and community life was about the "spiritual". "We send nursing sisters to you", the mother house told the authorities, "but you pay us for their services". Such is the economic functioning of the development of hospital congregations. But for unknown reasons (stakes of power, negotiations on the modalities of establishment of the nuns), it was necessary to wait another 20 years at the Freiburg hospital (March 14, 1779) from the moment the idea of replacing lay people by religious nuns was raised and before serious contacts were established with the *hôpital de Sion* (Sion hospital) (Canton of Valais). In fact, since 1771, the hospital of Sion has employed nursing sisters, the nuns of Sainte-Marthe de Beaune[20].

20 This congregation was founded in Beaune on August 4, 1443 by the Chancellor of the Dukes of Burgundy, Nicolas Rolin and his wife Guigone de Salins. A lay aristocratic couple thus founded, with their own fortune, a private religious establishment of pontifical right. The vows are simple, temporary and revocable vows.

Since the care of men posed a problem for (female) nurses in connection with the vow of chastity, there was talk on March 22, 1778 of "paying a man in the hospital to give care to patients of his own sex". This was achieved. Here was the reason for male participation in care. Claude Veber was then hired as the nurse's assistant "especially in charge of caring for and helping to bandage the men, as well as having the inspection on the poor passers-by". On April 11, 1778, abuses were also noted in the allocation of the portions of food prescribed by the doctor, which then forced the executive room "to order the nurse to accompany the doctor to each bed and to write on a card the diet of each person in order to have it carried out punctually" [NAD 93]. Here we have the beginning of what would later become the ritual of the medical visit.

NOTE.– Attention should be paid to language. In French *infirmier* (nurse) is not simply the masculine form of the term *infirmière*. Not being able to form a masculine term, the nurse was in fact the male servant of the nuns. The form of the word *infirmier* that can be found in ancient texts is always the unqualified helper of the nurse or the governess.

This changed with the entry of the first boys into secular schools in the mid-20th Century. This differentiation between the nurse's helper and the nurse existed until about 1972–1975 in the hospitals run by the nuns, in particular the sisters of Sainte-Marthe de Beaune who lived, for example, in the *hôpital de Porrentruy* (Porrentruy hospital) (Switzerland). So, let us not be mistaken! When the radical Georges Favon wanted to stigmatize the nurse profile, he declared before the Geneva Grand Council in 1897:

> What was that nurse a few years ago when the deaconesses were brought into the hospital? He was a man who was going to be taken from the back room where he had been a store boy, from the stable, from the plow where he was a farm boy, who was offered a salary about the same as that offered to a country valet, who was chosen simply because he was robust and willing to change his state, to earn five francs more per month, and who was faced with a task that would have required an education, culture and special knowledge that he did not have. [DRO 92]

That's right! But beware of the meaning of the words and the induced representations. Georges Favon was talking about an "unqualified helper", not a qualified man or a graduate. This did not exist! Politicians always found it difficult to grasp the qualities required to carry out a role they do not know! The nurse was always the nuns' male servant, the handyman of the hospital governesses or "the master of the low works" as they said in the Romont hospital in 1733 and who helped the hospital caretaker [NAD 12b]. And no one rushed to run for office, take care of the estate, ensure the domestic dynamics and do the heavy work necessary to maintain the house! Whenever the word "nurse" appears in texts before the 1970s, it is either a religious brother or an assistant of the sister-nurse that is mentioned.

In 1779, the shortage of domestic carers at the Freiburg hospital was a matter of great concern. At all costs, it was necessary to find more stable caregivers than laymen and those "assigned by state to the service of the sick". This was the case of the nuns.

> The difficulty of finding servants careful and intelligent enough to serve the sick properly has made it difficult for the *Messeigneurs* to find stable nurses, as in any well-run hospital, who are attached by condition to serve the sick; and it has been deemed necessary, in order to achieve this long-desired goal, to turn to R.P. Schüler for help[21], director of the Sion hospital, to ask him, in accordance with the offer he made to *Monseigneur* the President of Montenach[22], to send the Superior of his Gray Nuns both to acquaint herself with the interior of our hospital and to prepare the way for this new establishment, and to choose the people likely to take up his instructions; asking him, moreover, to ask him if it would be possible to have them trained in Sion. [NAD 12b]

On May 27, 1779, Father Schüler, both professor at the association and director of the Sion hospital since 1763, offered to accompany the Mother Superior of the nursing community (Marie-Barbe Anthamatten, originally from Saas) to Freiburg "to study with her the reformation and corrections to be made in the hospital. A car will be sent to pick them up in Sion and since M. Schüler wants to have someone to witness their journey, the hospital master will go to pick them up" [FON 71-82]. On June 13, 1779, the Grand Chamber received Father Schüler and the Mother Superior and entrusted them with a study "on the details to be observed and on the abuses to be reformed and to draw up a memorandum to be presented afterwards for discipline, cleanliness and economy" [NAD 12b].

The arrival of the Catholic nurses (not qualified for the time) in the lay hospital resulted in a new distribution of the architectural space and a change in the living

21 Ignatius Schüler (or Schueler, Schueller), a Jesuit from St. Gallen, managed the hospital in Sion from 1763. He introduced nurses (hospital nuns) to the hospital, notably the Superior Mother Barbe Anthamatten, a Valaisan woman trained in Pontarlier (France).

22 François-Frédéric de Montenach, President of the Grand Chamber of the hospital.

conditions of the dormitories[23], the hospital master and his family. In order to make room, the *dormiaudes* were evicted and the benefits received by the hospital master and his family (a six-room dwelling) were taken away. In addition, the hospital could not stay open as it has been so far. They were closing!

From this month of June 1779, R.P. Schüler was asked to make proposals that led to a complete reorganization of the Freiburg hospital including a new conception of space and time. New statements were made. The sick room became the "infirmary" according to the new language brought by the Superior of the nurses of the Sion hospital and R.P. Schüler. The other parts of the hospital continued to receive the same population as before. The hospital closed down and closed itself off a little more by eliminating exchanges with the outside world. It was even necessary to "close the storeroom in accordance with the rest of the building" [NAD 93]. The expelled *dormiaudes* now came under the jurisdiction of the "rescue office" of the city of Freiburg. The health sector transferred its beneficiaries to the social services. In order to maintain a certain degree of autonomy, the *dormiaudes* were also given some furniture and kitchen utensils and fir wood for heating. In case of illness, the hospital said it was ready to receive them free of charge in the infirmary. The development of a religious language in a secular universe that ignored the terms "*infirmière, infirmier, infirmerie*" (nurse in its male and female forms and infirmary) until then was being witnessed.

On September 29, 1779, a cloth was taken at Sion and the novices were sent to be formed in Sion and neighboring France in Pontarlier in the same community (Sisters of Sainte-Marthe de Beaune) at the expense of the hospital. Already on July 28, the Grand Chamber of the Freiburg hospital agreed to "pay a pension of four and a half crowns per month and per nurse, in addition to the extras, to go and do their postulancy and novitiate in the Sion community". The hospital then bore the cost of training its staff. The two nuns who took their postulancy in Sion, Anne-Catherine Furer and Marie-Judith Meschler, then went to Pontarlier to do their novitiate for two years. The costs for board and lodging amount to a total of 1,008 pounds 10 sous and were paid by the Freiburg hospital.

In 1781, Marie-Catherine Marx, 22 years old, from Tourtemagne (canton of Valais), was appointed superior nurse at the Freiburg hospital for a period of three

23 Inhabitants of the *dormiau* (*drumiau*) the dormitory. These places were occupied by able-bodied (alms) people who worked outside (sometimes even in the hospital itself) and who came to the hospital to receive, according to the agreements made, bed and board for life. As soon as the nuns arrived, the *dormiaudes* were given an annual pension of 30 crowns 9 batzen, out of which they were given an advance of 40 pounds for their board and lodging in a place they had yet to find.

years. On July 12, 1784, during his first canonical visit to the nurses of Freiburg, Bishop Bernard-Emmanuel de Lenzbourg, Bishop of Lausanne, adapted the rules of action brought from Sion to the circumstances of Freiburg. These rules, under the title "Our Lady of Seven Sorrows for the great hospital of Freiburg in Switzerland" were "confirmed to be observed, in their form and content, for all civil and temporal objects relating to the service of the hospital". They were ratified by the "Sovereign Lords of the Supreme Senate at the Assembly of the Grand Chamber on 18 July 1790".

The nurses of the Freiburg hospital were then constituted as a religious community. It was composed of three postulants and five nuns, including the Mother Superior [NAD 12b].

Responsibilities still needed to be assigned to the nuns. This was done on July 19, 1785, when the Chamber of the hospital took note, confirmed and ratified the distribution of the workload among them.

A new superior was appointed and the distribution of responsibilities was as follows:

> After the deliberation of the House in the last assembly, concluding that the nuns agreed among themselves to plan how the other offices, besides that of the Superior, could be distributed among them, the said nuns presented the following arrangement:
>
> – novice mistress, sacristan, first cook and spendthrift[24]: Sister Judith Meschler, Superior;
>
> – apothecary and linen: Sister Catherine Furer;
>
> – nurse to the men's ward: Sister Marie-Catherine Marx;
>
> – nurse to the women's ward: Sister Marie-Ursule Dupond, novice under the inspection of the apothecary sister;
>
> – second cook: Françoise Blanc, postulant;
>
> – first baker and gardener: Sister Claire Ackerman;
>
> – second baker and cook: Sister Anne-Marie Bürbaum;
>
> – children's governess: Sister Françoise de Marret.

24 The one who is responsible for "the expenditure" (in Old French), that is, the central store or food reserve.

NB: Sister Françoise will stay in the kitchen until she is handed over the care of the children. Françoise Blanc will go to the kitchen, only when the Superior is there, until then she will remain in the foyer.

Sister Anne-Marie Bürbaum will stay in the kitchen in the meantime and could be in charge of the care of the hemp. For passers-by and shut-ins, the one who will have the time while waiting to be provided otherwise.

Which aforementioned arrangement my honored Lords have confirmed and ratified in all its contents. (July 19, 1785, Manual, 1782–1792 in [NAD 12b, p. 106])

NOTE.– The hypothesis we made concerning the language contained in the supplement of September 13, 1771 to the hospital regulations of 1759 is confirmed. It was indeed a question of introducing a major change in the organization of the hospital. A new hierarchy of role specified by the language and affecting both lay and religious personnel appeared. The superior-nurse was the superior of the religious community. The nurse replaced the lay governess and the term sub-nurse was then applied to the sisters' lay handmaid, who became in the 20th Century the nurse's assistant (formerly a small handmaid).

The arrival of nurses in a lay world and the new language that accompanied them changed the meaning of the values linked to hospital activity and organization. But this did not take anything away from the daily care that remained to be done! The nuns also had, over a long period of time, many conflicts with the authorities of the city of Freiburg who wanted to keep their power over the functioning of the institution (on a temporal level). The nurses had to obey the Superior of the congregation, possibly the hierarchy of the Church, but not necessarily the hospital's Board of Directors; whereas lay servants and governesses previously owed individual obedience by taking an oath before the hospital hierarchy. According to the values and rules (which already represented a kind of care theory) of the Catholic Church advocated by private charity, the nurse's daily activity followed the recommendations and rules approved by the bishop of the diocese. Thus, religious culture was gradually taking its place in the hospital and remained there as long as there were vocations. In terms of knowledge, one passed from lay knowledge to "sacred" nursing knowledge, the knowledge of which, translated into daily action, was carried by the nursing rules and the knowledge learned during the novitiate under the authority of the "novice mistress"[25]. While this could give rise to reflection today, as we can see, the nurse

25 The mistress of novices "must be exemplary, punctual in her duties and of a well-regulated exterior, because actions are more persuasive than words" [REG 84].

was therefore not the one who simply entered a school of nursing or the faculty of nursing. She was above all a person who completed the novitiate in order to obtain the status of hospital sister in exchange for the individual spiritual and celestial benefit of her action.

On the content of the writings, we do not see great changes between the care given by the sisters and the care practices given by the lay handmaids. To get an idea of this, it is easy to compare the extracts from the texts of the hospitals of Geneva and Freiburg in 1744 and 1759 (see the quotation p. 90–92 of this work), the Carrère's text in 1786 (see the quotation p. 97-99 of this work) and the regulations of the hospital of Freiburg of September 13, 1771 (see Box 3.1). The text below, which dates from 1784, mentions doctors and surgeons. Carrère's text (1786) also mentions doctors and surgeons to whom the nurse had to submit. However, medical scientific language did not yet occupy the entire hospital speech space. In fact, the lay servants at that time also strengthened their collaboration with doctors and surgeons. We have not discussed this so far and reserve this point in section 3.5, devoted to "city physicians".

However, in substance, new values linked to the practical charity of the Catholic Church and to the esprit de corps that marked religious communities were mobilized in daily action, as mentioned in the Rule of the community of the Sisters of Sainte-Marthe de Beaune at Freiburg hospital in Box 3.2.

"There will be at least one nursing sister in every room. Their care will extend to the inpatients and sick passers-by. They will care for all the sick with the utmost accuracy and charity, complying punctually with the prescriptions of the doctors and surgeons, either for the diet or for the administration of remedies, giving them at the prescribed time and in the prescribed manner and never leaving the remedies at the disposal of the sick. In order to better comply with the orders of the doctor and surgeon, they will always attend their visits and change of dressings.

The most convenient time for these visits is in summer, from six in the morning until quarter past seven in the morning, and in winter, from seven in the morning until quarter past eight in the morning. In the afternoon from one to four thirty. In extraordinary cases, they may also take place from seven o'clock in the evening until eight o'clock at night.

The doctor's visit will take place at the same time or a little before the surgeon's visit, in order to consult on the state of the patients and to be able to carry out in time what he will have ordered.

Each nurse will accompany them in her department, from bed to bed, with their respective patients, reporting on the states and symptoms she has noticed in them. At these visits will also assist the sister in charge of the pharmacy with the prescription book, the nurse will carry the diet book with the writing case so that the doctor or surgeon can see both the diet and the remedies prescribed the day before and order from the patient what he will find out about it.

When the visit is over, the nursing sisters will inform the cook of the quantity and quality of the meat prescribed for the sick patient's meal; the apothecary will take care to prepare the remedies and have those she does not have ready.

If, since the visit, there is any change in a sick person or some unforeseen accident, they will contact the Superior and do what she advises.

Everything that is intended or presented to the sick and what is for their relief, will be laid out and practiced with all care and cleanliness: dishes, beds, linens, clothes, basins and spittoons, in a word everything will be in the decency and cleanliness required for a service rendered to the sick and who have the honor of being members of Jesus Christ.

First of all after meditation or even before, if it is necessary, the nursing sisters will go to their patients to inquire about their condition, empty the basins, make the beds, change the linen, if necessary, sweep the rooms, change the air, take on the task there.

After giving the holy water, they will take morning prayers with them, admiring the remedies and serving lunch.

They will spend the day in the hall, either to give the sick all the assistance that their condition requires, or to ensure that good order is observed.

When there are sick passers-by, they will visit them often and take the same care of them as the sick people in the halls.

They will not lose sight of those who, because of insanity, have the misfortune of being locked up and sequestered from other patients. They will take great care that they always have something to drink, since their condition requires a copious amount of drink.

They will try to do good and charitable service, to make their sad lot more bearable and will take advantage of the good intervals they notice to make them do acts of contrition, faith, hope and charity, even if these good times last for some time, they will notify the chaplain, to make them confess, if there is a way.

They will invigilate with great care that nobody gives the sick anything, especially that the visitor who will come at the permitted hours, visiting the sick, will not bring them either drugs or food, let alone wine or other drinks. If, in spite of their vigilance, something is slipped to the patients, as soon as they notice it, they will take it away to prevent the unfortunate consequences and prevent the inconveniences that may result.

> They will take care to occupy the sick, especially convalescents, for a little work, as much as their condition will allow, both to amuse them and to banish their idleness, the source of many ills, even among the sick.
>
> They will remove the bandages, strips and other cloths from the patients, wash them or have them properly washed, iron them and hand them over to the surgeons.
>
> At meal times, they will go to the kitchen to collect the food for the sick, which they will distribute, taking care not to exceed the quantity and quality of meat prescribed, unless circumstances require otherwise.
>
> They will say blessing with the sick before the meal, and after serving, they will give thanks.
>
> They will also say evening prayer with them and recite the points of the examination of conscience.
>
> When there will be sick people to be cared for, they will inform the Superior early so that she can provide for them. She will have many sick people to look after, and from time to time she will employ people from the hospital whom she finds capable, to relieve the sisters.
>
> In order that the sick may not remain without help during the absence of the Sisters and especially during the night, there will be a nurse in the men's ward and a sub-nurse in the women's ward, whose duties will be marked below" (Règles, 1784, pp. 63–69).

Box 3.2. *Excerpt from the Règle 1784 of the Sisters of Sainte-Marthe de Beaune for the large hospital in Freiburg, Switzerland*

The administration and organization of care, as well as the service rendered to the medical profession and the sick was newly specified, sometimes in great detail, as can be seen in this 1784 text. Was this a political alliance between the Church and the medical profession? What was also new in the text was the reference to "members of Jesus Christ", "meditation", "holy water", "prayers", "acts of contrition", "faith", "hope" and "charity", "benediction", "evening prayer" and "examination of conscience". These elements of language, which appeared as the result of two years of novitiate training preceded by several months of trial (probation, postulancy) and which were formalized by the Rule, were added to the existing language. In fact, the tasks to be done on a daily basis remained. One just adds spirituality to the existing temporal nature. We almost have an advanced practice before the letter. It is not because the sisters brought with them spiritual knowledge that the nursing staff in place naturally started to exercise a "feminine vocation". They did not become "parareligious" for all that! Neither was it because the sisters took possession of the work spaces that everything went well. Since they also had to fulfill their spiritual obligations, pray in the chapel and read good books, they had less time to do daily work. They were assisted by the lay people in place. Recurring tensions then arose with the existing lay governors.

With the arrival of the nurses, religious culture took possession of the hospital as long as public opinion was "unanimous in recognizing the Sisters' specific qualities such as lack of political ambition, professional competence, moral integrity and also the low cost of the services provided" [LAN 84]. In 1784, a nurse was someone:

- of impeccable conduct;
- of great vigilance and foresight;
- of profound humanity;
- of an ever-active charity;
- with an ardent zeal;
- with a welcoming modesty;
- of compassionate tenderness;
- of heroic courage;
- of a virtue consumed (Règles, 1784, p. 63).

Ninety pages thus dictated the conduct of the nurse for human care (the spiritual), in caring for the group as well as for herself (community life) and in the care of the domain (the temporal). From a trilogy of care in the lay age (*Domus–familia–ad-hominem*), we move on to two categories of sacred knowledge in nursing. Indeed, with community life, *ad hominem* and *familia* were in the same group on the spiritual level. *Domus* or taking care of the estate remained in the temporal. Taking care of others has never been easy and it is understandable that the theories of religious care aim, as Ricoeur said, "to desire the obstacle in order to tend positively to the difficult as a good and to the pure pleasure of overcoming" [RIC 88].

With the arrival of the nurses, the identity at work of lay governors also changed. There was a shift from the individual identity of the governesses and servants to a group identity. Lay governesses and servants were not structured as a professional group, had no common identity and no common knowledge. "Each individual was in total dependence on leadership" [LOU 00]. With the nursing community there was a community of nuns who had the sister identity, with common knowledge and skills (the Rule), who were united in the exercise of charity in two parts "one of which looked to God and wanted them to be united with him through prayer and interior perfection; the other united them with their neighbor through works of hospitality and mercy" [FON 84]. The nursing community also had a uniform, a form of training (the novitiate), initiation rituals, an expansion of the community which took place according to the "biological model" metaphor (from mother cell to daughter cell[26]) and means of control and punishment in the application of the knowledge and behavior prescribed according to Catholic tradition (the Chapter).

With the formation of a nursing community, the activity that was until then, according to Guy Jobert's typology, an individual occupation in an institutional setting, thus became a profession, since the community had common methods that were passed on to new recruits [JOB 85]. But attention should be exercised here, as it was especially a spiritual profession recognized by the Church which was emerging, not yet a temporal profession recognized by the state. Individual domestic work was being replaced by work done by a social body, a community. With the arrival of the nuns in the lay hospital, the "Body of Christ" was introduced as a Church in which the hospital activity was above all "a profession, an oath and an ordination; it was the profession of the monks' faith which designated a life choice, a way of ensuring his salvation" [DUB 05]. As we can see, the change for lay personnel, as much for the nature of the knowledge as for the dynamics of the hospital, was then of very great importance!

For the hospital authorities, community life prepared the nuns to assume all the duties and roles of the former collective household as it existed before 1784. In Quebec, the phenomenon was relatively similar. The "officers" of the Hôtel Dieu du Précieux-Sang (1639), generally Augustinian nuns of the Misericorde de Jésus from Dieppe in the wake of the Jesuit missionary fathers, had various duties divided into offices and offered so-called general care (reception of the sick, toilets, beds, meals, maintaining order, assistance to the dying, etc.). They were assisted by converse nuns for the maintenance of the rooms and equipment. "The hospital master then formed the center of the organization of care. All questions relating to the hospital, whether professional or scientific, were within his competence (…) the hospital rectress thus permeated the whole hospital with his personality (…), his authority extended also to lay employees (…), the philosophy of caring for the sick was transmitted from master to apprentice, from generation to generation" [VIO 05]. Like the Sisters of Sainte-Marthe de Beaune, the first hospital mistresses of New France received their training in France. "The Augustines de la Miséricorde learned their trade at the Hôtel-Dieu de Dieppe, while the hospital nuns of Saint-Joseph (Hôtel-Dieu de Montréal as early as 1659) did their apprenticeship at the Hôtel-Dieu de La Flèche".

26 This daughter cell became a mother house, which again led to a new establishment of nuns (daughter cell) in another hospital and so on.

Also in France, the place of origin of most hospital masters in the Catholic regions, there were an impressive number of hospital congregations. According to Knibiehler, in 1878 there were still 20,000 nuns in 225 congregations. In Paris, 485 nuns commanded 2,791 supervisors and servants in the hospital establishments. “In the hospitals, they essentially exercised a supervisory role over the male and female personnel of miserable condition, who performed the men’s and women’s dirty work” [KNI 84]. As in the French-speaking part of Switzerland, they directed the lay personnel in place at the time of their arrival, who were then demoted to the position of sub-nurse. Moreover, as Claude Langlois points out, “the female congregations enabled Catholicism to maintain close contacts with the ruling classes and to extend its hold on the working classes more widely” [LAN 84]. On this subject, the nurse’s rules of action specified:

> Nursing sisters consoled the sick with good discourses, instruct them in the principal mysteries of religion, teach them the acts of faith, hope and charity, contrition and good intention, which they often exercised, and made them wise in the practice of good confession and communion, of suffering with patience and of conforming with great resignation to the will of God. If the nursing nuns noticed among the sick, passers-by or others, some who were not instructed in the duties of a Christian and did not want to let themselves be instructed by them, they would then inform the spiritual father so that he could undertake them. [FON 84]

States supported by sympathizers of the Roman Catholic Church were beginning to ask how best to organize hospitals, secure their revenues and apply the principles of practical charity of the Catholic Church. Incidentally, the ongoing dechristianization needed to be prevented[27] and the hold of Catholicism on the working class needed to be extended. Among the post-revolutionary texts acting in this direction, that of Cabanis seems to us to serve as an illustration. During the winter of 1789–1790, the physician Pierre Jean Georges Cabanis, then a member of the commission for the reform of Parisian hospitals, published his arguments for developing nursing corporations:

> Men are in no way fit to serve the sick. Nature seems to have reserved this honorable function for women alone, as well as the care of children. See a man with the sick: if he wants to talk to them, he

27 “In the face of the dechristianization that continued in the 19th century, the clergy, however, did not want to renounce the practice of bringing the mass of believers back to practice, even if it was on their deathbed. This was the role that is increasingly assigned to the hospital masters, both traditional and new” [LAN 84].

> makes them dizzy; if he wants to shake them, he shakes them; if he gives them a drink, he pours half of it onto the sheets. His emotion is always delayed and his help never arrives in time. Put a woman in his place: her tender pity guesses, prevents needs; she does everything in a timely manner and without haste; with what skill she moves a suffering body! What cleanliness in the details of service! (…). The free association of the Sisters of Charity is, without a doubt, the best institution for the service of the sick. It is to be hoped that the government will entrust to them the care of hospitals for the sick and that it will seek natural and just means to increase the number of these respectable hospitals. [CAB 89]

With an identity proper to the Catholic Church, hospital nuns were thus the only ones to legitimately call themselves "nurses" [TUR 89]. It is therefore understandable why the term appeared at the moment when the authorities of the city of Freiburg began to evoke the possible arrival in the hospital of "these respectful hospital nuns". "The only place where women were deliberately prepared for a professional life" according to the church's doctrines of practical charity, the novitiate. To leave the novitiate is to enter working life. Two years of intellectual and spiritual training to prepare for action. This was the training of the hospitable nun. For Yvonne Turin, "without any complexes, the nuns extended their territory most naturally in the world, neither considered nor occupied it, much less conquered it. They assumed with tranquility and assurance the role they chose for themselves" [TUR 89]. After all, as we have seen with the Freiburg hospital, the nurses did not impose themselves. We came to find them!

We now find ourselves discussing the 19th Century. The sacred knowledge of the lay period spread throughout society. About a century after the Catholic regions, the Protestant Church, in turn, imitated the Catholic Church. Together with its sister deaconesses, it gradually took over the speaking space in the lay hospitals of the Protestant regions. On October 15, 1836, in a small German town, Kaiserswerth-on-the-Rhine, near Düsseldorf, the young pastor Theodore Flidner laid the foundations of an institution of deaconesses, which was not only to spread rapidly in Germany and in the Christian world, but also to lead to the creation of the institution of the Saint-Loup deaconesses, above the village of Pompaples, in the canton of Vaud (Switzerland), on December 19, 1842.

This indelibly marked, as we will see in Chapter 6, the entire later history of nursing, directly by its many ramifications [SEY 33] and indirectly by the chain of numerous reactions in Protestant regions (Switzerland, Great Britain, France) that it aroused.

It was also about "infiltrating Christianity into society" [CHA 79]. Indeed, there was no reason why the Catholic Church should be allowed to touch believers even on their deathbed. Fliedner noted that only Catholic charity had the means to develop educational and healing works. The theory put forward was that "we lack religious orders dedicated to practical charity; the Reformation went too far when it destroyed them all; Catholics rightly reproach us for not having any, let us have some" [DEG 54].

The development of communities of Protestant nuns was carried out as in the case of Catholics, in other words, according to the metaphor of the biological model from mother house to daughter cell, from community to community. In 1844, there were 55 consecrated deaconesses and 34 novices in Germany, 11 hospitals served by Protestant nurses. "They were sent all over Germany, some were sent to St. Gallen in Switzerland, three sisters went to London, others went to St. Petersburg". A motherhouse was established in Pittsburgh, Pennsylvania, and one in Jerusalem. "Wherever there was a Prussian consul, there was eagerness to foster an institution. In Constantinople, Smyrna, Beirut, at the request of the political agents of Prussia and at the King's insistence, Kaiserswerth sent nuns" [DEG 54].

After St. Gallen, Zürich and Bern, they arrived in French-speaking Switzerland on December 19, 1842. First in Échallens[28] (Canton of Vaud), then in a village called Pompaples (about 20 kilometers from Lausanne). They were then called the "Sisters of Saint Loup"[18]. Protestant religious houses developed from this mother house in the canton of Geneva, 76 houses in the canton of Vaud, 24 houses in the canton of Neuchâtel, 19 houses in the canton of Bern and 3 houses in the canton of Freiburg. Abroad, 17 houses were built. Pastor Haerter, founder of the deaconesses of Strasbourg in 1842, was pleased with "what Protestantism showed to the Roman Church corporations similar to those of Rome" [DEG 54].

28 Valérie de Gasparin's husband (founder of the world's first school for lay nurses), Count Agénor de Gasparin, returned from a trip to Germany where he had just visited Fliedner's work. Not having yet realized that the German nuns resembled "those in Rome", he proposed on August 10, 1841 to Pastor Germond to create an identical one in the Protestant region of Echallens. During the annual meeting of the Lausanne Evangelical Society, in which Germond participated, Count Agénor de Gasparin "took the podium and demonstrated with his own enthusiasm and artistry that the churches of French-speaking Switzerland were the best placed in French-speaking Protestant Christianity to undertake similar work" to that of Fliedner. Louis Germond, then in the assembly, "stood up to announce that the creation of an establishment of deaconesses in French-speaking Switzerland was decided and that the establishment would not be long in opening" [VIN 42]. Count de Gasparin even made a donation on June 30, 1843, of 172.50 CHF to support the work of Pastor Germond during a subscription [NAD 93].

The Protestant Sisters also gradually replaced the governors of the lay patients in several hospitals in French-speaking Switzerland. In the hospital landscape, they were in fact an addition to the Catholic nuns already at work in the Catholic cantons. The widespread idea that care was now linked to vocation and to the nuns partly erased the fact that this care was above all the work of the working classes and the servants in the public hospitals. In the 18th Century, women were generally excluded from any professional status. But the nature of the knowledge related to care did not change. Politicians did not believe that special training was needed to train the carers that would be needed in the future. There were no schools to train lay people, it was simply a case of calling upon the nuns who did the novitiate, that is, who submitted themselves in obedience to the spiritual initiation ritual of learning.

As long as the hospital was not overly medicalized, the domestic knowledge and assistance of the people being cared for in daily activities remained associated with the running of an ordinary household. Admittedly, a complex economy of assistance already existed within the hospital. This economy remained at a representation level, an ordinary activity, a family, household and state dynamic. The knowledge at work remained that of the lay period around the triptych of knowledge linked to "*domus–familia-homo* or *ad-hominem*". It was not easy to carry out this care activity. Today's natural caregivers are well aware of this and can testify to it. Let us add to this additional knowledge related to community living and the spiritual order. Deaconesses needed to respect their religious obligations and since they could not do everything, priorities for action were necessary. As for the Catholic nuns, they began to delegate to their helpers, lower level care and provided supervision. Let us add to this the growth of therapeutic knowledge which progressively completed the knowledge already in place as soon as doctors (more and more numerous in this half of the 19th Century) entered politics to develop the health system and bring the medical knowledge linked to the advent of the clinic (from 1790 in Freiburg[29]). The amount of knowledge required to be increased! And as hospitals in the 19th Century also tended to transform themselves to take into account both the increase in the number of patients and the accompanying technological progress, it was still additional knowledge that needed to be mastered by the nursing staff.

29 For example, while the Helvetic Republic had just been established after the entry of the French revolutionary troops, a national prefect had to be appointed to administer the Canton of Sarine-et-Broye. It was Jean-François Déglise, a doctor and notary from Châtel-Saint-Denis, who was appointed prefect. It was under his authority that on July 22, 1798, "the first Health Council was created to fight effectively against epidemic and epizootic diseases that threatened towns and countryside, man and beast". From this period, the government's control over the organization of health, the medical profession and its legislation became more evident [NAD 93].

However, the development of religious communities within Protestantism unleashed passions and a huge surprise that no one saw coming. These passions resulted in the creation of institutions of a completely new kind compared to the existing religious novitiates (Catholic and Protestant) at an international level. The first lay schools for women who wanted a care profession and no longer vocation saw the light of day (see Chapter 6).

3.3. Nurses (*enfermières*)

But what does the term "nurse" mean when it comes to religion-based nursing? Why is this term exclusive to the Catholic Church? Why was the legitimacy of bearing this title exclusive to religious nurses since lay women were not and could not be nurses?

Etymologically speaking, the term "*infirmière*" comes from the ancient French word *enfermerier*, *enfermier*, *enfermière,* which indicates that the one who bears this name, usually and by profession, is confronted with that which relates to the bad, to the stench, to what is "weak", "sick", "unhealthy", in other words to Hell, to the power of darkness, the dwelling place of the damned. Amazing! How can a nurse be led to promote health under these conditions? We hear today's nurses say that they are involved in health promotion, but at the same time it does not bother them to be recognized with an identity that relates to hell, to evil, to bad health. The profession does not seem to be more affected by this paradox and etymology alone is not enough to recover the meaning of the term.

The term "*infirmier*" is a reflection from Latin and Old French. By succession of time, we have taken up the Latin "i"; for we say today infirm, infirmity; "infirm", "infirmity" have received a special meaning in the language which Latin does not demonstrate [BLO 75, GOD 84]. The term "*enfermier*" seems to have two six-letter roots, of which the first five letters "*enfer*" are common to several formulations and indicate a relationship with hell in the French language. The origin of the terms "*enferm*" (bad, unhealthy) and "*enfern*" (place from below, dwelling of the damned) is not entirely consistent in ancient French dictionaries. So what is this "special meaning that Latin does not demonstrate" made of?

The combination of these two terms *enferm*[30] and *enfern*[31] was in use in the medieval religious hospital, which fell under the private practice charity of the

30 Infirm, sick, frail, bad [SAI 56, GOD 84].

31 "Hell in ancient mythology, a subterranean place inhabited by the shadows of the dead, one region of which, Tartarus, is reserved for the wicked; in the Christian religion, a place reserved for the torment of the damned, as opposed to purgatory and paradise" [GOD 84].

Catholic Church. The term "nurse", after several forms of adaptation, *infirmus, infirmitas, enferm, enferme* on one side and *inferi, infernum, infernus, enfern* on the other, was built around the common radical *enfer*[32], and *enfers*[33]. One says *enfermerier*[34], *enfermmier, enfermière*[35]. It symbolically designated a person from a religious world (nurse) who was confronted with the unhealthy and the bad. As mentioned in the historical dictionary of the French language, the term "*infirmier*" is borrowed from derivatives or compounds of the etymology (most often Latin, for example *infirmus*), but reserves some surprises in its use through relationships that are nowadays erased [REY 92]. The term "nurse" does not, therefore, qualify a person who takes care exclusively of lay patients, nor does it derive solely from Latin, as the majority of the French-speaking nursing community thinks today. What is the link with hell? We have to go back in time!

We often see the date 1288 or 1398 as proof of the first use of the word "nurse", then spelled "*enfermier*". But already in the Middle Ages, the term was used by the Order of Saint John of Jerusalem. At that time (1135–1139), the term *enfermier* or *enfermerie* was used in Old French, that is, in the Romanesque language. For example, we see in the writings left by Catholic communities of hospital masters, especially in the hierarchical statutes of the Order of the *Hospitaliers* of Saint John of Jerusalem and according to the Rule of the Temple according to the Manuscript of Provence, seven articles concerning the Friar *enfermier* of which we present below two extracts (excerpts) in langue d'oc (Old French):

> *190. Le frère enfermier doit avoir tant de discretion que il doit demander as frères mesaisiés, qui ne pusent mangier, e nen osent, de la comunal viande de l'enfermerie, l'enfermier lor doit demander de quele viande il porront mangier, et il le doive dire puis qu'il lor demande; et il lor doit faire apareillier et doner tant que ils puissent mangier de la comunal viande de l'enfermerie. Et noméement as frères foibles et mesaisiés et relevés de maladie doit si come il est dit dessus.*

> 190. The friar who is a nurse must have so much discretion that he must ask his fellow friars, who cannot eat, or dare to eat, the common

32 A symbol of suffering as a keyword in popular Christianity [REY 92].

33 "An evil inferno that has badly wounded the horn" [GOD 84].

34 "And to lock up, know what it will be used for. His patients must visit, for their illnesses are social (…) and lock them up with care" [GOD 84].

35 "An *enfermier* is a religious person who takes care of the sick. The convent owes bread and wine to the convict and secretary, when they have the houses of their offices repaired. How madam", says the prisoner, "you are my homicide" [SAI 56].

meat, the local meat, must ask for the meat they will be able to eat, and he must say so and then he must ask for it; and he must have it prepared and given as long as they can eat the common meat. And by name as many of the friars as faithfully and soberly and sickly must if as it is said above.

196. Le Comandeor de la maison doi trover au frère enfermier ce que mestier li sera a la table de enfermerie, et a l'enfermerie la ou li frères gisent malades (a l'enfermerie des frères); et doi metre a son comandement la bouteilrie, et la grant cuisine, et le four, et la porcherie, et la galinerie, et le jardin. Et se le Comandeor ne veaut ce faire, il doit doner au frère enfermier tant de monoie que il puisse (a table de l'enfermerie et en l'enfermerie des frères) en l'enfermerie faire avoir ce que mestier y sera. Le Comandeor de la terre doit faire avoir as frères ce que mestier lor sera, et ce dont ils achèteront les mecines que mestier lor auront.

196. The Commander of the house must find for the nursing friar what he wants to be at the nursing table, and at the nursing house where the friars lie sick (at the confinement of the friars); and he must put at his command the cellar, and the kitchen, and the oven, and the porch, and the gallery, and the garden. And if the Commander does not want to do this, he must give to the friar as much money as he can (at the nursing table and in the friars' home) by nursing him, making him have what he wants there. The Commander of the earth must make his friars have a use, and they will buy the medicine that will be used.[36]

The friar in charge of the nursing home watched over the sick or wounded religious brothers. For Duby, the male nurse was even one of the seven dignitaries mentioned in the rules of the chapter by Archbishop Imbert in Arles in 1191 [DUB 88]. What seems to mean all the same is that providing care and helping one's neighbor to live in the midst of a religious community was not an insignificant role as one might perceive it today as long as it gave rise to a useful and worthy form of recognition.

In theology, we rather see the nurse in relation to the body as the receiver of the bad behind the wounds that swarm with worms or the stench that comes out of the

36 Official regulations of the Order of the Temple. Extract 190 and 196 of the Rule of the Order of the Temple, available at: http://www.templiers.net/ (page consulted on June 9, 2011).

human body and which gives the soul a virtue superior to that of the body, which is therefore dearer to God. The proof is in the writing:

> The nuns who are hospitable out of humility, as the foundation and principle of all their movements and actions, should believe themselves unworthy of the honor they have to serve Jesus Christ in for the poor person whom they serve; reflecting on the corruption, baseness and infirmity of human nature, esteeming little of everything that seems healthy and beautiful and great in the world, since it hides only rottenness, continual sources of shame and pain in both body and spirit. In approaching the wounds that swarm with worms, the rubbish and stench that come out of the human body, judging from within the rottenness and corruption of the sick, the hospitable nuns will find continual subjects to lower themselves to and confuse themselves.
>
> They will make themselves commendable with great purity of morals, by a faithful correspondence to graces and by a great contempt for all human respect; they must free themselves from all attachments to creatures, considering them with indifference; they will study to overcome incessantly all the repugnance that nature has for suffering and for disgusting, low and stifled jobs.
>
> It is also a question of assisting those being cared for "all the more so in what concerns the spiritual, since the soul is dearer to God than the body (…). The nurses will take even greater care and pay more attention to the good of their patients' souls than they do to their bodies." [FON 84]

A Catholic nun was a nurse, therefore, at a time when there were still no schools, she was confronted with stenches, with wounds swarming with worms, with the powers of darkness[37]. So she was not the one who originally trained in a nursing school or in a nursing faculty. The discipline today also calls itself "nursing"! But what knowledge are we dealing with?

The myths of evil also refer to a demonic etiology of certain illnesses fought with therapeutic prayer, holy oil and holy water. Thus, in the prologue of the book of

37 To darkness is connected the color black in English before the 17th Century "evoked, according to the Oxford English Dictionary: filthy, defiled, dirty, foul. To have dark or criminal purposes, evil. Referring to – or evoking – death and morbidity. Dark, disastrous, sinister. Inexistent, atrocious, dreadfully bad. Marking dishonor, shame, punishment, etc." [ZIN 14].

Job (Job 2:6–7) and in the words of the Apostle Peter, "how God anointed Jesus of Nazareth with the Holy Spirit and power, and how he went around doing good and healing all who were under the power of the devil, because God was with him" (Acts 10:38), [LAR 91]. It is then, that:

> The disease is produced and reproduced, extended, developed, multiplied and strengthened and sometimes even incarnated by the powers of darkness and wickedness, the devil and demons, who then become one of the principal sources of disease, manifesting themselves most often indirectly through them, but also sometimes without mediation as in cases of possession, occupying then themselves in man the empty place of God. [LAR 91]

It is always the devil and the demons in connection with disease. We know that the two characters of the myth in general are that it is a word and that in it the symbol takes the form of the story. Ricoeur invites us to go beyond the narrative and to see with the phenomenology of religion, that "the myth-telling would be only the verbal envelope of a form of life, felt and lived, before being formulated; (…) it is in the ritual more than in the narrative that this conduct would be expressed most completely and the mythical word itself would be only the verbal segment of this total action" [RIC 88]. In this regard, the holy water that was still in the pharmacy of some of the care units of a small hospital on the Neuchâtel coast, run by nurse deaconesses in 1970, accompanied the ritual and remained a symbol for driving out the demons responsible for the disease and for warding off the fate that befell humans in order to purify them. "Gestural imitation and verbal repetition are but the broken expressions of a lived participation in an original act which is the common copy of the ritual and the myth" (*Ibid.*). Exorcism also occupied a special and traditional place among religious therapeutics, in the same way as the use of holy water or the sign of the cross. "God redeems sinners and restores the health of the body if it is useful for the soul; ungrateful people risk hell. It is not surprising, in this context, that the faithful seek to protect themselves in hospitals from evil influences". Perpetual masses in some parishes became a form of therapeutic exorcism to protect one's soul, body and possessions "from devils both on earth and in the air" [BRO 98].

Nor is it forgotten, following Collière [COL 82], that the word "*mal*" (evil) "is the translation of death: *maladie*, that which is a sign of death, that which makes one die". Therefore, what could be more normal than to still link to *enfermiers* those who are confronted with evil and demons and who support death.

Let's keep going back in time to the earliest civilizations. We already find hell and demons associated with man's illnesses and those who care for him. Thus, the reference to hell and demons is not surprising in establishing the link with diseases in the second millennium and was already part of a kind of theological mythology.

The link between sickness and hell and those who dealt with it is highlighted in the Sumerians and Babylonians in the third millennium. Through ceremonies, sometimes reaching the dimensions of solemn liturgies, "the rulers of the world were asked to command the demons and evil forces to stay away from the impetuous or to withdraw from them with the evils with which they had burdened them". According to Jean Bottéro, demons then became "the gendarmes of the gods, charged with executing their criminal decrees and bringing evil and misfortune as punishment to those who had offended their principals by some sin: some transgression of their will" [BOT 87].

Faced with these gods and in order to explain the evil of suffering as it is called, another series of personalities were forged, inferior, certainly to the creators and rulers of the Universe, but superior to their victims and who could freely cause the misfortunes that poisoned their existence. Such was the conception of the demons. In this conception, "the disease (*dimitû*) has risen from hell, and the demons that bring it, falling upon this abandoned patient of his protective god whom he had offended, have wrapped him in it like a coat! Evil is considered here as a material reality brought from outside ('hell') by the 'demons' and deposited in the patient's body, who was exposed without defense to such a danger by his god, whom he had offended and who thus delivered him to the executors of his vengeance" [BOT 84].

The role of the demons around disease, death and those who approach it "has been closely related to hell, from the moment they were imagined to play essentially the role of executors of the high works of the gods irritated against men". This principle is still relevant today and seemed perceptible in Europe in the 18th Century, when syphilis, for example, "was perceived as a divine punishment for sin. It could be attributed to the wrath of God, who allowed the disease to fall on mankind to curb their lust" [BRO 98]. Three axioms contributed to the identity of a nurse:

– the first was the demonic etiology of certain diseases fought with therapeutic prayer, holy oil and holy water;

– the second saw the body as a repository of evil, whether through the wounds that swarmed with worms or through the stench that came out of the human body, thus giving the soul a virtue superior to that of the body, which, because of this, "was more dear to God";

– finally, the third consisted of the nurse's consent to seek "the difficult as good" [RIC 88] from a paradisiacal perspective, which conferred exclusive ownership of what was called the eschatological promise of the hospital nun or gray nun.

So, the nuns were indeed the only ones who were legitimately nurses (*infirmières*). Their withdrawal from the world, their spiritual activities and the vows they made gave a specific meaning to their actions. They maintained exclusivity of their actions. But it was by no means on these axioms that the nursing discipline as it stands today was built. Saying, as we do today, that care is "nursing" or that thinking is "nursing" provokes a utopia of identity, bearing an aporia, that is, a rational difficulty that seems to have no way out, which brings with it a proliferation of theoretical models that have nothing "nursing" about them. Hence, the conceptual problem posed to the care discipline.

We previously noted that "nursing care did not exist" in contemporary times [NAD 03b]. The statement concerned the identity of the lay people. It is not meant to suggest their elimination or disappearance, quite the contrary. It is just to draw attention to the fact that the term nurse is correctly conceptualized for nuns, but absolutely not adequate for the contemporary lay practice of care. Why lay one value system on top of another? Talking about nursing does not tell the whole story about the evolving nature of a living language, and does not explain the skills required to practice it. The word "nurse" today is a symbolic image charged with ancient representations. It remains a verbal tic or myth. For 40 years, attempts have been made to define, reject or clarify this term, to explain its nature or to find a place at the heart of the discipline of the same name. Something else will have to be found to give meaning and a strong identity to the care discipline, which is much more complex than we can say. Admittedly, this complexity has yet to be demonstrated, whether based on personal knowledge, expert knowledge or scholarly or even scientific knowledge, if we want to talk one day about a *Bachelor of Science* delivered to female students of the universities.

What could be more natural for medieval theology than to take up the principle of this theological mythology of the third millennium and to continue to conceptualize the world of care and of humans in their relationship with God, with sickness, evil, unhealthy, demons, the powers of darkness and hell as the dwelling place of the damned. With these words about hell and the *enfermier*, the evil, the demons and the mythological environment of the sick, we can guess that we are moving directly on the linguistic level, so to speak, from a pre-Christian theological mythology to a medieval theology of sickness and "the nursing home", even influencing the writing of the rules of religious nurses and beliefs. The term nurse has not yet faced criticism. It has just been imposed on caregivers without anyone being in a position to challenge it.

3.4. Nurses and *gardes-malades*

The term "*garde-malade*" (*krankenpflege* or *pflegerin* in German or *sick-nurse* in English), in contrast to the term "nurse", is primarily a lay term. It is mainly used to describe a person who provides care in the home. We can find its use in the countryside of Freiburg in 1778. However, it is also present in certain documents at the Freiburg hospital from 1790. With time and the representation of uses, the vocabulary became more precise. It can be seen that the woman who was called "*gardienne de l'hôpital*" in the 18th Century later became the "*garde-malade*" between about 1750 and 1790. Society then became aware that the guardian of the premises (with what is inside) became the guardian of the sick (with what is around). The representations were reversed!

Prior to 1859, a *garde-malade* sometimes referred to an unqualified person as a caregiver or someone "taking care of..." With the development of training as of 1859, it was established particularly in the Protestant and French-speaking regions to describe a person who had attended a nursing school. From 1910 in Switzerland, it described a person who was a member of the *Alliance suisse de gardes-malades* and who had a certificate from the Alliance. In Switzerland, the term "*garde-malade*" also competed with the term "*infirmier*" until 1944[38]. It distinguished between the religious nursing profession of a Catholic or Protestant nurse and the lay nursing profession in Protestant regions. In a Freiburg health law valid in 1979 (since amended), the terms "*infirmier*" and "*garde-malade*" were still used as equivalents in the text (see Article 88). They demonstrate the equivocity of the role as a historical after-effect, which gave pace to the influence of representations on care and their knowledge.

> Article 88[39]
>
> (1) *Infirmier*, *infirmière*, *garde-malade* shall mean any qualified person who, for profit or free of charge, professionally provides care for the sick, injured, infirm, women in childbirth, infants.
>
> (2) A qualified *infirmier, infirmière* and *garde-malade* shall work only in collaboration with and under the direction of a licensed physician.
>
> (3) They must strictly comply with his requirements. [NAD 12b]

38 This year corresponds to the dissolution (May 6, 1944) of the *Alliance suisse de gardes-malades* (ASGM), which has a sick-nurse only in name, since its leaders were statutorily doctors and officers of the Swiss Army (Red Cross). By their position, they had the power to direct the health system and the knowledge expected from their "auxiliaries".

39 "*Extrait du Règlement du 16 mars d'exécution de la loi du 6 mai 1943 sur la police de santé et textes annexes*" (*Grand conseil du canton de Fribourg*).

No one in the nursing profession today remembers that the term *garde-malade* referred to the lay care group in Protestant regions and that the term *infirmière* represented exclusively the Catholic denominational group. The deaconesses, for their part, sometimes hesitated in their identity. Sometimes they were called "*la sœur*" (the sister), sometimes "*la diaconesse*" (the deaconess), rarely "*l'infirmière*" (the nurse) according to the use made of the term in popular vocabulary.

As for the English term "nurse", it is mainly related to the representation of the maternal role of women and the care they give to her child. Nursing is a symbolic figure of the living forces of the fertile woman. "To nurse, to give life, to suckle, to feed, to nourish and, from there, to soothe, to comfort" [COL 82]. Florence Nightingale, who changed her opinion several times about the tasks of nurses and the definition of the qualities necessary for the best, specified that she "used the term nursing because she did not have a better one" [BAL 93].

3.5. City physicians

In the 17th Century and until the middle of the 18th Century, doctors and clergymen did not yet reside in the hospital and only occasionally intervened in it. Interventions varied from one hospital to another. Of course, the hospital master, the governesses and their servants were confronted with medical language, even though their presence was not yet generalized throughout the hospital. They also needed to understand what they were saying or what they wanted. "The barber surgeons came to *try*[40] the sick and *meygier* (carer in Old French) those who suffered from illnesses. The hospital paid the barber surgeon for every treatment separately". They undertook a wide variety of cures: amputations, the healing of fractures, the care of wounds, the healing of skin diseases [NIQ 21]. In the 17th Century, the medical service was completely organized in the Freiburg hospital. As early as 1643, the hospital had its own doctor. Next to this doctor were two surgeons, the doctor supervised the operations that these two practitioners undertook. The oldest known physician in Frieiburg is Pierre Azon, who was established as a "city physician" as early as 1311. It was also in 1653 that the authorities of Freiburg created the position of hospital surgeon (*Spital-Wundartzet*), separate from the duties of "physician or city surgeon". But caution should be exercised here; this did not mean that there was a department of medicine or surgery in the hospital. In fact, doctors were asked to intervene promptly inside the establishment when they were overwhelmed by diseases and in case of epidemics or death in particular. At the Geneva hospital, the 1744

40 Examine whether they had leprosy (*a Peterman barbeir por esseier 2 malades de mesalie*) [NIQ 21].

regulation provided that "there shall be for the service of the hospital three doctors who are members of the faculty of that city[41], one for the poor who are housed in the house itself, the other two for those who are housed elsewhere and who receive assistance from the hospital" [FON 44]. The hospital master, on the orders of the doctor[42], went to the apothecaries of the city to get medicines. The hospital governesses familiarized themselves with these products. After receiving the doctor's instructions, the hospital master had them applied by the servants.

The governesses and servants then learned some knowledge about the use of these products: knowledge that was added to existing knowledge. This new "medical-surgical" type of language was linked to remedies, to new knowledge from the birth of the clinic, from the order of nature or from the different medical schools (naturalists, vitalists, nutritionists, etc.), to which hygiene knowledge was added. General hygiene first, hospital hygiene later. This medical language used by the nursing staff of the time preceded the permanent presence of the practitioner in the hospital and was the subject of a progressive learning process on the job of the nursing staff already in place (hospital staff, governesses, maids, servants, guards). In the large hospitals, around the middle of the 18th Century, the nursing staff were asked to render service to the medical profession by making sure that the patients took their remedies and followed the prescribed diets:

> The doctor who will see the sick who are in the house will be obliged to see them at least once a day and he will warn the people who will treat them about how to regulate their food. The governess will take care to make the sick take the remedies, and also the broths. [FON 44]
>
> The doctor will prescribe daily to the *gardes-malades* the remedies and food to be given to the sick, and will be made aware of the effects they have produced, so that he may be better able to direct himself accordingly. [SER 90]

One point needs to be made here. In this excerpt, we see that medical science depended on the layman's point of view. Without the service rendered to the medical profession, without the caring role of "data collector" for medical use, it is clear that the doctor was somewhat helpless and sometimes blind or deaf to adapting his therapy to the patient's condition. The caregiver was doing the medical profession a service by enabling it "to be able to direct itself all the better

41 Note: at that time, the faculty was not a university department, but only the corporate grouping of physicians, masters in surgery and pharmacy who thus had an intellectual rallying point.

42 The first doctor mentioned in the hospital archives is *Dominus Johannes, Gebennensis, sacerdos et physicus*. This priest of Geneva origin practiced medicine in Freiburg in 1312.

accordingly". This role was not always properly evaluated. The doctor did not live permanently next to the inhabitants of the hospital and needed representatives to process the information[43]. This was still quite convincing in 1903 in the Protestant infirmary of Bordeaux, where the student "hospital *garde-malade* was entrusted with the monitoring of several patients and had to provide the doctor with all the data he needed to effectively carry out his role" [DIÉ 90]. As Yannick Barthe points out, "the knowledge of experts can be, in certain circumstances, partial, but it is, by construction, partial. Once the incompleteness of scientific knowledge is brought to light, it becomes possible to interpret the opposition of laymen to the discourse of authority held by experts as something other than the manifestation of ignorance" [BAR 99]. We can also deduce from these excerpts from the texts the skills required of governesses, servants and maids to do what was to be done and required by the prescribed action:

> And since the proper administration of remedies is as necessary as their good quality, apothecaries will be exhorted to have them taken from the sick in the time that will be marked by the doctors; for this purpose they will be careful to carry them or have them carried when the patients themselves lack the facilities to send for them and to have the enemas given by their servants. [FON 44]

Traditionally, a certain kind of medicine was practiced among the few patients in the hospital. Language was an obligatory part of the practice. The lay nurses had been accustomed for some time to observe the effects of certain therapeutics delivered from time to time by the city doctors (*physicians*) and to assume sometimes the undesirable medicinal effects of certain drugs or compound medicines. Let us think of purgative drugs, for example. With these few examples of medical prescriptions, the nursing staff could do nothing but handle, store, sometimes package and administer them. At the Freiburg hospital, medicines were sometimes supplied by the doctor himself; but, more often than not, the hospital master, on the doctor's orders, obtained them from the city's apothecaries, because the Freiburg hospital, like other large establishments, did not have its own in-house pharmacy. "In the 16th century, for example, barber surgeons undertook a wide variety of cures at the Freiburg hospital: amputations, the repair of broken bones, the treatment of wounds and the healing of skin diseases. They were assisted in the operations by their own servants". The governesses took over in case of absence. The accounting documents from the 15th to 17th Century discovered on the hospitals that disappeared in Switzerland reveal that in 1635, for example, at the Freiburg hospital, products considered to be remedies were used, such as: "plasters, ointments, pills, distilled water, scorpion oil, medicinal herbs, catholicon, coloquinte, rhubarb, jalap (julep);" […] "the sick were also given lemons, oranges,

43 Argument still relevant at the time of writing!

honey, jams" [NIQ 21]. These are all requirements of knowledge that appear in the first manuals of care, more and more frequently in the second half of the 18th Century. We note the content of the prescriptive discourse given to the hospital masters, then newly appointed "*gardes-malades*" in 1786 according to the medical point of view:

> The administration of the remedies prescribed by the people of the art and the preparation of those which can be made at less expense to the sick are still part of the duties of the *gardes-malades*. The former requires a great deal of accuracy, either so as not to change the nature, combination and order of the remedies, or so as not to neglect the timing of their delivery. The latter requires special knowledge, skill and intelligence which can be acquired through habit. The *gardes-malades* are neither physicians nor surgeons of the sick; their roles are limited to helping the sick in their needs, reporting to people on the art of what they have observed, and using the remedies they prescribe. They are to be regarded as mere instruments to be used in administering to the sick the help they deem necessary. They need, therefore, a great deal of accuracy in the account they give to the physician, a great deal of attention to what he prescribes, and a great deal of docility in following his advice. [CAR 86]

After observing, transmission was necessary, that is, possessing a specialized discourse in order to report particular observations and information to the doctor. This required the lay hospital servant of the time to learn about the advancement of her practices and new linguistic and cultural norms, so that the meaning of the message was not too far removed from the reference system of the person for whom it was intended. This principle is still valid today. This system of values linked to medical science (values, ideologies, knowledge), gradually delegated to the servants as a now legitimate language, steered the discourse and actions demanded by what is sometimes still called today, a delegated or medico-delivered function of the professional role. There were still no schools for caregivers. It was through contact with the doctor or by reading his texts that carers internalized the biomedical language. In the interdependence that existed between them and the physician, the caregiver, although not yet scientifically literate or trained, needed to become familiar with the official professional language, the legitimate language of medical knowledge. However, just because a medical language was added to the existing language did not mean that it should take on greater importance than the knowledge already at work. When the doctor arrived in the hospital, new medical knowledge arrived and new languages were added to the existing languages.

From the end of the 18th Century to the 20th Century, this cognitive instrument imposed in the face of a hitherto effective autonomy in the rules of action of the lay carer supported the caretakers in their passage from domestic service to the service of the institution and the sick, to this new position of servant and doctor's assistant. The first two roles, the institutional role which first prescribed in writing what the nursing staff (*Domus*), whom we shall later call SC1, needed to do, and the caring role (*familia–ad-hominem*) (later called SC3), did not disappear. The language proper to the triptych *Domus–familia–ad-hominem* was completed. It was a fourth role (medico-delegated function) (SC2) which was added in writing to the previous ones, but in second position as far as writing is concerned.

Under these conditions, and as Knibiehler and Fouquet point out, 20th Century training "shaped new staff, changed behaviors, gestures and moral attitudes. Teaching needed to inform by eliminating any overview, any possibility of synthesis. The purely utilitarian knowledge of the nurse needed to remain subordinate to the coherent science of the doctor. A pure and simple executioner, any initiative remained forbidden to him. Trained by and for the doctor, she remains at his service. Her role did not include any specificity" [KNI 83]. However, being at the service of someone is not the same thing as being of service to the latter and that what used to be the knowledge of the nursing staff's experience did not suddenly disappear by magic because new knowledge was added to the previous.

In this dependent role, the hospital servants and governesses then became a "double agent" who rendered service to the medical profession: an agent "collector" of data without power over the logic and purposes of the operations and an agent "applicator" of prescribed therapeutics without control over the relevance of the prescription. It was indeed a service rendered to the medical profession. With the development of the clinic and the progress of scientific medicine, this double agent role only became stronger, but without taking away the primary skills of the lay era demanded by the implementation of *Domus–familia–ad-hominem* knowledge. It took time for the nursing staff to become aware of these positions and language issues. Especially since "the social service relationship was not only a relationship of interpersonal exchange based on the functional utility of the service. It conveyed, in various forms, relationships representative of the organization and hierarchical structure of society" [DEL 87].

Thirteen practices[44] of service to the medical profession that are still part of the practices at work today were already identified at the time of lay knowledge. In this "double agent" practice, observation and communication with an understanding of learned languages are demanding skills. They range from 13 to 18 practices in the

44 Eighteen of these practices are mentioned in the publication of the nursing conceptual model (nursing activity, the cultural intermediary model) [NAD 13].

results of an international scientific research (Switzerland-Quebec) conducted in partnership with the Faculty of Nursing at Université Laval in Quebec City in 2002 by the research and development unit of the Haute école de santé de Frieburg[45] [NAD 03b]. These groups of practices merit in-depth research today to provide additional details to fully understand what is being done or what is known to implement the ordinary and daily practice of "service to the physician and surgeon".

At a time when there was still no structured professional training, the doctors gradually took up a position paid for by the hospital needed to rely on the existing staff and force the nursing staff to follow imperatively and linguistically what they advocated in terms of health (medical order). However, the symbolic power of the medical discourse used to enslave employees could not be denounced enough, and this enslavement (or paternalism) was all the greater in the status of the knowledge in question and the more effective the performative enunciation. Even though in the 20th Century, nurses were led to believe that they were the "disciplined but intelligent colleagues to the doctor and the surgeon", as stated in the circular of October 28, 1902 addressed to the Prefects in France by Émile Combes, then Minister of the Interior and Religious Affairs, one should not be mistaken about the purpose of such an assertion. Can we really speak of "collaboration" when it is in any case asymmetrical, or is it only a euphemism intended to hide certain power issues associated with the languages used?

In addition to her ordinary activities related to "caring", the nurse gradually became more and more a "double agent" providing services to the medical profession: on the one hand, a data collector for medical analysis (observation, evaluation of the patient's condition and transmission to be made in the legitimate language); on the other hand, an agent applying medical prescriptions. This clearly demonstrates here the power that the one who completed studies had over the one who could not. In this way, the physician had the power to delegate knowledge to those he inexorably considered as his auxiliaries, knowledge understood as a fragmentary or residual part of his knowledge and his art. What are the differences between this dual agent function and the advanced nursing practices of the nurse practitioner specialists who still demand access to new knowledge today?

From the end of the 18th Century to the middle of the 19th Century (and even after), caregivers gradually witnessed the medicalization and the stakes of this game and had to adapt or experience the arrival of a new language, that of the medical culture. In this adventure, they sometimes took over certain languages or techniques that lost their prestige for medicine (e.g. the control of vital signs: pulse, blood

45 Research financed by the *Fond national suisse de la recherche scientifique*, Nadot *et al.* Project No. DO-RE 01008 and CTI 5545 FHS, *Mesure des prestations soignantes dans le système de santé*. Research and Development Unit, Haute école de santé, Freiburg, 2002.

pressure, temperature, breathing or injection techniques, etc.). But the rules of action that they needed to then apply were delegated to them by doctors and surgeons who, gradually, contributed to writing manuals "for the use of nurses" as the formula of the moment required (see Chapter 7). These rules of action which they needed to henceforth apply were delegated to them by the doctors and surgeons, the latter seeking to discover, in part of the clinic, the disease in the patient in a systematic and orderly manner and which, in the face of "known, probable or hidden" causes, should lead, after having stated the prognosis, to "vital, curative or palliative indications" [FOU 88]. In fact, this was already provided for in the Ordinances in Geneva in 1697 for those seeking the *agrégation de médecine* (Aggregation of Medicine, seeking tenure as physicians). It was necessary to "discuss the causes, signs, prognoses, indications and cure of the disease" [LOU 00]. Seeking tenure as physicians is perhaps to be put into perspective, because we also know that the examination of medical theories towards the end of the 18th Century showed that their level was rather low. The same subject came up very often and it even happened that the text of a thesis reproduces almost exactly that of a previous one. This was more of a ritual and corporate ceremony than a scientific examination [NAD 12b].

Access to therapeutic language in the 18th Century was insidious and gradually became part of hospital practice. To indicate how this therapeutic language entered the hospital, we give as an example a list of written prescriptions found in the archives[46] of Romont hospital for 1795–1796. The "*gardienne*" of Romont thus become familiar with the prescribed medicines and how to administer them. In the caring discipline, it was all about language and communication. There was still a lot of knowledge to be acquired! The accounts of the remedies of the surgeon Martin show, for example, that:

– December 22, 1795: given to Béline Grivet, who remained in the hospital, a jar of laxative opiates;

– January 15, 1796: given to little Défferard, a chicory syrup made of rhubarb. Given to Bélot, the caretaker, a laxative package;

– January 24: a box of purgative pills, a packet of sudorific woods;

– March 12: given to Béline Grivet a jar of pectoral opiates;

– March 14: ditto, a pectoral julep;

– April 3: ditto, pectoral tablets;

46 Archives of the city of Romont: account of the remedies of surgeon Martin, Romont hospital, 1796–1797, approved and ordered for payment. Administered on April 5, 1799, signed: Wullieret Secretary.

– April 5: given to a patient coming from Valais, a large packet of herbal tea;

– April 8: given to a patient in hospital, a packet of herbal tea (2 batzen) and a very composed medicine (10 batzen, 2 sou);

– April 10: given to a woman who was also in the hospital and similarly discomforted, a medicine like the previous one;

– April 11: given to Béline Grivet a pectoral julep and a package of herbal tea;

– April 16: given to Mrs Bélot, the caretaker, a packet of ypécacuanum powder;

– May 10: ditto, a package of herbal tea;

– May 11: ditto, a very composed medicine;

– July 6: gave a patient in hospital a pectoral and balsamic syrup;

– August 5: given to Mrs Bélot, a bottle of Goulard water;

– August 18: ditto, a jar of purgative opiates and an aperitif. Given to a stranger, a jar of red ointment;

– August 22: given to a poor feverish stranger, laxative opiate. Same for two of his sick children, laxative opiate;

– September 20: given to the caretaker Mrs Bélot, a bottle with calming and carminative results;

– November 11: a bottle of the same nature and a blister plaster, etc.

The arrival of medical culture did not eliminate the traditional tasks to be performed. Even in the face of the "doctor", the care of the human being, the care of the group and the care of the field, not only remained, but reinforced with the new treatments that made it possible to limit, for example, hospital infections. In order to survive, one did not need to receive care. But when there was treatment, attention, precautions and care increased, as Marie-Françoise Collière said in 1996 [COL 96]. In insidious and progressive ways, the arrival of the physician, the development of scientific medicine and technological progress only added complexity to an already existing complex feature. The caretaker of the hospital became a kind of specialized practitioner before the latter. Similarly, the new architecture or technological advance of a hospital was never insignificant in terms of the development of new skills, new knowledge, behavioral change or the proliferation of multiple languages.

Faced with all the new languages that were being introduced into the hospital, the risk for the caregivers was that they cast aside their own usual language, that of life support and care, which became, if not illegitimate, at least insignificant. The mental burden, however, increased. Gradually, the medical and therapeutic language exogenous to the hospital penetrated the latter and is reinforced daily through the statements. With the remedies distributed by the caretaker of the Romont hospital in 1799[47], skills increased. This was somewhat the case in several countries. It was necessary to learn the language of these treatments. There was a necessity to discover the usefulness of the treatment and how to store, distribute, conserve or store these products.

Nobody at the end of the 18th Century was still thinking of giving professional training to the carers of the lay age. Caregivers who were in the hospital twenty-four hours a day, ahead of doctors, were not empowered to speak with authority. "Necessarily, because in the place where acoustics were best, there was no room for everyone: it was precisely the possibility of access to it that played a role as hierarchical discrimination within the order, as a stake in internal struggles, as a criterion for success and as a badge for belonging (the diploma or degree). Intellectual power was the fact of being there, of controlling access to it and maintaining the monopoly" [DEB 79]. Without access to training, until the middle of the 19th Century, caregivers were not yet in a position to produce their knowledge (therefore no discipline), to control access to it and to maintain a monopoly on it. These constituted important conditions for the development and recognition of a discipline. But this concern was not yet on the agenda.

47 Account of the remedies of Surgeon Martin, Romont Hospital, 1796–1797, approved and ordered to be paid. Done in administration on April 5, 1799, signed: Wullieret Secretary.

4

Practices and Knowledge

To be able to identify some care practices carried out in hospitals and demonstrate the link between yesterday's and today's practices, it is necessary to have some clues as to their existence over time. Caregivers do not write, but we write about them. There is a before! Before hospitals took on the dimensions as we know it today, before there were schools to ensure the transmission of language traditions, before the doctor was in residence in the hospital, before the church colonized the hospital in order to impose new values on it, caregivers with a status close to servitude and domesticity exercised care that was quite contrasted from one place to another. In this lay period, knowledge was sometimes transmitted "on the job", from practical experience to real practice without ever leading to an abstract system of knowledge or theoretical discourse. On the one hand, those who had access to the nature of the phenomena (church, medicine, aristocracy), on the other hand, those who, being insufficiently educated, had no strong professional status, especially women. As Marie-Françoise Collière rightly points out:

> It is on the basis of sacred knowledge, and then on the basis of knowledge inherited through writing, that the gulf will widen between those who profess doctrine and hold instruction and those whose practices will be judged to be of a lay nature because they are carried out by matrons, old women and healers considered ignorant because they are illiterate. Yet it is their knowledge that has fed the manuscripts and now provides the manna for anthropological works. [COL 96]

At the end of the 18th Century, ordinary "scholarly" expertise in the hospital setting "was based on a given conception of humankind, social relations, behaviors and values. The reasoning and thinking skills of lay people were generally largely ignored or underestimated" [WYN 99]. Since all practice is cultural, it is therefore closely linked to local knowledge. Indeed, the caregivers who performed their duties (right or wrong is not the question) generally referred to the surrounding knowledge and local experiences in their field. And as Wynne mentions in relation to a study conducted by Van der Ploeg on Andean farmers, this practice "then refers to truly dynamic knowledge systems that involve a constant negotiation between manual work and mental activity, a continual interpretation of production experiences. This leads to a highly complex knowledge system and an adaptive, flexible culture that does not easily lend itself to standardization or planning" [WYN 99].

Because this knowledge is not codified by writing or appears as a group standard, it remains in the form of individual know-how. This lay knowledge is rarely recognized as such. This is quite the case with the nursing knowledge of the lay period, or even with the ordinary contemporary work of the woman or the housewife. It is only a short step from this to explain why the simplicity projected on lay knowledge cannot compete with the complexity of scientific knowledge. Like the lay knowledge described by Van der Ploeg (quoted by Wynne), the knowledge of care in the lay era was also "complex, reflexive, dynamic and innovative, nourished at the same time by material, empirical and theoretical aspects (…). They were charged with implicit cultural models, a conception of the human subject, of action and responsibility" [WYN 99].

4.1. *Domus* or looking after property life

Caregivers who worked in lay[1] hospitals often needed to have experience of community care knowledge to be hired (experience in middle-class homes, farms, inns, hotels, agricultural colonies, work colonies, etc.). There was nothing shameful or reprehensible in this function. In the 21st Century, the nurse is still the "housewife" in the care unit. Indeed, even today, it is still necessary to perceive the information transmitted by the care environment and to find a balance between organizing, coordinating, anticipating, controlling, evaluating care activities and managing the human and material resources available to provide the expected services.

The activities useful for caregiving in the property were the first to be delegated to the caretakers by the hospital authorities. It was necessary to keep the house alive. These activities required the ability to guide the care action (*Domus*) or to take care of property life. This function of the professional role was one of institutionalization delegated to the "maids" of the past by the hospital authorities. The implementation of these capacities in rules of action required skills to organize the hospital dynamic and to make the institution function.

1 This should not be confused with the Hôtel-Dieu.

The practice[2], a term widely used in nursing, but probably commonplace in today's language, is a human action controlled and guided by symbolic elements included in a cultural system (knowledge, values, ideologies). The practices that can be detected in ancient hospital documents constituted the objective aspect identified by those who observe and write about caregivers. It is a kind of "compromising process" integrating both the prescribed action and the action carried out. Visible today within health institutions belonging to the tertiary sector, that of services, these practices as sensible action are "services" delivered by the carers. Meaningful action is therefore "in one way or another, governed by rules. The meaning of the action depends on the system of convention that assigns meaning to each action". One can even speak of "symbolic mediation" to underline the public nature, from the outset, not only of the expression of individual desires, "but of the codification of social action in which individual action takes place. These symbols are cultural and not only psychological entities" [RIC 86].

The first system of values prescribed to the carers and which subsequently guided the caring action (*Domus*) or caregiving sector related to the institutional purposes and the modalities of the respect of discipline, order and coordination of work, management of time and space, principles of management of the domestic economy, transmission of knowledge and institutional law. This function of the professional role was one of institutionalization delegated to the "maids" of the past by the hospital authorities. This function still exists today. It is a matter of adapting newcomers to the house or making them adapt to the established rules of action. This function of institutionalization requires knowledge and skills to communicate, transmit written and oral information (with several interlocutors with multiple statuses), welcome, reassure, inform (new residents and new staff), supervise people in training, control (the performance of delegated tasks), to be accountable for what is consumed (to those in charge of the establishment, to the accounting services or to the various public prosecutors, bursars), to manage equipment (stock control, stores, maintenance, replacement), to control the movements of the hospital's "inhabitants" (admissions, discharges, transfers, commitments, resignations) and to ensure the domestic economy (organization, financing and logistics).

Through language, a representation of the activity described within the retrieved documents began to form within the living environment of the people being cared for, based on words such as beds (bedsteads), sheets, blankets, quilted blankets, armchairs, sleepers (bolster), cleanliness, toilet, bathtubs, clothes, linen, towels, tablecloths, starch, soap, water, hot, cold, eating, eating lean or fat, sleeping, washing, hemp field, meadows, cleaning, dishes, airing, brooms, sweeping, toilet

2 Definition already mentioned in the introduction.

facilities, latrines, stools (putrid miasmas), vermin, infection, combs, dressing, walking, moving, working, vomiting, blood, illness, healing, remedy, convalescent, food, firewood, urine, blood, candles, diapers, wine, water, pain, screaming, whispering, silence, crying, death, dying, coffin, prayer, serving, swearing, inventory, poverty, bed keeping, infirmary, relief, salary (salt), laundry, soap, attics, etc.

These words (here extracted in bulk), placed in the sentences that give them meaning and indicate their use, call for knowledge and are formed progressively and continuously in the environment of care (*Domus*). Knowledge takes shape! In the long term, they will gradually constitute the lay knowledge of hospital maids and servants with their tacit knowledge for action, before becoming part of the professional language of care in the strictest sense of the word. From space, the verb springs forth! Moreover, the hospital environment seems to protect those who live there from the events that accompany the changes experienced by society. "If the hospital has been a mirror of its social, political, economic or cultural environment during all the eras it has lived through, it benefited in the past from a certain gap, a privilege conducive to stability and reflection (a haven of peace during wars or an object of support in spite of financial crises)" [DON 03]. In fact, by giving responsibility for organizing the house so that people can live in it and provide care, hospital authorities expect housekeepers and maids to organize space and manage working time in such a way as to meet institutional goals. Do as you wish, promise to do your work well and that everything will be clean and tidy! This is the message more or less implicitly conveyed to the hospital maids and their servants. This service to the institutions will go through the centuries and adapt to the institutional changes that the hospital will undergo.

Twenty-seven practices[3] for caregiving in the estate (*Domus*) and offering a service to the institution with the required knowledge in hygiene, management and housekeeping (in continuity with lay knowledge) were thus identified in the results of international scientific research (Switzerland-Quebec) conducted in 2002 by the research and development unit of the *Haute école de santé de Fribourg*[4] [NAD 03b].

3 Eighteen of these practices are mentioned in the publication of the conceptual model of nursing (nursing activity, the cultural intermediary model) [NAD 13].

4 Research conducted in partnership with the Faculty of Nursing at Laval University in Quebec City, funded by the Swiss National Science Foundation [NAD 02b].

4.2. *Hominem* or looking after human life

We retain "Hominem" in its phonology to qualify this group of practices. We should have said *Homo*, *Homines* or *ad-hominem* to be precise and respect the Latin terminology. "As soon as life appears, there is care, because we must take care of life so that it can remain. Hence, one of the oldest expressions in the history of the world: to take care of..." [COL 96]. This quotation by Marie-Françoise Collière is emblematic of the care profession and of the activity of caring in all the spaces and times of the planet and for all eras of knowledge.

Caring was first and foremost an ordinary part of life. This activity, often based on tacit knowledge, developed in the private sphere of the family and was dependent on the conditions of urban or rural habitats. When daily care could be provided in the family, there was no need to institutionalize it through a hospital. If a mother, for example, took care of her children, her sick spouse or the elderly grandmother or aunt who lived under the same roof, kept her home cleaned, prepared food for the household, prepared food for subsistence, cultivated the vegetable garden, put away household effects, did the laundry and ironing, disinfected common wounds, prepared herbal tea, maintained good relations within the family or neighborhood, managed household goods, participated in correspondence and accounts, and because she could read and write, also participated in the education of her whole little world, she did not need to go to an institution to receive care.

This care was given in all classes of the population, both among the common people (servants), among the ordinary people (working classes) and among the clergy and aristocracy (educated classes), who generally had the means to hire tradesmen for the activities of daily life. This was, for example, the case of Florence Nightingale, the aristocratic heroine who allowed the educated class to enter the care environment without necessarily entering religion.

One has to look at the job descriptions of non-religious hospital staff in the 18th Century to perceive the knowledge they had to mobilize to take care of the human population. Below, we present an extract from the hospital prescriptions of Freiburg in 1759 and Geneva in 1744[5] as an emblematic figure of the care activity. This is not the only document in our possession. Others, found for the hospitals of Bulle and Romont, resemble this one and have already been published. We therefore refer the reader to these, particularly in the work on the "nursing myth" [NAD 12b]:

---

5 "*Règlement pour la direction de l'Hôpital général de Genève en 1744*", found in the *Archives de l'Etat de Fribourg* (AEF), handwritten work in French, *Fonds de l'Hôpital Notre-Dame*, 83 pages, 330 mm × 224 mm, 600 g. As this document was not listed at the time of our research at the *Archives de l'État de Fribourg* (1990), we describe it precisely.

The choice of people to serve and care for the sick is of no less importance than that of doctors and surgeons. For on them depends the cleanliness of the beds and the apartment to keep them free from infection. On their attention very often depends the promptness of healing; real cleanliness, robust complexion, readiness to give help, compassion with courage, are the qualities with which persons in such a job should be gifted, as well as an attentive and judicious mind to be able to give an account to the doctors of the condition of the sick. [REG 59].

You will always try to take for the service of the sick all that is best in these respects, and as the Board of Directors will invigilate on all matters, you will be particularly careful about how to serve the sick, you will also order the Moses whom you deem the cleanest and most suitable [REG 59].

The housekeeper of able-bodied women and girls will be given as many servants as necessary to keep all the rooms clean, and these servants will be responsible for making the beds, sweeping the rooms daily with great care, having the hospital master provide them with the brooms they will need, and marking the time at which the poor must be lifted in all seasons (*sic*) [FON 44].

The housekeeper and her servants will take care that the poor have combs and all that is necessary to keep themselves clean and free from vermin, and that their clothes are likewise as clean as possible (p. 59). They will also be careful to keep the windows open as often as possible [FON 44, p. 70].

She will take care to keep her rooms very clean and to remove the bed linings from her rooms three times a year, beat them and clean them well so that no insects are born in them and to expose the quilted blankets to the sun as often as possible [FON 44, p. 59].

The housekeeper of the sick, both men and boys and women and girls who are welcomed into the house, shall take care to keep her rooms very clean as well as the sick, and when it is a question of getting up at night to look after a sick person, she shall be diligent in giving him what he needs for his relief. She will take care to make the sick take their remedies, as well as their broths, and help them to make their beds. She will have to take the food and broths for the sick from her rooms to the large kitchen, giving each one his portion, being helped in

> this by her servant. The said housekeeper will be obliged to help herself to spread the washing and soap in the attics and also to help herself to fold the cloths after they are dry. She is forbidden to receive or attract anyone to her rooms to eat and drink.
>
> She shall take an oath at the beginning of each year to faithfully discharge her employment and to render an account of all that is entrusted to her by signing the inventory of the effects that will be handed over to her and for which she will be responsible [FON 44].
>
> In the sick men's room, there will be two women to serve them. In the sick women's room, there shall likewise be two women to serve them, and if it is necessary for the relief of the sick both men and women that the number of persons to serve them be increased, it shall be increased [FON 44, p. 72].
>
> When a person who has been welcomed into the house out of poverty falls ill with a sickness that forces him to stay in bed, he will be taken to the sick room so that the sick are not mixed with the healthy and the whole house is not an infirmary.
>
> The sick will be treated as sick people and for this purpose there will be a special pot for them to have broth, barley or oat groats which the persons destined to serve them will give them at the proper times.
>
> The rooms where the patients will be held will be kept very neatly by those who will be in charge of them, and the hospital will spare neither sheets nor the other cloths necessary to keep them clean.
>
> When a patient is convalescent, he will return to the room from which he came out, and if he cannot yet go down to eat in the canteens, he will be fed in his room in the same way as the doctor orders, not according to his fancy [FON 44]; see also in [NAD 93, p. 67].

The actions or words required by these excerpts require a minimum of knowledge, if not about health, at least about what was part of the lifestyle of the time, practical knowledge, experience and gestures, which were themselves dependent on the cultural context in which they took place. We do not think that it is necessary to wait until hygiene became a common and popular habit to attribute its practice to the hospital's caregivers. In his analysis of the regulations of the Geneva hospital in 1712, the forerunner of the 1744 regulations, Cahier-Bucceli reports that:

> The clothes of the sick and the rooms is the object of careful care. The sheets of the poor are changed every three weeks or a month, their shirts are changed every eight days. All have the right to their personal comb to keep themselves free from vermin. No bed linen or towels are spared for the sick.
>
> In the refectory, everyone must sit in their assigned place, the old separated from the young. All the dishes are made of pewter. Each guest has his or her own plate, cup, picholette and cutlery. The serving dishes contain portions for four people. The tables are covered with tablecloths large enough to take the place of napkins. The same brown bread is served to all, half a pound a day, not counting the bread for the soup. Twice a week, we eat lean food. Everyone drinks the same red wine, the quantity of which varies according to whether the wine is abundant or scarce. [CAH 85]

We also see in the preceding text that hospital servants and maids needed to have notions (applied or not) about domestic, individual and collective hygiene, as well as personal hygiene, without omitting the opposites, about the experience of dirt, vermin and grime. Before becoming part of either a civility manual or a medical manual, cleanliness was rather part of a customary practice, perhaps not very systematic, but highly differentiated according to where it was practised. Generally speaking, hospitals in Bern, Lausanne, Neuchâtel, Geneva and Freiburg "were kept very clean" [LOU 00]. Before witnessing cleanliness in writing, it seems to us that cleanliness was more of a gesture. To "keep the sick very clean", in the absence of explicit knowledge, it was necessary to have implicit knowledge about the gestures to be made and the equipment used. The maids and servants of the lay period of knowledge were generally constrained but willing to live with and for humans. They were therefore also confronted with the uncertainty of their reactions, their behavior, their motives for living or dying and their desires.

We also see that when it was a question of getting up at night to care for a sick person, the housekeeper "was diligent in giving him what he needed for his relief" [FON 44, p. 60]. Here, diligence required, at the very least, attention to others, tact, a certain celerity, all based on what we would call "a relationship with the other". It is hardly possible to enter into a relationship without being confronted with elements of the culture and personality of others, especially if the caregiver must live this relationship almost continuously. Let us recall that the hospital received people of both sexes at different stages of life, beggars, passers-by, strangers and the sick. This situation could not avoid confronting the servants and housekeepers with the experience of multicultural and social diversity. For there to be a "caring" relationship, there had to be two fundamental characteristics of care, namely, the notion of proximity and permanence. Proximity inhabited by ways of doing things, inhabited by observation, by the use of our senses to understand the needs of the person,[6] the object of this relationship.

As for permanence, it seemed particularly demanding in the 18th Century, since the servants and housekeepers lived in the hospital and had to share their living conditions with the residents. Twenty-four hours a day, they were obliged to be present. According to the management of the Swiss Red Cross, this presence was still required in 1933 for student nurses, since they had to be present at all times:

> The nurses were also given the opportunity to live in the hospital itself, to learn about the day and night shift and to be constantly available to the head nurses. [NAD 93]

Sharing the living conditions of hospitalized patients and the poor contained in the hospital space, it was also through proximity and permanence, in addition to the sharing of smells and noises (breathing, moaning, whining, snoring, crying, monologues, shouting, insults, etc.). Through the perception of these multiple languages, the daily encounter of those who shared the hospital space and time, the experience of a bond, which we sometimes know to be subtle and deep, as well as fleeting, could be born. Every time a third party intervenes to facilitate a relationship or the understanding of a situation, we speak of mediation. In the context of care situations within the healthcare system, we talk about health mediation.

The notion of "relief" in the service of the sick also appears frequently in ancient texts. A language of manifest expectations on the part of society translated into hospital regulations, these values related to relief were translated into gestures and words in lay knowledge. In the expression "she will be diligent in giving him what he needs for his relief", one may wonder what meaning is attributed to the word relief and what knowledge is associated with the word? Is it the relief of suffering? Is it relief related to the functions of elimination? Or simply and generally speaking, the meaning given to the word, in the reworking of the ancient French word *soulas*, consolation, and the Latin *solacium*, consolation, softening of pain? Since man has lived, it would seem that it is more the fear of suffering, which would then be, according to Ricoeur, "the motive to integrate, to reject or accept this suffering. Endurance is to continue to suffer if the idea demands it" [RIC 88]. Behind the complaint made is often hidden a suffering generally linked to existential events, a

6 Even 250 years before the writings of Virginia Henderson, who popularized the notion of needs in one of the first care theories on the subject, the notion of the needs of the people being cared for was known and verbalized.

state of sadness, professional, family or emotional torment. The relief of this suffering required those who were entrusted with the mission to discern its natural, supernatural or social origin. And, if they could not discern its origin, the caretakers of the 18th Century had, at the very least, experience of the manifestations of this suffering.

As for the relief related to the elimination functions, it is for us a notion close to that of comfort and assistance. Assistance in an activity of daily life that a person could no longer perform alone and that the caregiver could try to make as little unpleasant as possible by her actions and knowledge. It was not uncommon to find in *Ancien Régime* hospitals a bedridden elderly person who, in spite of himself, had transformed his bed into a place of comfort during a salutary diarrhea that pushed the morbific matter out. A situation that was neither specific to time and space, since the person had been feeding himself, it was necessary to "go" in order to carry oneself properly, and this too could be learned.

The caregiver, in her condition, may then have been called upon to share this "slice of life" with those who depended on her for sustenance or hope. Faced with this example of diarrhea (a very good example to give concrete information on the simple and complex, but daily acts of life), she would have to ask herself how to lift the adverse condition that affected both the institutional and personal life of this patient. The meaning given to the "how to do something" was then significant of the knowledge mobilized, linked to the complexity of the situation encountered. Was it necessary to start by washing oneself or changing the bed? After having made a decision, which if possible required thinking correctly, another question arose and so on, until the patient regained a state of cleanliness and comfort close to the initial pre-diarrheal state. If she decided that it may be good (for whomever) to change the bed, she may have still wondered whether she would turn the patient to the right or to the left, depending on the patient's impotence, or whether she would tell the patient to raise themselves up or get up, depending on his or her physical, cognitive or socio-affective resources. Many other questions may have continued to arise and all of them required a decision to be made. While it was hoped that this decision would be as good as possible for the patient, it was also hoped that it would be as good as possible for the caregiver and her immediate environment. And, even then, deciding not to make a decision would also be equivalent to decision-making.

If washing the bedridden old man's toilet was the servant's first choice, her experience would tell her that in some situations it was better to start by washing the cleanest part and move on to the dirtiest part, and that in other situations it was the other way around. To wash the whole body of a person who could no longer do it himself was a caring action. But during this action, the thought could also escape and continue to question the servant's judgment. During the (complete or partial) washing of the bedridden old man, the servants may still have wondered whether she should lecture and punish him (because he gave her work and this was not the only thing she had to do) or whether she should take into account the expression of his shame and guilt which in fact summed up the expression of his suffering of being dependent on others? Faced with an apparently simple, banal or taboo action, such as that of washing someone other than oneself, we perceive all the complexity of the gesture from the very moment when the reflection turns to the action in order to attribute a meaning to it. Caregivers of the lay era as well as those of today (the scientific era of care knowledge) are still confronted with the same uncertainties and other mini-decisions.

Doing our daily wash, for which we have been educated, washing our children where education is less obvious; washing unknown, yet dependent people, entering into their intimate sphere, does not belong to the same aims, the same representations, the same gestures and the same knowledge. The acts related to helping in daily life are relatively simple once they are internalized, we have learned them anyway. They are of a more complex degree when it comes to providing them to others. Let's not forget that each person is different in their physiological aspects, their culture, their beliefs, their reactions to the action of which they are both the object of care and the subject of care. These acts of daily life, which may be ordinary, are already a little less so for the human being who is then deprived when he cannot perform them alone. The servants of the 18th Century could or needed to consent to provide this care in order to obtain their own means of subsistence.

This assistance or relief also required the servants to know how to use specific equipment. In 1711, 18 commodes were ordered among the carpentry works of the Geneva hospital, and Carrère mentions in his 1786 work for the relief of the sick when they were in bed, to pass under the patient "flat basins, covered with skin patches or made with a thin and worn towel" [CAR 86]. In 1760, the latrines "of the patients' apartments" in the Geneva hospital had to be repaired. In fact, "the conveniences were placed as they should be at the end of the corridor, behind the patients' room, and for those who could not walk, chairs with holes were available every two beds" [LOU 00]. The notion of relief from the function of elimination and the knowledge it required existed. Functional disorders related to senility, including temporo-spatial disorientation, also existed. They were not the prerogative of the 20th Century. We will also notice, in relation to this notion of relief mentally linked to the elimination function, that not only did caregivers have to transmit certain knowledge or tricks of the trade to each other in order to accomplish their task, but also find a way to preserve their strength, used to lift a bedridden patient, for example, in order to slide under him the commode mentioned above and to remove it when necessary. And what about the experience of smells? Along with practices related to hygiene, cleanliness (or dirt), it was also an approach to the body that was required of the caregivers. Often from a social background close or identical to that of the people they were caring for, the maids and servants could develop a relationship with the body (touch, language) that allowed them to know so much about the stakes that the body and its health represented in their daily lives.

The third meaning of the word relief that we can try to pinpoint is that of consolation, the easing of misery and sorrow. By being relatively close to the residents of the hospital, the servants of the sick were called upon to establish a relationship based on a notion that may seem obvious, but is not at all so. The notion of sharing, a sharing which in turn imperatively required that a relationship of trust be established between the caregiver and the person being cared for. The health mediation thus established was "a metalevel that organizes the relationships among men" [DES 19]. The means that we perceive as daily means, used for this sharing in the age of lay knowledge were: listening with one's counterparts, silence and whispering, prayer, meditation, self-pity, solicitude and compassion. On the consequences of sharing, little is written in nursing. However, even if, as Diébolt points out, "what is not said, written or expressed is certainly as important and more important than what is said, written and transmitted" [DIÉ 87], the nature of sharing cannot be perceptible, because it seems to us to be of the order of an implicit secret and confidence.

As a shrewd observer of both the imperialism of some servants and the skill and dexterity of others, Carrère mentions that:

> Those who care for the sick are often the necessary witnesses to minor internal harassments, family divisions, business circumstances: they must get used to keeping the deepest silence on everything that happens before their eyes. Discretion is especially necessary to them in particular illnesses or accidents which may be of interest to the honor of families or individuals. [CAR 86]

Since maids did not have access to writing to describe their working conditions, let us turn to those who had the power to observe their work to get an idea of the skills projected on them. Thus, Joseph-Barthélemy-François Carrère, Medical Adviser to King Louis XVI, after having verified that the work of[7] a German doctor who had preceded him had nothing in common with the one he proposed to publish, specified:

7 May M., *Introduction pour les gardes-malades*, Manheim, 1784. Warden translated here from German makes a good reference to lay people, as there were no Protestant nuns (deaconesses) in the country yet.

> Witnessing the frequent inconveniences (*sic*) of the imperialism of sick nurses, the unfortunate consequences which result from this, and the fatal outcome of illnesses which sometimes follow, I have long wished to see the formation of establishments from which they could draw useful instruction, and the establishment of a police force relating to their duties (*sic*). [CAR 86]

He then proposed a work "especially intended for the sick nurses", including 215 pages. We now find ourselves in 1786!

> The care of the sick often contributes as much as remedies to the cure of disease; it requires special knowledge, which alone can make it useful; but this kind of service is usually given to a class which is devoid of enlightenment and which neglects and is even powerless to acquire it. The government has not yet made its views known on this subject; we have no institution designed to provide the persons who care for the sick with an education that will lead them into a career they do not know [CAR 86].

He then mentioned a few recommendations that still seem to be relevant for today's caregivers. They can be identified in the following excerpts:

> It is important to gain the trust of the sick; it is the means of obtaining from them many things they sometimes refuse to do: the art of persuading them can lead to their tranquility and healing.
>
> Illness often changes or alters their character, giving them moments of mood or caprice, movements of impatience, even sometimes of brusqueness; only gentleness and patience should be opposed to them; annoyance increases their restlessness and aggravates their ills.
>
> The sick nurse must always be ready to go to their aid, to foresee their needs, to help them or relieve them in their movements. Small care and special attention flatter them and contribute to their tranquility. But they should not be multiplied too much; they may become tiresome and uncomfortable.
>
> There are some who like to be cared for; there are others who want to care for themselves who want to be left alone, and who would be inconvenienced by hasty care. One must behave according to one's knowledge of their way of thinking, and vary the kind and extent of care according to the desires of each individual.

> One can report here the skill and dexterity needed by a sick nurse to arrange the sick in their beds, to place them in the situations that are most convenient for them, to help them in their needs. These two qualities do much to lessen the fatigue that the slightest movement causes in major illnesses, and give the sick a momentary feeling of well-being that pleases and relieves them.
>
> The administration of the remedies prescribed by the people of the art and the preparation of those which can be made at less expense to the sick are still part of the duties of the sick nurses.
>
> They are neither doctors nor surgeons of the sick; their duties are limited to helping the sick in their needs, reporting to the people of the art of what they have observed, and using the remedies they prescribe. They should regard themselves as mere instruments to be used in administering to the sick the help they deem necessary. They must, therefore, be very accurate in the account they have to give to the physician, very careful in what he prescribes, and very docile in following his advice.
>
> They must win the confidence of the sick, to always use the path of gentleness and persuasion, to bear with patience the mood swings that are often the effect of illness, to inspire courage and resignation against their ills, and confidence in the use of remedies, to avoid harboring the rather ordinary fears among them about the consequences of illness, to keep an inviolable secret of everything that happens before their eyes, to be always ready to give relief from illness and to redouble their care and attention in view of the circumstances. [CAR 86]

At a time when the psychology textbooks "for nurses" of the 1970s were not yet written and distributed, it is pleasing to read that the idea of "studying and skillfully dealing with the character of the sick" was already popular. Caregiving "in accordance with the individual's wishes", that is, trying to individualize care, was also seen as a desirable practice in the 18th Century. Moreover, assisting with the needs of activities of daily living was already apparent in the discourse of this care manual in 1786. This reference to meeting needs had long been part of the care activity. However, this assistance in the prevention or satisfaction of the individual's needs was not yet qualified as "nursing care". Nor did this language wait for the work of Virginia Henderson, an American theorist who, in an anthropological theory of deductive care, portrays the person being cared for as having 14 basic needs. She had a great influence in France, and even in the international nursing community for the teaching given in nursing schools from the 1970s onwards[8].

The followers of "nursing's own knowledge" from the nursing discipline today can always object that Carrère was a doctor and therefore does not represent the point of view of the nursing discipline. But was Carrère more distant from the knowledge possessed by the nursing discipline than Florence Nightingale who has not yet been born? In fact, and without wishing to prejudge the importance of his work, why should the words of Florence Nightingale, who, as an aristocratic woman, did not have the same status as that of hospital maids and servants, be more legitimate than those of Carrère so that Florence Nightingale might be recognized for having founded "modern nursing"? And even if we disregard the words of Carrère, in what way are the contributions of Florence Nightingale superior in importance to the contents of the texts found in the French-speaking hospitals of the *Ancien Régime*? The hostile maids and servants of the *Ancien Régime* in French-speaking Switzerland cared well before her while belonging to the "servant" class and not to the "educated class", bourgeois or aristocratic. And as already mentioned, the hospitals in Bern, Lausanne, Neuchâtel, Geneva and Freiburg were kept very clean. The working conditions and atmosphere in the lay hospitals of French-speaking Switzerland in 1750 seem to us to have nothing to envy to the working conditions and atmosphere of the London hospitals in 1850. Except perhaps that the hospital was more medicalized in 1850 than a century earlier. We know that at Florence Nightingale's Training School, they only provided:

> a very rudimentary apprenticeship, with very little instruction and no notion of general knowledge. It was also led by a real guard dog (Shara Wardroper), a soulless woman, devoid of any pedagogical sense. As for the only teacher, a doctor (R.G. Whitfield, resident physician), he was mostly drunk, renowned for his questionable morals, to say the least. (...) For a long time Miss Nightingale was not kept informed of what was going on at the training school. And when she was informed, she adopted an attitude that could be considered reprehensible. She tried by timid tinkering to put things in order, while

8 "Through multidisciplinary exchanges at Teachers College Columbia University in New York City, where she frequented both physiology and social science teachers, she adopted in her work the notion of 'need' that was widely used in academic work at the time, including that of anthropologist Ralph Linton". She also met the psychologists Edward Thorndike, Abraham Maslow and Carl Rogers [COL 94]. Drawing also on other anthropologists, the 14 needs of Virginia Henderson's (1950) care theory can also be compared to the 14 needs found in Bronislaw Malinowski's work.

> at the same time she gave instructions so that the general public would not know about it. [SIN 08]

In what way were the values and means available to the aristocracy more specific to the discipline than the knowledge of action mobilized by the "women of the people" of the 18th Century? Moreover, Florence Nightingale's media promotion has nothing to do with that of the hospital maids and servants of her time. The latter simply did not seem to have had by far the chance to benefit from the political support and reports that appeared in *The Times* for 22 months and that surrounded Florence Nightingale during the Crimean War.

In fact, it is probably more in terms of social class than in terms of knowledge (at least in its early days) that Florence Nightingale's work has scored points. By opening up the field of care to the educated classes, the aristocracy and the bourgeoisie, Florence Nightingale offered women access to a field which, until about 1860, was rather for the underprivileged, the working classes and the servants. Unless they withdrew from the world, entered a convent and became a hospital nun or deaconess within a religious congregation, it was almost impossible for a woman of the educated class or girls from a good family to share the living conditions of the hospital staff and to confront the maids and servants of the sick. The knowledge that can be guessed from the hospital texts of the 18th Century has little to envy the knowledge promoted by the writings of Florence Nightingale, especially from 1860 onwards[9].

Besides trust and listening, it seems to us that the servant girl also had to "take upon herself" evil or suffering. No or little possible exteriorization of what she was experiencing was offered to her. This servant had no other way out of her burden than resignation and interiorization. The risk was great for her to sink into routine, sadness or melancholy. It was necessary to be able to dominate the evil coming from the other, not to let it overwhelm her. It was then again this act of "life or health mediation" presented in our nursing conceptual model that appeared. Not only did this act of life mediation through language and sharing seem to require confidence building, but it also demanded taking on oneself, assuming, making one's own, that is, consenting. When, faced with adverse conditions that could threaten the life of an individual, the power that for Ricoeur [RIC 88] "ensures the essential tasks of life before any reflection or effort, he will then find in front of him a care worker with a style of consciousness that will distinguish her from all others and who, in her motives for care, also had to consent" in order to practice health mediation.

9 Nightingale F., *Notes on Nursing: What It Is, and What It Is Not*, Harrison and Sons, London, 1859.

Mediation between the person being cared for and the servant by means of her own thought, a mediation that would claim, in our opinion, the experience of being "between" oneself and the other, the other and others, mediation between the body, time and space, mediation between the senses given to the contradictions of the present, mediation between social life, the natural world, the sacred and death. "To be between" requires understanding the meaning of sharing, the meaning of the mediation of life and health, the meaning given to proximity.

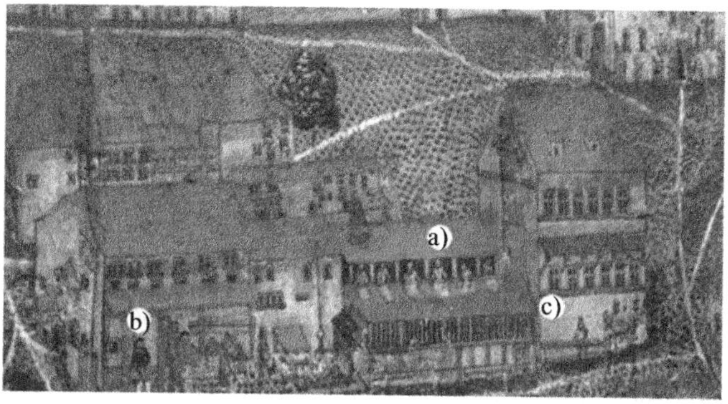

Figure 4.1. *In this picture of the Freiburg hospital in 1582, we can see clues to hospital activity[10]. For a color version of the figure, see www.iste.co.uk/nadot/nursing.zip*

COMMENT ON FIGURE 4.1.– a) Maids or servants airing bedding, b) carpenters making coffins and c) residents maintaining a social bond by meeting at the hospital pub (source: G. Blokinger 1582, Indian ink and tempera on paper, Musée d'Art et d'Histoire de Fribourg, photo: B. Rochat 2008).

"Language is symbolic mediation, as it organizes the relationships among men and allows them to represent symbolically the reality that they perceive" [DES 19]. Relationship is the first act of care. In the 18th Century, as in the 21st Century, it was always present, due to its timelessness. These life mediations were also knowledge acquired through experience and therefore represented even in the absence of writing, part of the "caregiving" already internalized in the lay era, as shown by the image of the care activity and collective hygiene practice (Figure 4.1).

Forty-eight practices for caring for and serving humans (*hominem*) with the knowledge required to establish a professional relationship and help them live (in

10 Illustration from Michel Nadot's course on "The Foundations of the Nursing Discipline" at the Faculty of Nursing at Saint Joseph in Beirut, Lebanon, in 2016.

continuity with lay knowledge) are thus identified in the results of contemporary international scientific research (Switzerland-Quebec) carried out in 2002 by the research and development unit of the *Haute école de santé de Fribourg* [NAD 03b]. A beautiful continuity of knowledge!

4.3. *Familia* or looking after group life

The term *familia* refers to the group of familiar people with whom the carer is in contact within an institution. *Familia* is derived from *famulus*, "servant". "The Roman familia was etymologically the set of *famuli*, slaves attached to the master's house, then all those who lived under the same roof, master and servants, and over whom the authority of the *pater familias*, the head of the family, reigned" [REY 92]. All those who lived under the same roof in the age of lay knowledge included, in the hospital environment, all the inhabitants of the hospital as a group (residents, sick or not, the hospital master (or rector) and his family, the institutional hierarchy, various servants and hospital employees)[11]. Some were more in contact than others with the hospital maids and servants. This was the case of the existing professional relationships within the care teams. However, many were likely to come into contact within the institutions with other professions or to meet episodically with other staff members.

Caregivers were then in daily contact not only with patients, but with "sociological" women and men with different statuses, roles, functions, desires and powers. Communicating with this "small world" presupposed knowledge to understand the languages used and the issues at stake, while at the same time one needed to identify useful knowledge to be able to integrate into the group or to distance oneself from it according to needs. In fact, the hospital space itself became a "social actor, because the relationships it created contributed greatly to creating solidarity between people" [WAL 94]. This is still the case today! *Familia* concerns life in the community (care teams) and the demands of the latter. Caring for the life of the group determined practices and languages of experience that generated benefits for both the hospital staff and the residents who lived there or the "day laborers" who passed through the hospital. This was quite observable in the 15th Century for the Yverdon hospital (Switzerland) where, as a community hospital, it had a strong base in the region:

> In fact, all the relations it has with third parties show that they do not exceed 8 to 10 km around the city. Whether these relations are

11 "The rector, his family circle and the servants, together with the residents, form the hospital's *familia*. The residents who stay for a certain number of days also belong to the *familia*. In contrast to pilgrims or other passers-by (*euntes and redeuntes*) who are set apart" [ROD 05].

> commercial, legal or social. In fact, the staff, whether permanent or temporary, probably originate from the same regional area. This also applies to regular boarders who are part of the *familia* and are clearly distinguished from mobile, transient, *euntes* and *redeuntes*. [ROD 05]

Caregivers in the lay era were daily confronted with multiple languages that needed to be coordinated and evolved in the midst of people with very different statuses depending on the size of the institution. As the hospital evolved, expanded and modernized, the space changed and the risk of encounters increased. The "pub" of 1582 at the Freiburg hospital (see Figure 4.1) was no longer the same as the hospital cafeteria in the 20th Century. But there was still a place where the local community found a way to meet.

At the end of the 18th Century, with the gradual arrival of medical language in the hospital, *Hominem* and *Familia* practices tended to come together in the same group (care activity), as they had to be distinguished from the new languages that were emerging. As "cultural intermediaries", caregivers were already confronted on a daily basis with the multiple collaborators intervening in the hospital. Divided between serving and caring, they had to make choices, because it became impossible to do everything in the hospital and satisfy everyone. Of course, we know today that beyond a certain number of human interactions, we no longer see the other person within the group as a unique and interesting being, but as a "number" who must be served. Who then benefits from the selective attention of caregivers?

Confronted with the group, lay caregivers in the era still remained alone and isolated in their tasks in the face of the world around them. We could not yet speak for lay caregivers as a community with shared values, as a constituted professional group or as a structured corporation with a common identity. Lay caregivers seemed to lack a class consciousness. Yet caregiving was not yet an occupation[12] or profession[13]. It was a low paid and legitimated occupation with individual activities

---

12 "When the number of people working with common methods, passed on to new recruits, is large enough, we can speak of occupations or groups of occupations" [JOB 85].

13 According to Guy Jobert, the status of a profession, compared to that of an occupation, is differentiated "by the possession of a certain number of attributes whose constant component is that they tend to confer on the activity an autonomy, a power of self-control explicitly recognized by society. The control exercised by the profession over training must not only be exercised as a transmission of knowledge and a certification of its possession, but must extend to the constitution of this knowledge (specific knowledge that is not the lower level of a dominant knowledge). This knowledge must also be recognized by the elite of other professions, the public and governments; it must be possible to transmit this knowledge to the highest level of the education system" [JOB 85].

integrated and not isolated from all the acts of collective life and which took place in an old institutional framework while corresponding to a social demand.

It has long been known that “the advantage of having good nurses is not desirable; they are, in a way, the support of the hospitals. Without them the service languishes, the efforts of administrators become futile, the care of physicians is unsuccessful”. This statement, taken from the Parisian dictionary of medical sciences by Panckoucke in 1812–1822 and taken up by Louis-Courvoisier to characterize the central place of nurses in the Geneva hospital, “sums up in itself the central importance of the nursing staff of a hospital, a real pivot and relay for the influences of the various protagonists of health” [LOU 00].

Today, this *familia*-type practice makes the nurse a specialist in the coordination and synthesis of the multiple languages that surround her in the institutions in which she works. It is on the basis of these languages, the meaning given to them and the writing that makes them exist, that the nursing discipline is constituted through its different models. As Foucault reminds us, “knowledge is what can be spoken about in a discursive practice that is thereby specified” [FOU 69]. Thus, knowledge only exists from the relationship between language and actions in the field of a given social practice.

Taking care of the life of the group (*familia*) – a practice associated with the culture specific to the nursing discipline – means entering into and maintaining relationships, preserving the identity of the people being cared for, maintaining social links, coordinating the language of a team, recalling ethnicity or ensuring links with the entourage (including sometimes with pets). It also means serving, sometimes regulating visits, reassuring and comforting, taking into account the status of the visitors (children, parents, husband, spouses, lovers, neighbors) or their culture (Mediterranean or Nordic, for example). It also means managing lack of privacy (too many sick people) or isolation (own bedroom, bathroom or at the end of the corridor because there is no more room). It means supervising the servants, assistants and auxiliaries on all sides, the trainee personnel or the personnel starting in the service. It means assigning a work place in the service to new members of the *familia* and making sure that the work is done according to the rules of the occupation or those of the moment. It means communicating with the various stakeholders (doctors, technicians, administrative staff, police officers, ambulance attendants, all kinds of specialists, etc.), called upon to intervene in the institutional environment.

The practice of traveling within groups was also used to transmit information or objects from one place to another (a bed, for example) or to accompany a person on a trip. This movement connected the different spaces of an institution and the people who lived there, or even united the institution with the city or living environment of the person being cared for. In the 20th Century, the practice of relocation also included leaving the ward with or without the person receiving care and was dependent on the topographical and architectural structures of an institution.

Practices such as today's coordination practices were once called "order and discipline" in the texts of the lay age of knowledge. These were activities that affected the management of time, space and movement necessary for the management of personnel and the organization of work, as well as the management of people present in the institution in order to avoid chaos. It required both language coordination and social control. It also required control of the culture delegated by the carers to the staff who assisted them in their roles, as well as the management of the people being cared for and their visits. It also required the establishment of informational as well as cultural or environmental mediations.

Finally, the *familia* group of practices also aims to prevent or manage human conflicts and dysfunctions in the organization through the regulations it operates. This serves to maintain the balance between production energy and recovery energy in nursing activity. Without taking into account (common in the 18th Century) this practice of regulation, institutional dysfunctions and increased risks can occur. In addition to supervision and the processes of reinsurance or conflict management, this practice includes various breaks and possible moments of relaxation, which were very lacking in the 18th Century (and never in the 20th Century) to cope with the tensions and constraints of professional practice. This type of practice, and the knowledge that goes with it, preserves the productive power of service provision. Without taking this regulatory practice into account, we are witnessing a predominantly emotional overload which wears out the care staff and may lead them to resign or become demotivated. It is therefore vital to the smooth running of a healthcare institution. Without energy for regulation and recovery, we cannot hope to achieve production energy[14]. The working atmosphere within healthcare teams today is partly dependent on this type of activity.

Through their practices of moving around within the space belonging to the group, the caregivers can also bring together various interlocutors and spaces that would not exist without their intermediary. Space leads to movement, and movement also leads to both closeness and distance. It is through connections, affinities, awareness of a force in the group, questioning and the perception of common interests that caregivers gradually began to come together, have intellectual rallying points and later create various professional associations or groups (in which

14 See on the subject: Rosnay J., *Le macroscope*, Le Seuil, Paris, 1975.

the group would also be cared for) that emerged between the end of the 19th Century and the beginning of the 20th Century.

Twenty-four practices for taking care of the group (*familia*) and offering it a service with the required knowledge of coordination, regulation and organization of the activity (variable, but in continuity with lay knowledge) are thus identified in the results of the contemporary international scientific research (Switzerland-Quebec) already mentioned [NAD 03b]. The context changes, the words remain, the modalities evolve!

4.4. Never enough time to do everything

By grouping the three forms of caring in the lay age, we already realize the difficulties of coping with the ordinary demands of caring. The complex economy of relief was already well established and required the mobilization of a variety of mundane but indispensable knowledge. Caring for department life meant ensuring the orderliness and hygiene necessary for a satisfactory environment. This was reflected in "the clothes of the sick and the rooms needing to be as clean as possible". It was also necessary to ensure "food and a food service". It also meant ensuring the logistics of the service. Taking care of the human being meant helping to live and establish satisfactory relationships with humans at all ages of life. It meant establishing bonds of trust, it meant "studying the character of the sick and lending oneself to it with skill". It involved "administering remedies". It was "going to the aid of the sick", "to foresee their needs", "to relieve them in their movements". Let us not forget also that death was still part of life. Taking care of the dead also meant accompanying them in their final moments, communicating with the burial directors "who would not demand anything from the relatives of those who were buried, and if we were willing to give them something, they received it as a free gift and shared it faithfully among themselves" [FON 44]. It also meant advising whoever was entitled to do so, so that the visitor "who would ordinarily be at home and prompt to visit the dead bodies as soon as he was required" [FON 44]. And there were dead bodies in the hospital! As the hospital master Abraham Joly from Geneva said, "the hospital does not kill, but it buries". In a report on the hospital in 1789, the hospital master noted that the mortality rate there was very high. Between 1760 and 1769, for example, there were 343 deaths. In general, the body had to be prepared (mortuary) and sometimes transferred to a coffin on the second floor of the establishment. This body would remain up to "twelve hours in bed in the Geneva hospital so that the parents could see it" [LOU 00]. Observing death was still for the carers to mobilize tacit knowledge from emotional experience, spectacle and smell.

Taking care of the group meant ensuring coordination at work, allocating staff according to their skills, making regulations to avoid institutional chaos, dealing with organizational contingencies, informing the interlocutors with whom one needed to collaborate. In fact, with the combination of the roles of "mother", "carer" for the sick, "maid" both in the rooms and in the department, "housekeeper" to welcome guests and the new staff, "housewife" to ensure order and cleanliness, it was impossible to rely solely on the representation of feminine stereotypes to ensure the daily hospital life of the lay age. Caring, caretaking, is much more than that! And social representations are not to be outdone in continuing to produce their share of prejudices. "It takes ten years to train a nurse, as a member of the *Conseil général du Doubs* claimed in 1792, or one hour, as the contradictor asserted, because there is not a girl who, on entering this sector, has not already served her father, mother or sick brothers a broth and herbal tea" [LOU 00]. As if that's all it takes to be cured! Hence the thought that when one carries out domestic chores that requires no knowledge, it's only a step away! Even when we know that the demands placed on the staff were much more focused on caring for the patient himself than on caring for the illness (which is right)[15], we cannot claim without any other form of analysis that "the emphasis on the patient cannot be learned, at least not in a theoretical way. Only individual aptitudes, enriched by years of experience, can lead to adequate patient management" [LOU 00]. This is a complete disregard for the requirements of caring according to the triptych of *Domus–familia–ad-hominem* knowledge outlined above. The sick are not the only beneficiaries of healthcare services and have never been the only ones. There has never been enough time devoted exclusively to the sick. But the caretakers have never explicitly perceived the service rendered to the institution and the service rendered to the group in their daily activities.

The task related to the three facets of caring became excessive with the development of the *maison* (home) (the hospital) and the slow but steady growth of scientific knowledge. Busy with multiple tasks, the maids and caretakers of the *Ancien Régime* never had time to devote exclusively to the people they cared for, whether sick or not. They often moved from one activity to another within the house. As can still be seen in 1849 with a nurse who cared for the mentally ill in the Geneva hospital. "She first worked as a nurse for the mentally ill, then as a wash boiler for the sick, then as a washerwoman in the large kitchen, and finally as a maid in the sick men's room" [LOU 00]. Yes, many actors already benefitted from the services of the maids and servants. Nothing reprehensible in an institution represented as a "big house" and at a time when there was still no structured training

15 As a reminder: "The way of seeing nurses is more focused on the condition related to the disease than on the disease itself and is oriented towards assistance that will allow the day-to-day control of impairments resulting from health disturbances" [ACA 07].

or corporation. This reminds me that when I was the director of a small hospital on the Neuchâtel coast in 1971 (about 120 beds), there was a brave "anesthetist, nurse, gardener" named Alfred on our staff. He went from the garden to the operating theater and to caring for urinary tract care in men without any other difficulties. So, yes, there was sometimes role versatility among the caregivers, as well as a plurality of knowledge. This was often the case when there was a lack of staff, means or activities to fill a single position.

It is sometimes understandable that in some hospitals we find ourselves in the presence of a real muddle of people specializing in the miseries of the world when we try to distinguish between the caring activities. In addition, everyone is watching everyone else and as a result, many people pass each other in the rooms. Thus, at the Geneva hospital in 1744, the bursar:

> Every day after supper, he visited all the rooms of the house to see if everything was in order and if the poor were removed at the proper time. He took care to see that no accidents related to fire occurred and prevented smoking in the house. When in the daytime he was not busy outdoors, he made the rounds of the house and the court of discipline to bring the idlers back to their work. He kept the books of the goods and those of the works or supplies of the locksmith, tinsmith, blacksmith, blacksmith, glazier, saddler, lantern maker, boilermaker and wheelwright. [FON 44]

Hospital authorities often required that caretakers be both in the service of the general estate as in a private dwelling and in the service of the poor who lived in the house. Thus, in 1733, the caretaker of the Romont hospital (Switzerland):

> He took care of the things which the Receiver of goods gave into his hands, as well as of the poor, as well as of the fire, made and cultivated the garden, took care of the beds and other furniture which remained in the hospital, and served for the sole use of the poor, as well as the gardening, and what was his dependence. For their benefit and relief was applied all the duties of a servant and all that was ordained for them and given sufficient security.
>
> He was delivered for his maintenance three sacks of wheat by the Receiver of the Granary, and a bag of oats to feed and maintain a few hens for eggs for the sick, in addition to a pair of shoes and ten small crowns for his wage (*sic*). [VIL 33]

This type of regulation was reviewed from time to time to adapt it to the hospital's environment and evolution. Thus, in 1774, the working conditions of the caretaker of the Romont hospital were slightly broader and more precise than the previous regulations and made it possible to see what was required of the nursing staff:

> Regulations made for the Caretaker of the Charitable Hospital, with regard to his establishment and his salary. The caretaker shall be given somewhere to sleep only for five years, behaving properly and performing all duties and charges which she is required to do, and shall not be expelled[16] in any time whatsoever. She shall receive for her wages ten small crowns, three sacks of wheat, no oats; two pounds of meat per week; twenty coins for a pair of shoes. For the wood for her use, she will have four white gold coins a year, but if any poor people come to the hospital and she is obliged to heat the stove in their room, she will be provided with wood from the hospital which the hospital master will pay for, and for putting their pot on the fire.
>
> For what retribution and salvation the Caretaker will be obliged first of all to care for the poor and apply herself to their relief. She will have to cut and spin all the hemp coming from the Charitable Hospital, she will take care of everything that will be handed over to her according to the inventory that will be made of it. She will not lodge or receive any poor people in the hospital without notifying the hospital. (*Registres du Noble conseil de Romont*, *Minutes of the Conseil général de la ville*, September 1774, *Archives de la ville de Romont*)

Governors and maids did what they could while sometimes trying to escape their particularly difficult conditions. In some hospitals, they were close to slavery or domestic servitude. But let's not look for signs of medical activity under the *Ancien Régime*; there was little or no such activity. "In terms of properly technical or medical care, the qualities required were extremely rare. Only once, the sources mention the preparation of medicines by the maid of the sick women's chamber in 1813" [LOU 00]. And why seek a medical activity for a discipline located in the human and social sciences and not in the natural sciences or medicine? Once again, it seems that we are faced with a confusion based on clichés and stereotypes that persist.

16 Drive her out, evict her.

In other hospitals, housekeepers, maids and even the hospital itself also did what they could, but with some support from the hospital authorities or the complex relief hierarchy. Let us remember that the hospital world was extremely contrasted. Some hospitals seemed to function well; others had no means left to carry out their mission or were falling into ruin. There were even plans to help the governors of the Geneva hospital by hiring more people. They were thinking of giving the maid "as many maids as she needed". This "maid-servant" binomial was quite common in the organization of work in the hospitals of French-speaking Switzerland in the 18th Century. This prefigured hospital work in Switzerland in the 1960s and 1970s, when the registered nurse was frequently assisted by nursing auxiliaries. Nurses and nurse's aides, an important pair in modern times! It should also be noted that there was so much work in some hospitals of the lay era that the able-bodied sick or some elderly people were called upon for certain jobs. This was still sometimes the case in some old people's homes at the end of the 20th Century, where the able-bodied sought to keep busy and give a helping hand to avoid boredom, to maintain a certain mobility or because they simply want to help.

5

A Return to Image: Minion Syndrome

The lay age of knowledge saw the establishment of an institutional space of speech (the hospital) in which care was provided. After the fire, the fire place, the house, the estate, the household, the space and time of care in which one took care of life in the community became the hospital. It was designed for those who were out of the home, and those who no longer had a place to stay. Caring or "caregiving" was then situated in a three-dimensional field inseparable from the hospital environment which gave rise to the first languages and foundations of the nursing discipline. It was indeed necessary to take care of the life of the property, to take care of the human being's life and to take care of group life. That is, taking care of a form of life in all cases. As we have surmised, a whole scholarly adventure began, and not necessarily the simplest one. In the lay age of knowledge and in general, the nursing staff was therefore an essential factor in the understanding of a hospital, particularly because of its continuous presence with the people being cared for over several centuries and the communicative role it played between them and the other players in the institution.

As we have seen, with *Domus*, you have to take care of property life. This first system of practices guided the care action in a prescriptive way. It related to institutional purposes, domestic economy and professional succession. It was necessary to take care of order, discipline, personnel management, the squaring of time, space and movements and to transmit one's knowledge orally. This function of the professional role was a function of institutionalization delegated to the "maids" of the past by the hospital authorities. It was also a case of ensuring that the hospital's inhabitants complied with institutional rules (schedules, clothing, spaces, behavior). They were entrusted with the running of the institution. Today, female students are confronted with the demands of this function from their first internships in an institutional setting. Already in the past, this institutionalization function required skills such as communicating, transmitting written and oral information, welcoming, reassuring, informing, reporting on what was consumed, managing equipment, controlling the movements of the hospital's "inhabitants" (entries, discharges, transfers, resignations, commitments) and ensuring the transmission of knowledge. Because of their movements associated with group life (*familia*), the nursing staff also has the ability and skills to move simultaneously from one space and level of communication to another, from one area of sociability to another. It is the field of thought, the mental effort and the nervous load that widens during these movements. Data occupy a large place and this, because of their density, all the more so as they can be contradictory, unexpected, heterogeneous, hybrid or polysemic. Let us think, for example, of the information sources that capture the attention of nurses today and how they appear in space and time. This information can be: undergone or sought; verbal and non-verbal, audible, visual, olfactory, gustatory, kinesthetic; telephonic, bureaucratic, documentary, computer, sound, musical, esthetic; it is also a question of familiarizing oneself with noises, continuous noises, respiratory noises, noises associated with a fall, external noises (arrival of an ambulance, a police car). This also includes familiarizing oneself with noises coming from a specific space and time (in care services, small, large, suburban space, monobloc space), noises of a group (team meetings or medical visits, for example) or a network, noises of an individual at all ages of life, noises of the work environment or external to this environment, language of egalitarian or hierarchical, political or strategic positioning, etc. It is still necessary to become familiar with the smells of the work environment. This information often has difficulty complying with protocols and routines presented as reassuring, since in care, we never know the nature of the message, its intensity or the moment when it will be delivered. Hence, the temporo-spatial imbroglio denounced by some observers of the hospital scene between the Middle Ages and the *Ancien Régime*.

With *Familia*, you have to take care of group life. This second set of practices refers to life and the demands of working in a community. Today's students also develop these types of skills during their internships in health institutions. Taking care of group life today implies meeting with various interlocutors, managing and coordinating information in space and time, coordinating movements, coordinating and regulating languages between various healthcare professionals, promoting order, preventing chaos, controlling, supervising and, if possible, resolving some relational conflicts. Taking care of the group is not an "accident". It is already an ordinary regular activity that requires experience and skills.

Finally, with *Hominem*, we must take care of human life (assisting survival, facilitating institutional life). It is a very old relational activity of proximity, educational and sanitary. It is imperative to take care of human life when the adverse conditions of life appear threatening. Ensuring survival, preventing illness or helping to overcome it, supporting in death, helping to regain strength and dignity, helping to regain hope and self-confidence, helping to maintain links were already skills demanded of carers in the lay age of knowledge. They remain so today, but how much are they worth economically? Offering comfort to caregivers and having the skills to sustain both life and purpose has always been at the heart of the profession. This *hominem*-type practice is one that the nurse carries out on her own and can delegate to her auxiliaries. This group of practices is usually referred to as the independent function of the professional role. This service is provided 24 hours a day, regardless of the age, pathology, culture or gender of the person being cared for and regardless of the health organization on which the person depends.

NOTE.– In this basic triptych of the nursing discipline, *Domus–familia–hominem* does not depend on a medical prescription or any medical mandate. Dependence is only related to the mission of the institution and to the needs of the person being cared for.

5.1. Even more knowledge

The initial triptych of knowledge is supplemented by the requirements and skills of the medical culture when it enters the hospital. It was only at the end of the 18th Century in French-speaking Switzerland that doctors followed by surgeons gradually introduced a new language related to remedies and new knowledge from the order of nature or from naturalistic or vitalist medical schools in the hospital. Medical language preceded the practitioner's work in the hospital and was the subject of "on-the-job" learning by the care providers in place (maids, servants, caretakers). With this new discursivity, which made institutional care a medically oriented "care", the carer needed to familiarize herself with a culture and a language composed of knowledge, values and ideologies, enabling her to exercise what we today call the "medico-delegated" function of the professional role.

In addition to her ordinary activities related to "caring", the carer still had to gradually become a "double agent" in the service of the medical profession: on the one hand, a data collector for medical analysis (observation, evaluation of the patient's condition and transmission to be made in the legitimate language) and, on the other, an agent applying medical prescriptions. This double agent role was imposed later (from 1860) during training. And this, with care manuals or works "for the use of nurses" according to the established formula. This clearly shows here the power that the doctor has to delegate to the person he inexorably considered as his auxiliary, a fragmentary or residual part of his knowledge. Whenever new knowledge was to be delegated to caregivers, the medical profession consulted and gave its opinion on the limits and new responsibilities assigned to caregivers. However, fragmented or residual medical science knowledge added to the existing nursing knowledge was not enough to make those who had access to this knowledge paramedical actors. The existing initial knowledge could not be overlooked. As the hospital expanded or transformed, new knowledge about the institutions, their legislation and financing was needed: new knowledge to take care of human beings and their needs and new knowledge related to the management of working groups (cooperative work, coordination of activities, conflict regulation, prevention of organizational chaos, etc.).

As medicine developed and the hospital received more patients, the language structuring the medical-delegated practices occupied the hospital space and became more specialized, increasing the workload and quickly taking precedence over other languages and practices. Unable at the time to value the various aspects of its function in their entirety and complexity before the advent of writing and the appearance of the first theories of care activity, the nursing profession was obliged to hide behind the privileges, hopes and "magnitudes" carried by public health thinking, which were irremediably linked to the contexts in which services were produced.

With the development of health systems, the social and technological revolution of our societies, the increase in costs and the commodification of healthcare, institutional care today is increasingly complex. A large part of the healthcare activity is carried out in the tertiary sector, the service sector in which we operate. It is financed economically on the basis of, "it goes without saying", a reason which could explain why relational care practices are not taken into account in institutional analytical productivity and its costs. The knowledge of the lay era was produced by extracting experience and practice and fed daily into the occupations of staff who, in the early days, did not respond to a "female vocation", a trade or a profession. There was no collective thought and no recognized standards of knowledge. These were individuals engaged in voluntary servitude in order to exist and survive.

With the emergence of lay knowledge, this was Year 1 of the knowledge carried today by the nursing discipline. Local knowledge is closely linked to practices, which do not easily lend themselves to standardization. This not only reminds us of the difficulties in finding the characteristics of knowledge linked to the foundations of the discipline in the lay era, but also, in a way, challenges us on the difficulty of highlighting knowledge today from a perspective specific to nursing sciences. "This knowledge is oriented towards experimentation and is flexible, non-dogmatic and open. Whatever its qualities or defects, it is epistemologically alive and substantial" [WYN 99]. The lay foundations for "caring" were already at the heart of the hospital, long before medicine arrived or the Church found a way to rechristianize a society in the process of de-Christianization.

In the early days of caregiving, caring was an ordinary practice that, economically speaking, was nothing special, somewhat like the ordinary traditional work of women in popular cultures, much like mothers, wives or spouses today. While it was "relatively simple" to maintain order in an eight-bed house in the days of the first hospitals, it is quite different today, with establishments full of technological innovations, inhabited by many actors with heterogeneous statuses and sometimes with more than a thousand beds. We are no longer in the Middle Ages. Care activities are made up of a set of details. As it was sometimes enough to forget a detail within a family project, for example, to cause the failure of an educational activity (with children), logistics (supplying the household or repairing the accommodation), representation (welcoming visitors or family members) or the continuity of the couple (marital conflicts, divorces), let us imagine the repercussions of forgetting a detail in our gigantic and complex modern institutions. In the complex relief economy of the 18th Century, as in the services provided today, everything is made up of a multitude of details. And it is not uncommon, as the popular saying goes, that "the devil is in the detail".

This explains why the terms "domestic sciences" appeared in nursing knowledge at the end of the 19th Century in the United States[1] or "household sciences[2]" in Europe at the beginning of the 20th Century to describe the orientations of "caring". It was a question of giving "scientific" value to a shadowy activity that wanted to prove its social usefulness. Even if the student nurse in the psychiatric institutions of Neuchâtel still had to pass the floors with iron straw in 1967 with the blessing of Mr. "L'Économe" and the graduate nurses of a famous private clinic in Lausanne, cutting a piece of trout on a plate for tray service in the men's rooms according to methods worthy of a hotel school today, let us not deduce that the nursing discipline can only refer to knowledge that participates in the "minion

1 19th-Century feminism in the United States sought to "professionalize women's traditional roles" [EHR 14].

2 Even if these representations are now forgotten among *Bachelor of Science in Nursing* students, the language and skills required still persist in the care environment, whether in or out of hospital. Household sciences were making their voice heard at the beginning of the 20th Century in French-speaking Switzerland. Thus, schools and "the courses set up for the training of women as housewives had to be considered as corresponding to the professional schools of further education and higher technical schools in terms of their didactics and organization" [BRU 02]. However, it was only in 1994 in the French-speaking part of Switzerland that nursing schools reached this official higher professional level. For a hospital director in 1908, "a good hospital worker must first be a good housewife. Nurses possess the difficult art of the housewife: they will need it as hospitallers, not only to command and train the staff, but to put their own hands to the task when needed" [DIE 90]. Today, this may still be a necessary condition for the supervision of work in the care unit. And again, in the 1970s, if a candidate for nursing school had attended housekeeping school after compulsory schooling, she had a good chance of being accepted into the school. But beware! Let's not say that a nurse's major skills are limited to domestic, maternal or household activities. This shortcut may be a necessary condition to identify the tacit knowledge at work, but not a sufficient condition to decipher the requirements and knowledge of the nursing discipline today.

syndrome"[3]. Instead of fleeing from these clichés, nurses should integrate them as part of their knowledge heritage, the one that characterizes an era in the development of their discipline, and include them in the original professional collective memory. It is indeed around the domestic activity and the qualities required to run a household, including taking care of one's own during illness and welcoming visitors, that the institutional adventure of care began. But it was by no means an ordinary domestic activity, especially at a time when women were not allowed to associate. Institutions shaped practices and the hospital institution by its aims and its multiple challenges were of course more complex than a private household. Similarly, religious institutions also shaped their practices. We saw this with the arrival of nurses. To the lay hospital servants, servants of God were only added at the time when certain religious congregations were called upon by the politico-religious authorities to serve certain hospitals.

5.2. The economically unnecessary provision of services

It is true that it is often difficult to find the particularity or specificity of one's own activity for services that are sometimes presented without formally recognized economic values. According to Adam Smith, one of the founders of the liberal economy, "what is wise for the head of a family cannot be madness in the management of an empire". He believed that work is the only universal measure of value. And since "it is not easy to find an exact measure of either the difficulty or the ingenuity of work, the adjustment, that is, the bargaining and transactions of the market, is made according to that sort of approximate equality which, though not exact, is sufficient to carry on the affairs of ordinary life" [DUB 05]. For J.-B. Say, for example, another thinker of the liberal ideology of the early 19th Century, who is still sometimes influential today, the state of domesticity did not imply the accumulation of human capital such as that used by the doctor. "The science of service is nothing or little, and since the application of the servant's talents is done by

3 Evoked during the main conference of the second international congress of the Faculty of Nursing at St. Joseph in Beirut on November 18, 2016 to denounce a habit worn by some nurses. The theme of this congress was: "The nursing profession, at the heart of the health care system". As stated by the journalist Julien Arlandis, in the *Grand soir* of June 20, 2010, "in an individual, the minion syndrome is a pathological behavior aimed at systematically defending the most privileged classes to the detriment of those from which it originates. This syndrome diminishes the minion's capacity for analysis and results in a psychological blockage that encourages him to act preferentially against his own interests to the benefit of those who exploit him. The minion ends up identifying with his masters by imagining that he belongs to the social body that exploits him" (source: juliendusud, available at: http://www.dailymotion.com/video/xes!). Hence, explaining why nurses in some countries sometimes identify with medicine from the point of view of knowledge is only a step away.

the one who employs him, the servant is left with little more than servile execution, which is the least of the operations of industry" [DEL 87].

This could explain why some nurses who are indifferent to the past of their knowledge seek to identify with the characteristics of medical science. And this point of view remains valid for hospital servility, even with the arrival of the sisters in the hospital. Servitude persists. As much in the hospital servant as in the nun, dependence on something remained. Instead of functioning with hospital servants, the hospital functioned with servants of God from the moment care became their responsibility. Sismondi, a member of the de Gasparin family, the very people who founded the first lay school for nursing sisters in the world in 1859 in Lausanne, added that "the nursing population produces nothing. However, the first caretakers at the end of the lay period of knowledge were the guardians of the hospital. They were entrusted with the running of the hospital (of the house). They were transformed into 'caretakers' during the 18th century. One can understand the difficulties that nurses have today to have 'strong care' recognized by the political class. "As the service that the carer class renders to society as a whole, however great, is felt by no one in particular, it could not be the object of a voluntary exchange. It had to be paid for by the community itself, by raising a forced contribution from everyone's income. The labor force of the beneficiaries is therefore paid by tax revenue" [DEL 87]. For Smith, too, the market cannot take over all economic activities, because some are not profitable for any company, yet they greatly benefit society as a whole. These activities, especially those of public services, must then be taken over by the state (taxes). It should be noted that this is still the case in many countries around the world for the majority of nurses' salaries. The triptych of basic knowledge, *Domus–familia–ad-hominem*, represents the foundation of the nursing discipline on which new knowledge, new roles and new statuses would later be superimposed. The purpose of nursing is therefore not only based on health and the care of the sick. It is much more subtle and complex than that! The lay period of knowledge came to an end. The protodiscipline period followed. With other structures, other places of speech and other elements of language, it is the school that came into being.

PART 2

Protodisciplinary Knowledge

6

From Hospital-School to School-Hospital

It was not until the mid-19th Century that protodisciplinary knowledge of the discipline developed quite unexpectedly. This knowledge took root with the creation of new institutions, which we shall call "schools". The latter demanded the questioning of the logic of exhibiting the knowledge to be implemented so that those trained could be useful to society. The institutional horizon was no longer the hospital, but the school. "Proto" then indicated a first element to be posed in regard to knowledge before the latter was gathered and distinguished to be constituted as a discipline within the university. This period was long before the writings of Florence Nightingale and the first care theories from North America. At this point, the knowledge of the lay age took the form of a prototype of heterogeneous knowledge that had not yet been completed. It was trial and error! Not only was there not yet uniformity in the discipline's frame of reference, but the very idea in the mid-19th Century that there might be a care discipline was not yet an idea of the moment. And it was not the hospital maids of the time who were going to create new schools, become teachers (instructors) or produce new knowledge and write the first care manuals! The logic of lay knowledge remained unknown. Training to be set up for a group in charge of caring for others when this activity seemed to belong more to the very nature of women and their tacit knowledge or to what was usually required in hospital domesticity was not really evoked in the mid-19th Century.

In this 19th Century, hospitals were growing, actors were proliferating and questions about the structures of the health system were beginning to challenge the ruling classes and the public sphere. From 1859 onwards, the first training institutions for female nurses were established. Knowledge became common to a group of people. Those who were students were able to share their experiences. Towards the end of the 19th Century, new teaching aids were introduced and care manuals written by doctors and clergymen were only part of the triptych of knowledge from the *Domus–familia–hominem* era. "To the empirical knowledge acquired through observation and learning of the things of life, was substituted the knowledge of instruction, knowledge taught by doctors for having transcribed and retranscribed it, without having practiced it" [COL 88].

However, there was no reason why the knowledge to be favored needed to make a break with the language tradition that came to the fore. The purity of the air in a sick room or the rules of hygiene to be applied were already part of the knowledge in force before Florence Nightingale. The response to the needs of the sick was also, as already mentioned, long before the writings of Virginia Henderson. In the mid-19th Century, the question began to arise as to what knowledge to teach in order to make healthcare practice efficient and to enable members of a community to share their knowledge and apply it in a standard form in appropriate situations. For what purposes should one be trained and with what autonomy of thought should one envisage action? We did not yet have a discipline. Only the foundations existing at the time of lay knowledge (*Domus–familia–hominem*) gave an orientation and pointed out the singular spaces in which holding a specialized language could give access to a profession.

The only existing training throughout the world to work in a hospital environment was those of the nuns formed in the novitiate as nurses according to the orientations of practical charity of the Church (Catholic or Protestant). All the knowledge that existed before the arrival of spiritual knowledge is almost forgotten today. It is as if it has no value. Yet it has managed to survive the centuries. Before the religious practice of charity, no country had the idea of setting up a training course for hospital maids, servants and lay governesses.

It was then that Joseph-Barthélémy-François Carrère, from whom we have already quoted some excerpts, Louis XVI's doctor, trained at the Montpellier medical school, was worried about it, because he was "witnessing the imperiality of the sick nurses". He did try around 1780 to show the French government that the care given to the sick "requires special knowledge, which alone can make it useful; but this kind of service is generally delivered to a class devoid of enlightenment and which neglects and was even powerless to acquire it. (…) It is a service to humanity to present them with a table of the most essential precepts from which they can draw some of the knowledge they need" [CAR 86].

But, "The Government has not yet made its views known on this subject; we have no institution designed to provide the people who care for the sick with education that will lead them into a career they do not know. I have even presented the Government with a table of reasons why it is necessary and the means of achieving it; but perhaps more important objects have hitherto prevented it from taking care of them" [CAR 86]. Carrère then published his care manual by making sure beforehand that his German competitor, Doctor Franz May of Manheim, who had just published a first manual *Instructions pour les gardes-malades*[1] in 1784, did not say the same thing as him. Noting that "the author enters in it long definitions of chemistry and physics that I avoided, as being above the knowledge of the people for whom this book is intended", he then remained faithful to a writing that avoids "all kinds of digressions; I have simplified and shortened the reasoning and I have limited myself to the precepts; I have even tried to be concise, to facilitate the reading of my work to the people for whom it is intended" [CAR 86]. He then published his manual (the second of its kind after May) and even though the government was not yet ready to put in place structured training for sick nurses, the book was distributed as widely as possible. Moreover, how could this government have set up training, having no recognized female experts around the lay foundations of this discipline that we have described so far? The basic triptych *Domus–familia–hominem* and the knowledge useful for caring of the time was either considered too common or completely unknown.

6.1. A non-religious form of training

It was then the Church and the call to the vocation of women that preceded the concern of Carrère. As we have seen, spiritual knowledge arrived in certain hospitals at the end of the 18th Century. It was to replace and dominate the knowledge at work in lay establishments until then.

The nurse returned to the novitiate and, with the help of the novice mistress, she was led to take her solemn vows. With obedience, respect for rule, many prayers, a uniform and the reading of good books, she directed the lay servants who were in place when she arrived and participated in temporal and spiritual care. The nurse was then confronted in her activity with the demonic etiology of illnesses, the power of darkness, the confrontation of the difficult as well as the good and the nun's eschatological promise.

Generally speaking, at the request of lay hospital directors, Catholic or Protestant religious communities were thus developing throughout the world according to the biological model described above. They offered services to the various establishments that called upon their services. They could be found in Ireland, Germany, France, Belgium, Canada, the United States, England and French-speaking Switzerland. In this region alone, 157 religious communities were founded in 1842 from the *Maison-Mère des diaconesses* in the village of Pompaples in the canton of Vaud. The religious communities took up most of the space, so to speak, but had to give way to the establishment in French-speaking Switzerland first, followed by

1 It is clear that the term "*garde-malade*", or sick nurse in English, was an exclusively secular term, because at the time of its use (1784), there were no Protestant nuns in Germany.

Great Britain later, of a lay training course for non-religious women who wanted to become nurses.

This invasion of society by religious communities was causing a reaction. But the reaction was partially ignored. As a philosopher of the time, Friedrich Nietzsche, would tell us, once again, "the devil is in the detail"! No less than four European countries were affected by the consequences of the beginning of the protodisciplinary period of nursing knowledge (Switzerland, Germany, England, France)[2]. The sister guilds that were developing both in schools and in hospitals in the Protestant regions of French-speaking Switzerland were beginning to provoke reactions in the population and in the press. Between 1849 and 1850, the publication of eight letters to the editor of a religious newspaper in the canton of Vaud called "*l'Avenir*", "fired the gun". For information, at that time, Florence Nightingale was 29 years old and she was not a stranger to Valérie de Gasparin who was 36 years old at the time. Valérie de Gasparin was the first to explain:

> I am writing against the introduction into our Church of an organization that modifies the great social laws, of which I find no trace in the Bible and whose frightening model I see in Roman Catholicism (January 1850, fifth letter to *L'Avenir*). [NAD 93]

The uniform and the title of "nun", which imitated the Catholic nuns possessed, the Protestant nursing sisters, as well as community life, fueled the debate:

> [The institution] calls eighteen-year-old girls into its heart, who wants them unmarried and employs them only as such; who subjects them wherever they go, whatever they do, to a central and sovereign authority; who imposes on them the renunciation of wages; who takes them from their families, who removes them from their natural duties, who robs them of the holy guidance of a father and a mother, who dresses them in a uniform, who endows them with a monastic name: sister. [DEG 54]

For Pastor Fliedner in Germany (founder of the deaconesses), the trial period lasted six to seven months, at the end of which the novice was solemnly consecrated. In 1844, at the consecration of seven deaconesses, Fliedner reminded the seven novices that, as Christian servants, they owed the pastor and his wife filial obedience:

2 In the 19th Century, the term "*infirmière*" (nurse) was used very little in Protestant regions. In general, nurses were presented as deaconesses or as "The Sister" or "*Schwester*". At the end of the 19th Century, deaconesses sometimes presented themselves as *gardes-malades*. The term "*infirmière*" exclusively remained a Catholic affiliation.

> May Jesus, the Sovereign Bishop and Pastor, give his yes and bring your declaration and vow! Come closer; hold out your right hand to me, extend it to the headmistress to confirm your promise. Kneel down on your knees. May the holy trinity, God the Father, Son and Holy Spirit bless you; may He give you faithfulness unto death and then the crown of life. Amen! The congregation prostrates itself: Father of mercy, who formed these maidens for your son, that they may give themselves to him as his own! You have now entered as servants of Christ, into his holy vineyard. [DEG 54]

But this type of solemn commitment did not fail to leave the Countess de Gasparin more than perplexed, who saw a great analogy in this religious promise with that of the Catholic sisters. It was shocking! The message did not go down well with this radical Protestant woman and her husband, Count Agénor de Gasparin, born in Orange, former student of the Louis Legrand high school in Paris, lawyer, deputy of Bastia, chief of staff of the Minister of the Interior (her father) in the Guizot government in France:

> It is enough for me to note that the Sisters are now really in charge of doing what others did before them, and as well as they (…) after having given the Sisters the hospital establishments themselves, we will not delay, rest assured, in abandoning to them the visiting of the poor and the distribution of alms. Then will come the schools as in Germany. [DEG 60b]

Valérie de Gasparin, as an emancipated woman, was opposed to the form of unconditional obedience exercised over women in the novitiates of religious congregations. This obedience "religious, monastic, permanent, exact, weighing with equal weight on the details of existence and on great events; this obedience, anti-biblical, maintains the individual in eternal childhood" [DEG 55]. The tone was set. This had the merit of being clear!

6.1.1. *Valérie de Gasparin*

Both born and dying in Geneva (Chambésy) on September 13, 1813 and June 16, 1894, respectively, she was the daughter of Auguste Jacques Boissier and Caroline Buttini (1786–1836), a great composer from French-speaking Switzerland. Her father, a great landowner, owned several estates: Le Rivage near Geneva and the manor of Valeyres-sous-Rances in the canton of Vaud. Her tutor was Pastor Louis Valette, who gave her an education based on stoicism. Great-niece of Madame de Staël, a pupil of Franz Liszt and a piano virtuoso, in 1837 she married Count Agénor de Gasparin, auditor at the *Conseil d'Etat*, Corsican deputy of Bastia (1810–1871), Protestant, writer and son of the Minister of the Interior of the bourgeois Monarchy of Louis Philippe d'Orléans[1], head of his father Adrien de Gasparin's cabinet, Prefect of Lyon.

The Gasparin couple lived in Paris between 1837 and 1846 and frequented the family of François-Pierre Guizot, then Minister of Public Instruction under Louis Philippe (monarchy of July 1830–1848). "She met many personalities of her time" [SMI 92]. Invited to the Tuileries by the King, Madame de Gasparin criticized the status of women at court. Valérie de Gasparin was also one of the famous female writers of French-speaking Switzerland in the 19th Century. Even if some people put Valérie de Gasparin in the "blue-stocking" category[3], no less than seven works about her were published between 1885 and 1902, to which must be added two works published for the hundredth anniversary of her death in 1994 in Lausanne by Gabriel Mützenberg and Denise Francillon, as well as the various historical booklets on her school: the *Haute école de santé La Source à Lausanne*, one of the sites for bachelor's degree in nursing at *la Haute école spécialisée de Suisse occidentale* (HES-SO). Sainte-Beuve "emphasized her sensuality, describing her as a Calvinist in celebration, with the devil in her body, a formalist who broke the mold" [SMI 92].

This rival of Florence Nightingale's in terms of values is completely ignored by nursing education institutes in France, courses in the history of the profession in Switzerland (her own country) or in nursing faculties in North America. Fortunately, she is well known in Pasadena (a suburb of Los Angeles) at the California Institute of Technology, where Annette Smith wrote a brilliant synthesis on her [SMI 92], or in Israel, where Michèle Bokobza has also written a doctoral thesis in philosophy for the University of Haifa, which is added to the works on Valérie de Gasparin, since it was published in 2018 [BOK 18]. Valérie de Gasparin was also an energetic campaigner against poverty and prostitution, the colonization of Algeria and Tahiti, the death penalty, the prison system and the founding of the Salvation Army. Her original role in setting up the world's first model school for women wishing to learn to care for others than by becoming a "nun" is probably not part of the history of nursing discipline!

Let us also note that it was Valérie de Gasparin who gave Henry Dunant the idea of founding an association in favor of wounded soldiers (the Red Cross), an event that often goes unnoticed when Henry Dunant's work is mentioned or when a film is made about his life. One only has to read the footnotes written by Henry Dunant in 1862 in *A Memory of Solferino* to be convinced of this. While the International Conference of the Red Cross, meeting in London in 1907, "honored Florence Nightingale as the inspirer of this same Red Cross", it is undeniable that it was Madame de Gasparin who had the honor of having thought of a neutral association (CICR) to help the military wounded on the battlefields, and not Henry Dunant, who only gave substance to the idea. Why is Madame de Gasparin obscured while Florence Nightingale is in the limelight?

Box 6.1. *Brief biography of Valérie de Gasparin*

3 A term adopted by conservative men and reactionaries to stigmatize women, such as George Sand, for example, who had literary or intellectual pretensions in the 19th Century.

But back to the organization of work among the Protestant nuns. We notice that it was almost the same as that seen in a Catholic hospital. The nursing activity that was to be done did not change according to the people who carry it out, but according to the aims and the institutional dynamics. The work plan was also the same; the care of people was entrusted to a nurse (also a non-qualified helper of the nuns). The arrival of the nuns did not suppress the activity of the lay servants, but the nuns had the privilege of directing their work and wearing a uniform. And it was not because there were nuns, for example, in Kaiserswerth, that the work seemed to be of better quality. Florence Nightingale, who spent three months in Kaiserswerth, had noticed this. "The nursing there was terrible, the hygiene was horrible. The hospital was certainly the most defective part of the institution" [KRE 32]. In fact, Valérie de Gasparin noted that to pass from the knowledge and rank of hospital servant to that of knowledge and rank of servant of God, it was above all an elevation of charity which was at work:

> [The nuns taking part in the novitiate] that contrary to the teachings of Jesus, there are two kinds of devotion for the sincere Christian: the commonplace devotion that concerns us all; the exceptional devotion, the sharing of a few elite souls. They will learn that there is an inferior holiness, that of the Church, and a superior holiness, that of the religious. They will learn that one reaches the perfect state by means of a special vocation; that it is this vocation, strictly speaking, that constitutes it. [DEG 54]
>
> God did not reserve the exercise of practical charity for one class of believers to relieve the other. [DEG 55]

For the Count de Gasparin, the habit, indicative both of the group to which he belongs and of the special consecration conferred on the Sister, "this charity uniform", was "a Pharisee's trumpet, which loudly announces professional devotion" [NAD 93], while for his wife, this conventional habit was a "leveling principle which lies at the basis of all religious orders" [DEG 55]. Little by little, a Mother Superior came to supervise the work.

When Mrs. Fliedner, who had been exercising leadership authority in Kaiserswerth in 1848, could no longer cope with the whole task, "the Sisters were invited to appoint one of them to the position of superior or, textually, first Sister. From house to house, the superior or mother abbess replaced the director with the female director. The primitive establishment was governed by a pastor and his wife. But very quickly, any new foundation would invariably be placed under the authority of a superior" [DEG 55]. Even when it was necessary to develop a mother house at the expense of another, it was the extension of the work that had priority, as Count de Gasparin noted:

> At the very time when the management in Paris complained that they did not have enough Sisters to care for the sick, they sent one to La Rochelle to found a school. Let it be done, and in a little while we will not have a single work without one or more sisters at its head. What was perfectly accomplished before they were invented, we will not be able to do it again unless we call them. [DEG 86]

As for Joseph-Barthélémy-François Carrère in 1786, Valérie de Gasparin in 1850, she simply did not understand why the existing lay nurses, those who already worked in English, German, French and Swiss hospitals, were not trained and why religious congregations were brought in their place, each order of which provided services and received money from the civil authorities, money which enriched the congregation and above all, which was not necessarily redistributed to the sisters[4]:

> Alongside the servants of the Lord, you need other servants, poor common devotees to whom no one sets up altars, who are not celebrated, who are not dressed in costume, for whom no monastic rule has been devised! It seems to me that we could stick to those we had on hand and to which we must return. [DEG 54]

Yes, there were common devotees in hospitals, governesses and lay servants. Why did we need special servants of the Lord (nurses) to care? The governesses and lay servants were on hand and we inevitably come back to them, because they were the ones the nuns needed. This was the cry of despair!

> I see very humble peasant women, untitled caretakers, who do not catch the eye and whose self-sacrifice with persevering love has nothing to envy the Sisters. Serving the sick in corporate hospitals requires a lot of patience! And if I have to say all my thoughts, I admire even more the lay helpers, those modest servants who in Paris, in Germany and almost everywhere, care for the sick under the direction of the sisters, than I admire the members of the corporation placed at the head of these various establishments. (…) We have sick nurses everywhere where the direction of the hospices is evangelical. It is not the workers who are lacking, they have rarely been lacking; what is lacking is the zeal to support them; that is our role. (…) Let us have hospitals that offer normal schooling for the sick nurse (…) it is not a question of changing the route, it is simply a question of walking faster on the one we are on. [DEG 55, 1st letter 1849]

4 For Valérie de Gasparin, "the services provided are paid for and the money makes a detour and passes through the director's cash register" [DEG 55].

Valérie de Gasparin, who corresponded with Mr. Baird, author of *La religion aux États-Unis*, also knew what was happening in this country. She noted that throughout this vast continent where arms were so scarce and servants were so hard to find and keep, "hospices for the sick were multiplying at will in the Protestant states of the Union and to meet the needs of all, there were nurses of both sexes, pious and devoted" [DEG 55]. There was no need to bring in religious corporations. While Mr. Fliedner has just escorted four deaconesses to the City Hospital in Pittsburgh, a letter from the Reverend Mr. Baird, written at the same time as Mr. Fliedner's arrival in Pittsburgh, mentions "we never had any Protestant Sisters of Charity until Mr. Fliedner arrived, the institution is too similar to Rome to suit our people. Mr. Baird was not mistaken" [DEG 54]. Deaconesses were thus growing in the United States as well.

Valérie de Gasparin first of all opposed the development of institutions that trained nuns for hospitals (novitiates). The places criticized were Echallens (Switzerland), Paris (France), Kaiserswerth (Germany) and Devonport (England). In a second stage, she turned her criticism to those who espoused the forms of religious vocation developed by institutions of the same kind, first Catholic, then Protestant. This was the case of Florence Nightingale. Later, she criticized women who allowed themselves to be "regimented" as "lay saints" to work at the Barrack Hospital in Scutari on the banks of the Bosphorus. These women were the ones who embarked for Crimea on board the *Vectis* on October 21, 1854 under the direction of Florence Nightingale:

> Miss Nightingale, called by the representatives of Puséism in the government, chosen in contempt of the evangelical Christians, who on all sides had asked for the honor of spending themselves for the love of Christ, Miss Nightingale accepted the mission conferred on her by the ministry; she composed as she pleased the phalanx of guards who accompany her, she brings in married women, we know it, women who receive an honorable salary, we know it. Her companions, too, taken in the common life, did not leave her, all this is true, and we bless God for it. But Miss Nightingale and the Pusyte[5] Party have, to the great sorrow of the biblical Christians in England, clothed these mere sick nurses in a costume proclaiming charity, but they suffered Miss Sellon to impose four of her sisters of mercy on them (…) grant the costume, you will be shown the need for leadership, the convenience of a salary, the practical utility of celibacy. [DEG 55]

5 Ritualistic movement which brought part of the Anglican Church closer to Catholicism and which was due to Edward Bowerie Pusey and his friends, canon of Christ Church, the great school of Henry III.

The nun's uniform, obedience to the director of monastic institutions or to a Mother Superior, the non-remuneration and practical usefulness of celibacy were inadmissible in the case of Valérie de Gasparin for the valorization of the feminine condition. This led her to propose, shortly before Florence Nightingale, other perspectives to women who wanted to provide care. Feminist before her time, with a passionate temperament, a liveliness and a conviction that emanated from her, she stood out in her literary work. Valérie de Gasparin shocked those around her for whom "a woman should not speak up and should keep herself away from public life, she should not try to free herself from the social conventions of the time" [MOR 92]. Not only did unconditional obedience to the Superior or the Spiritual Father pose a problem for her, but the uniform, the unpaid work that was unattractive and devalued, the imposed celibacy and the vows taken were for Valérie de Gasparin, obstacles to freedom.

6.2. Valérie de Gasparin and Florence Nightingale

Economists, religious congregations, doctors, statesmen and the aristocracy, with Valérie de Gasparin and Florence Nightingale and their respective entourage at its center, indirectly or directly shaped future nursing training. These ladies seemed implicitly condemned to inform each other and to think together, probably indirectly, but on the same subject. The main topic was to ask how and why to train women to improve care and hospital organization. Where should this training be organized? In order to tackle this topic, a sudden brief comparative analysis will have to be carried out to enable us to identify what we think are "strange coincidences".

Valérie de Gasparin and Florence Nightingale both received excellent educations. They were both polyglots, speaking at least four languages, even though Valérie de Gasparin started learning English late. Valérie de Gasparin was a virtuoso pianist (her mother, Caroline Boissier-Butini was a virtuoso pianist, composer having published with Ignace Pleyel in Paris and an ethnomusicologist before her time). Valérie de Gasparin was a pupil of Franz Liszt and Anton Reicha in Paris during the winter of 1831–1832. Florence Nightingale was also a pianist. Religiously speaking, both women belonged to the English-speaking Protestant movement and read the press on the subject: the Free Church of the Awakening[6] for

6 Evangelical Free Church of the Awakening: a movement of religious renewal led by John Wesley and his disciples. This movement, Methodism, with its very diverse sources and forms, was born in the Anglican Church during the 18th Century. A return to the sources of the Reformation, revolt against the power of reason, it was concretely the appearance of independent religious communities having broken with the traditional Protestant Church. Valérie de Gasparin joined the Church of the Awakening in 1836 on the death of her mother.

Valérie de Gasparin as early as 1836, on the death of her mother, the Unitarians[7] and Puseysts[8] for Florence Nightingale. Apparently, with two different religious orientations, they were not really made to get along. However, they both often referred to God in their writings. Valérie de Gasparin met Jean-Charles de Sismondi (historian and economist) in 1835 (at the age of 22). He wrote the foreword (three lines) to her book *Voyage d'une ignorante dans le midi de la France et l'Italie.* Florence Nightingale also met Jean-Charles de Sismondi in 1837 (at the age of 17) during a stay in Geneva. She came back to see him again in 1839. Florence Nightingale was also impressed by Augustin de Candolle (botanist) whom she met in Geneva in 1837 [SIN 08]. Augustin de Candolle happened to be a very dear friend of Valerie's brother Edmond, a great botanist and neighbor of the Boissier au Rivage family in Geneva. Another coincidence is that the two young women were both in Paris in 1838. Rue de Courcelles for Valérie de Gasparin[9], Place Vendôme for Florence Nightingale. When Valérie de Gasparin was in Geneva in 1839 (26 years old), Florence Nightingale (19 years old) listened on Sunday morning to Agénor de Gasparin's public lectures (up to 3,000–4,000 listeners)[10].

In 1848, Valérie de Gasparin traveled to Egypt, Palestine and Lebanon. In 1849, Florence Nightingale traveled to Egypt and Greece. The two women displayed the same personalities. It should also be noted that traveling in the East in the first half of the 19th Century was very fashionable for the aristocracy. It was a matter of "discovering emblematic places and thus offering themselves the luxury of a change of scenery" [TAN 15]. But these journeys also had a cost. For example, for the trip from Trieste to Alexandria via Athens, Valérie de Gasparin, her husband and two servants spent 560 French francs just for the boat (Lloyd), about the equivalent of the average annual salary that a servant or housekeeper received at the time. Valérie de

In Paris, Valérie took an active part in the work of the Evangelical Societies; she was the secretary of the Bible Society and contributed to the launching of the Œuvre des missions.

7 Unitarians: Christians who do not adhere to the dogma of the Trinity. This current refers to the anti-Trinity Protestant Reformation of the 16th Century. It is part of a Christianity of liberal and adogmatic theology.

8 Puseyism: a ritualistic movement that brought part of the Anglican Church closer to Catholicism. For Valérie de Gasparin, the Puseyist party and the congregations of Miss Sellon (Sisters of Mercy, recruited by Florence Nightingale and protected by the Bishop of Exeter) "play, among our Protestants drawn to Rome, the role that the Montanists had in the fourth century. She is the lost child of the monastic spirit among us" [NAD 93].

9 In front of the Queen of Spain Hotel [NAD 93].

10 According to some historians: Mützenberg G., *Une femme de style, Valérie de Gasparin*, Éditions Ouverture, Le Mont-sur-Lausanne, 1994 and Michèle Bokobza in Haifa, Israel (telephone communication of September 2, 2015 at 10:20 a.m.), author of the book *Madame la Comtesse de Gasparin, protestantisme radical, genre et pèlerinage au* XIXE *siècle*, L'Harmattan, Paris, 2018.

Gasparin had a stoic education given by a tutor[11]. From her rich and distinguished Protestant parents, she had a solid moral, literary, musical and scientific education and learned "double-entry" bookkeeping to manage her property [FRA 09]. Florence Nightingale also had a solid education (languages, history, philosophy, mathematics and music) given principally by her father. In particular, she took some advanced courses in mathematics and statistics and was the first woman in 1858 to be elected a member of the Royal Statistical Society. Finally, both women displayed a sharp sense of humor.

Valérie de Gasparin was closely following events in Crimea. On December 30, 1854, she proposed to bring a little comfort to the mobilized soldiers and wanted to create by subscription "a surge of solidarity so that the English and French troops besieging Sebastopol would receive pipes, tobacco and cigars as a token of affection for their New Year's gift" [MÜT 94]. This was the origin of cigarette packets distributed free to French soldiers with their sales still in the 20th Century. In 1855, she suggested in the press the foundation of an association for wounded soldiers to remedy the Army's shortcomings. Henry Dunant met Valérie de Gasparin at her home and followed her advice. After correspondence (until July 21, 1859), this led to the implementation of the first international relief mission on June 30, 1859. Under the leadership of Pastor Charpiot, a French doctor and surgeon, "a committee was set up, a precursor of the Red Cross committee, and the first international relief mission for the wounded was sent to Italy" [MÜT 94]. With the alliance of Valérie de Gasparin and Henry Dunant, supported by the Swiss Red Cross, the first "care and army" links were established. After the Church and medicine, it was the army and the Swiss Red Cross that "entered the fray". This may also explain the famous formula devoted to the place of manuals and nursing knowledge in the society mentioned by René Magnon: "between the army, the church and the faculty" proclaimed the latter [MAG 88b]. Thus, there was not yet any explicit knowledge of its own for the discipline. Only disparate elements of knowledge and historical sequelae of values related to the three dominant cultures. It also seems that Henry Dunant was not indifferent to the charm of Valérie de Gasparin, and it seems that the same was true for the other side (see Michèle Bokobza, Israël). Henry Dunant also seemed to have been inspired by the press releases on Florence Nightingale's action in Crimea.

Like Florence Nightingale's grandfather, Valerie's husband (Count Agénor de Gasparin, Corsican deputy of Bastia) was a strong advocate for the abolition of slavery. At the age of 17 (1830), Valérie de Gasparin had a failed romance following social incompatibility. Following this failed romance with a young violinist ("I will marry him or I will die", she said), a wall of incomprehension rose between Valérie and her mother. This lasted about two years. As a diversion, the family went on a

11 Louis Valette, pastor of the Lutheran Church in Paris.

trip in 1831 accompanied by four servants. At the age of 17 (1837), Florence Nightingale suffered a nervous breakdown and auditory hallucinations, "God calls her to His service". Not accepting that her mother was opposed to her religious vocation, she was in perpetual conflict with her. Her father mediated between the two. As a diversion, the family went on another trip in 1837.

Florence Nightingale was a prolific writer (two hundred documents, books, reports, notices). Valérie de Gasparin also. No less than eighty books would be published, most of them republished and translated into English. But we do not know exactly how many documents make up her private correspondence and various notes, as her archives are scattered among members of her family, the Geneva cantonal archives and the archives of the Haute école de santé La Source in Lausanne. With two distinctions from the French Academy (Prix Montyon), she became one of the famous authors of the French-speaking Switzerland literature. She also protested against the exploitation of the poor. Florence Nightingale too. In 1859, Valérie de Gasparin developed the first courses for visiting nurses. Florence Nightingale did the same later, but from a technical college [SIN 08].

Valérie de Gasparin read the works of George Sand (Baroness Dudevant) and found them fatal to the union because they awakened female egoism. Having also Franz Liszt as her teacher, she knew George Sand indirectly since Liszt and Sand were friends. In addition, and to distinguish herself from this woman, like George Sand who smoked a pipe in public, Valérie de Gasparin, always at ease with a certain form of provocation, sometimes signed her writings with "a woman who does not smoke". On the other hand, Florence Nightingale seemed strongly impressed by the works of George Sand, particularly in 1854 with the novel *Gabriel* [SIN 08].

Valérie de Gasparin used her own property to create her works, including boarding and tuition fees for her students (the first school in the world). With a view to perpetuating her work, she created a foundation in 1890 and left a substantial capital "to guarantee the training (lessons, boarding, accommodation, lighting, heating) of 16 boarding students per year" [FRA 09]. Like Valérie de Gasparin, Florence Nightingale also used her own funds to buy equipment for the Crimean hospitals. For example, the room next to her room "looked like a veritable souk where the most heterogeneous objects were piled up: towels, sponges, shirts, flannels, tea, sugar or bread" [FRA 09]. In her requests for equipment to ensure hospital logistics in the Crimea in 1855, there were thus: "1,000 pairs of socks, 10,000 flannels, 10,000 shirts, 2,000 underpants, 2,000 pairs of shoes, unlimited soap, chests of drawers for storing objects, knives, forks and spoons, coconuts, 100 cushions, combs and hairbrushes, razors, cologne and gin" [SIN 08]. In a letter to the Minister of War, Florence Nightingale wrote on January 8, 1855: "I am sort of a merchant of socks, shirts, knives and forks, wooden spoons, tin tubs, benches and tables, cabbages and carrots, operating tables, towels and soaps, combs, lice products, scissors, bedpans and stump cushions" [BAL 93].

The "modern nursing" mentioned in contemporary history books consisted, for Florence Nightingale, of introducing order in the organization of work and providing useful equipment to take care of the home according to the customs and hygiene of the aristocracy. With her money, she also financed the renovation of the hospital's floors. Never demanded a salary, since caring was a vocation. With important political support, she also raised a Nightingale Fund to meet needs.

As we have seen, Valérie de Gasparin received two distinctions from the *Académie française* (the *Prix Monthyon*) for her writings. In 1843, for *Le mariage au point de vue chrétien*, the *médaille d'or*, the *Prix Monthyon*, and in 1846, for *Il y a des pauvres à Paris et ailleurs*. Florence Nightingale was awarded the Cross of the Order of Merit by King Edward VII in 1907. This also shows us that we are dealing here with two distinguished women.

After these few coincidences where Valérie de Gasparin and Florence Nightingale seemed to meet furtively, let's review some disagreements and differences in values between these two ladies. Valérie de Gasparin had some grievances against the English. She wrote on September 26, 1847 (age 34): "For my part, I feel that I am everyone's neighbor, except the English; it is that, to tell the truth, they are nobody's neighbor. There is only one Englishman who leaves his great body lying on the sofa when a woman enters a living room; there is only one Englishman who keeps his hat on his head while sewing it; there is only one Englishman who thinks he is dishonoring himself by saluting someone he does not know; there is only one Englishman who, at once, with the beard of the universe, always and everywhere seizes the best. I am much less angry at them for being rude than I am at them for forcing people who have no desire to be so" [DEG 78]. Florence Nightingale was English.

The two women were opposed on the usefulness of religious congregations. As we have seen, Valérie de Gasparin was against "the introduction into our Church of an organization that modifies the great social laws, of which I do not find a trace in the Bible and whose frightening model I see in Roman Catholicism […]" [DEG 55]. And Florence Nightingale regretted not being able to enter the Catholic Church. "[It was] the best form of faith I have ever encountered", she said. She was even initiated into the care of charity by the Protestant nuns at Kaiserswerth-sur-le-Rhin for three months in 1851[12] and by the Catholic Sisters of Saint Vincent de Paul, Maison de la Providence, rue Oudinot in Paris, for three weeks in 1853 [NAD 93].

12 At this time, Florence Nightingale traveled "surrounded by five servants" [SIN 08].

One was in favor of marriage, the other was against it. Florence Nightingale was single and had no children. “People often say to me, ‘You can’t feel what it’s like to be a mother or a wife’. No! I answer, I can’t and I’m very happy about it!” She preferred to love humanity rather than love for a single being. Valérie de Gasparin, married, was in favor of marriage (her writings on the subject with a prize from the Académie française prove it), had no children, but raised her niece in 1849, Caroline Boissier-(Barbey), orphaned by her mother (Lucille Butini).

For Valérie de Gasparin, in marriage, there was male/female equality with distinctions of role: to women, the private sphere, to men the public sphere. She was 30 years old and had been married for six years when she wrote in 1843 in her three-volume work entitled *Le mariage au point de vue chrétien*: “Within a couple, power is given to the man and influence to the woman”. Finally, for Valérie de Gasparin, caring was an independent paid profession. But for Florence Nightingale, it was a vocation. One understands better the origin of the controversies which arose later on the subject. Florence Nightingale never thought of peasants and workers as nurses. This was absolutely not the case with Valérie de Gasparin.

Valérie de Gasparin seemed to have less prestigious political support than Florence Nightingale and did not benefit from the same sounding board or media attention for her achievements or positions. Indeed, Florence Nightingale benefited from extraordinary publicity in the media for 22 months during the Crimean War thanks to one of the first war correspondents (*The Times*) in the history of the press (William Howard Russel). In addition, she secured the benevolent approval of representatives of the three dominant cultures of the time. For the Church, Henry Edward Manning, Archbishop of Westminster; Arthur Penrhyn Standley, Dean of Westminster; and some Unitarians. For medicine, John Sutherland, member of the McNeill Hygiene Commission in Crimea, his own adviser; Henry Acland, University Professor of Medicine at Oxford; William Bowman, ophthalmic surgeon; William Farr, pioneer in medical statistics. For the Army, Sir Douglas Galton, captain and military engineer, and above all, Sidney Herbert, Minister of War who sent Florence Nightingale to Crimea.

While some classify Gasparin’s Butini, Boissier, among the philanthropists, Florence Nightingale “forcefully asserted that philanthropy was a sham. We treat the symptoms without attacking the source of the evil”, she said [SIN 08]. Moreover, while for Gilbert Sinoué, “Florence Nightingale prefigured socialist thought”, we also know that Valérie de Gasparin “saw red as soon as she was spoken to about socialism” [SMI 92].

Let us note again that Valérie de Gasparin tended to make an active missionary proselytism in connection with the Protestant Revival. However, Florence Nightingale “was profoundly opposed to all forms of proselytism, without distinction". For example, in Crimea, "the sight of a nun preaching the good word at the bedside of a dying man plunged Florence Nightingale into a state close to hysteria" [SIN 08]. Finally, one adored her mother; the other was in constant conflict with her mother.

It seems that Valérie de Gasparin was first spotted by Florence Nightingale. Was she intrigued by this woman? Did they meet in Geneva, Paris or London during social dinners? Did she read her writings? Did she hear about her during her stays in Geneva? Would she attend the conferences of Agénor de Gasparin who, as already mentioned, managed to gather, as mentioned above, three to four thousand people to listen to him? Anyway, in a second phase, Florence Nightingale then projected herself into a domain identical to that of Valérie de Gasparin by standing out particularly, but with a certain indifference from this rival in terms of values. Let us note that it was not customary either in the aristocracy and women of the educated class to openly and publicly criticize the contrary ideas of people of the same rank. But an absolute ignorance or misunderstanding between the two women seems unrealistic to us. Valérie de Gasparin and Florence Nightingale may never have met. But one of them must have heard of the other. Valérie de Gasparin explicitly referred to Florence Nightingale in her writings on several occasions. Florence Nightingale learned, as she says, to "weave between the Protestant booing and the Roman Catholic storm" [BAL 93].

As we have seen, Valérie de Gasparin distanced herself from the religious healthcare orders and wanted to give training to the "poor common devotees" already in place in the hospitals of the Protestant regions of French-speaking Switzerland. On the other hand, Florence Nightingale, who belonged to the educated Anglican class close to the Unitarians, was inspired by the values of the Catholic religious orders, supported in this by the sympathizers of Puseyism. She imposed the attributes and values of the religious congregations on lay carers and women from good families. Thus, the uniform imposed by Florence Nightingale on lay people aboard the *Vectis en route* for Crimea on October 21, 1854, similar to that of the Gray Nuns, was violently fought against by Valérie de Gasparin. On the other hand, for Florence Nightingale, "the nurses should not be tempted to make themselves elegant, whether in uniform or otherwise" [BAL 93]. Faced with these controversies, Florence Nightingale replied: "I hear that there is a religious war about my poor person in the *Times* and that Mr. Herbert has defended me generously. I don't know what I have done to be dragged out in front of the public in this way" [SIN 08]. "But I am glad that my God is not the God of the upper or lower Church, that he is not Roman, Anglican or Unitarian" [BAL 93].

For Valérie de Gasparin, to enter a religious novitiate for a woman was to follow an absurd ("abnormal?") school, to be protected from the constraints of life and to be withdrawn from the world. The "abnormal" school was religious and turned the woman away from the world. It positioned itself on the subject in a convincing manner. "You keep the individual under guardianship, as long as he is part of your corporation he renounces the government of himself. (…) The monastic institution is definitive, the brothers and sisters enter it as children, they remain children; the monastic institution keeps us in swaddling clothes, it wants us eternally weak, eternally minor; it establishes a holy and perpetual guardianship of souls, intelligence and wills" [DEG 54]. Let us listen to her about the novitiates used to form brothers and sisters in religious institutions:

> You feather your birds to keep them under your wings; the teacher training school throws its own birds out of the nest; it teaches them to fly by throwing them into the void. The employee receives his salary, marries or doesn't marry, but he is in charge of himself; he has a home where he will be able to spend his leisure time as he pleases, he is a man, he is like everyone else and that is why he is not called a brother, but simply a teacher, a nurse, a caretaker: there is nothing new, nothing special about him, he walks the common path. That is what makes a normal school a normal school and you are a monastic corporation. [DEG 55]

For Florence Nightingale and her mystical thoughts, "the life of celibacy is that of Christ" and "sex is synonymous with distress (…) a nurse was no longer a nurse from the moment she got married" [SIN 08]. One year after Valérie de Gasparin, she then reflected on her vocation to be trained in the practice of hospital care by placing this action as "a good for God alone". The English school was not a new construction. Located on the premises of St Thomas' Hospital in London, it was above all a place of apprenticeship in a hospital environment where the trainees were exploited under the authority of a "real Cerberus and soulless woman (Miss Sarah Wardroper) devoid of any pedagogical sense" [SIN 08], "who knew nothing and understood nothing" [BAL 93]. This school provided a "steady stream of dedicated trainees from good families, who were willing to work hard and provided cheap labor for the hospital" under the authority of an incompetent matron (Wardroper) and an alcoholic doctor (Whitfield) [BAL 93].

At the age of 58 (following the death of her husband on May 14, 1871), Valérie de Gasparin lived for two years in her Geneva property Le Rivage in Chambésy. Although she later withdrew into herself, she continued to write and maintain occasional relations with the pupils of her school. Described as a "sectarian or psychorigid" by some, she was also a woman of writing, a woman of words, a woman of polemics, a woman of commitment, a woman of action for others, in particular members of her family. Augustin Filon, a French literary critic, in 1889, saw Valérie de Gasparin as "a brave lady who was a little crazy".

At the age of 37, Florence Nightingale adopted a "catatonic" attitude and withdrew into herself for 54 years while continuing to write and give her opinion on issues that were close to her heart. In 1857, Florence Nightingale was unable to enter the Order and "took up residence[13] at the convent she had always wanted to enter". She was described by her relatives as unstable, tormented, nervous, devout, whimsical, hysterical and depressed. Marked by the figure of her father who gave her access to the knowledge of men, apparently sexually repressed in a puritan society, she devoted her life with exuberance and in the form of impulses. In 2005, Dr. Katherine Wisner, psychiatrist, epidemiologist, head of the psychiatric clinic at the University of Medicine in Pittsburgh (USA), mentioned that Florence Nightingale suffered from a "personality disorder, a bipolarity with a predominantly manic-depressive nature, bordering on schizophrenia" [SIN 08].

Valérie de Gasparin was convinced that there was no need to become a "nun" and withdrew from the world to be trained in care practices. While Florence Nightingale, for her part, saw no harm in taking up the values of practical Charity of the Catholic Church, putting on the nurse's uniform and convincing the lay people of their vocation.

In the period preceding the opening in Lausanne of the school for lay nurses (between 1837 and 1848), i.e. at an age between 24 and 35, Valérie de Gasparin lived a lot in Paris where she had the opportunity to frequent the Protestant bourgeoisie and the Court of King Louis-Philippe. She exchanged and discussed with the best families on the status of women in society and participated in various debates, notably on the teacher training colleges and the methods of mutual teaching discussed within the family of François Pierre Guizot, Minister of Public Instruction under Louis-Philippe, to whom Valérie was invited with her husband (Valérie de Gasparin was impressed by Madame Guizot (mother), "an object of veneration and attraction" [NAD 93]. Close to Protestant educational circles in France, Valérie de Gasparin was thus imbued with discussions about school, especially about model (normal) schools and mutual pedagogy (Bell, Lancaster, Carnot, Guizot). Moreover, the title "normal school that could serve as a model" appeared[14] in Article 11 of the Guizot law of June 28, 1833 on schools that served as models for primary education. But Valérie de Gasparin had no interest in imitating particularly teacher training schools or training teachers. In any case, in her home, the "*école normale*" did not refer to a school that trained teachers.

---

13 10 South Street.

14 Already in 1794, a first abortive attempt at an *École normale* (normal school) was made in Paris. Carnot took up the idea again on April 27, 1815 in a decree by which it was planned to open in Paris "a trial school of primary education, organized in such a way as to serve as a model and become a teacher training school to train primary teachers" (electronic edition of Ferdinand Buisson's dictionary, 1911).

It was a "model school" and not a school for teachers that she wanted to offer to civil society for training in care, particularly home care. It was therefore necessary to create a normal school that could serve as a model for civil society to provide care in the city and distinguish itself from religious novitiates. A new space of speech, a school, distinct from a hospital and open to women who did not wish to become nuns and withdraw from the world, saw the light of day. The origin of the term "normal school" deserves attention. It follows the evolution of the words of the norm family and begins with the Latin *norma*, which has the meaning of "setsquare" (which measures the straightness of a construction), then acquiring the figurative meaning of "line of conduct, rule". In the expression, *école normale*, the adjective "normal" has the meaning of the Latin *norma* (norm) "line of conduct, prescription, school that must serve as a model".

But it was also a question for Valérie de Gasparin to provide training for home care, in a liberal practice. There was a need to provide help within families and not send everyone to the hospital. This idea was already part of the reflections of her father-in-law Adrien, Prefect of Lyon, Peer of France, Minister of State for the Interior. In a report made to King Louis-Philippe on April 5, 1837, Adrien de Gasparin on page 16 of his report [DEG 37] wrote "it is certain that the hospital system has the disadvantage of destroying family ties". There was an idea of whether they should not be replaced by a better understood home emergency system. In this logic, hospitals would be kept for the sick and home care would be developed, especially for people who could not take care of the activities of daily living on their own, the infirm and the elderly. Valérie de Gasparin's intentions were better understood.

Valérie de Gasparin-Boissier, an educated woman and a great Swiss Protestant pedagogue of the 19th Century in her own way, was awarded the *medaille d'or* from the *Académie française* at the age of 30. With a project already evoked in her writings as early as 1854, she practically innovated by officially announcing the creation of her school on July 20, 1859. In a prospectus from Valeyres, the population learned "that an establishment had just been founded in Lausanne, to provide midwives and nurses to the populations of all French-speaking countries: the canton of Vaud, the cantons of Geneva and Neuchâtel, the Bernese Jura, France and Belgium" [NAD 93]. This establishment, which was a counter-model to religious houses, was thus the first model school for lay women carers in the world (Lausanne, Switzerland).

NOTE.– This was not a hospital-based training course. The training took place in a new building separate from a hospital structure. Spaces were changing! A new kind of model school was being created, not a hospital transformed for the occasion. The challenge was to introduce a major change of status in the training of nurses[15] and to enhance in particular the organization of home care.

The Valérie de Gasparin (and her husband's) school escaped the power of the hospital administrations and was then different from the training given in the religious novitiates. Valérie de Gasparin's conception of her school was already expressed in 1854 (Florence Nightingale was then 34 years old). For Valérie de Gasparin, a model school for the time was:

> A school where single, widowed or married men and women come to do their apprenticeship.
>
> The students of the school will not receive the title of 'sisters'; no special uniforms will be imposed on them.
>
> In a teacher training school, leadership is exercised only over those who are doing their apprenticeship.
>
> This learning does not last a lifetime, it is invariably limited to a limited amount of time in advance.
>
> The leadership fades away as soon as the pupil, sufficiently educated, leaves the house and goes to exercise his vocation in society.
>
> The teacher training school receives no wages for the work of those it has trained and who apply their strength to such and such a work in the world.
>
> The employee remains free; nothing is decided about him or for him; he goes out, he returns, he leaves the service of the work, he takes it up again as he sees fit; this service is not an extraordinary consecration, it does not in any way apply the enslavement of conscience.
>
> The employee receives his salary, marries or does not marry, but he is in charge of himself; he has a home where he can spend his leisure time as he pleases, he is a man, he is like everyone else, he is what every biblical Christian is and that is why he is not called a friar, but

15 Valérie de Gasparin, as a Protestant, never used the term "nurse", knowing that this term carried other values than her own and that it was exclusively linked to the practical charity of the Catholic Church.

> simply a teacher, *infirmier*,[16] caretaker: there is nothing new, nothing special about him, he treads the common path.
>
> Obedience is required in normal schools; but one goes through the normal school, one does not settle there; authority ceases as soon as the clearly determined hour of exit is reached.
>
> As soon as the apprenticeship period is over, the worker enters the common conditions of life and exchange.
>
> During his apprenticeship, he pays the school for the instructions he receives from it; when he leaves school, he in turn receives the salary he deserves for his work.
>
> Normal schools prepare the individual for self-government; invariably they return him to freedom; they emancipate him up to the age when he must measure himself against life.
>
> The school is a school, that is to say, an essentially transitory establishment; the pupils enter it at a very young age, complete an education which, when finished, leaves them face to face with all the duties and all the human rights. [DEG 54, DEG 55, NAD 94, NAD 12b]

It is therefore easier to understand why La Source was emerging as a model school for healthcare education worldwide. In the period of lay knowledge, as we have seen, the transmission of knowledge between maids and servants took place on a peer-to-peer basis. This transmission could even be financially rewarded by hospital management if the person who had knowledge to transmit agreed to do so. But it was still about learning on the job, an individual horizontal transmission, from individual to individual. There was knowledge, but it remained fragmented and non-standardized. Knowledge was transmitted locally, within the same hospital and not necessarily in neighboring institutions. At that time, women of the working class and servant women could not go to any vocational school. There were simply none for this kind of work.

16 We recall that the French masculine for nurse "*infirmier*" is not at the same linguistic level as the feminine term. The term "*infirmier*" was only attributed to lay men who helped the religious nursing sisters who were sworn religious to respect their vows in their work. The lay nurse also did not have the status conferred on religious friars in male communities (Order of the Hospital of St. John of Jerusalem, for example).

So, with the initiative of Valérie de Gasparin, the women of the working class and the maids were finally given the opportunity to learn a trade in the care field. A major initiative for the time! Teaching in a systematic and collective way the art of taking care of the estate (*Domus*), the art of taking care of the group (*familia*) and the art of taking care of the human being (*hominem*) was possible. In 1860, "so little was known about what was, and what was to be a sick nurse, that no one showed up, and that in order to have students, Mr. Reymond (director of La Source) was obliged to give lectures in the country" [KRA 95].

Two distinct training models were then put in place nine months apart. First, the School-Hospital in Lausanne. The Hospital-School in London afterwards! Thus began the protodisciplinary period of care knowledge. There was not yet a constituted discipline. There was only disparate and heterogeneous knowledge that tried to find a utility, a structure and a coherence.

So at the age of 46, on November 1, 1859, Valérie de Gasparin created with her husband "the evangelical[17][18] normal school[19] of independent[20] carers" in Lausanne (the original name of the school being the *École normale évangelique de gardes-malades indépendantes*). A new space of speech, totally independent of a hospital, was set up. On March 10, 1860, seven students began their training: "Two were from Paris, one from Lyon, four from the canton of Vaud. They were between twenty-six and forty-seven years old. Three were married, four were single" [DEG 60a]. This was also the second field of nursing practice, that of training practice, which began to emerge. As a reminder, the first field of practice, that of care, was established as we saw in the age of lay knowledge. The discourse at school was not necessarily the same as the discourse at the hospital. The school became a reference model, and students easily found work in several cities. In 1867, for example, they were in demand in France: Pau, Bordeaux, Nantes, Paris, Nîmes and

17 Model school.

18 By this term, Valérie de Gasparin "sought to preserve the religious principles that were integrated into the life of the boarding school run by an evangelical pastor" [FRA 09]. "Evangelical does not mean clerical or regimented". According to the director of the school in 1899, this term means "free, subject only to his own conscience, independent, capable of initiative and conscious of their responsibilities" [KRA 00].

19 From the end of the 18th Century, the term "*gardes-malades*" gradually replaced the term "*gardienne de l'hôpital*". It was a term of secular origin mainly used in the Protestant cantons. According to the Académie française dictionary of 1762, "to look after a sick person is to be assiduously with him to assist him in his needs" [ACA 62].

20 "As soon as the apprenticeship period is over, the worker enters the common conditions of life and exchange. During the apprenticeship, he pays the school for the instructions he receives from it; when he leaves school, he in turn receives the salary he deserves for his work" [DEG 54, DEG 55].

Lyon. In Switzerland: Geneva, Lausanne, Neuchâtel, St Imier, Le Locle and Tavannes. In 1899, they worked in Belfort, Mulhouse, Sèvres, Avenches and Montreux. In 1900, candidates for the school flocked from Italy, France, England, Holland, Germany, Russia, Bulgaria, German-speaking Switzerland as well as French-speaking Switzerland [KRA 01]. "Our little school, so much criticized in the past, is becoming more and more the model on which other institutions are being created everywhere, in Bordeaux, Paris, Bern and Zurich" [KRA 00].

For training purposes and on the advice of doctors in her circle, Valérie de Gasparin attached a clinic to her school on January 28, 1891 (in order to provide clinical teaching in particular). She rented to a doctor-surgeon (Charles Krafft, pioneer of appendectomy), then new director of the school, an old apartment which was transformed into a clinic (Beaulieu clinic) of about eight beds. In fact, in their early days, it was mainly in home care and in liberal practice that the student nurses of La Source ensured their reputation. With a clinic at its disposal to give complete care to patients in institutions, the school, as a school-hospital, allowed its students to be confronted with various pathologies and care integrating the knowledge related to the functioning of a medical institution. Thus, here could be found *Domus* and *ad-hominem* of the lay period associated with medical knowledge of the SC2 type, i.e. linked to the cultural system which was the second to delegate written prescriptions to the sick nurses. The delegation of medical knowledge was done in writing.

NOTE.– The school therefore had a clinic at its service as an exercise area where the caretakers could learn about the actual hospital care to be given to the patients[21]. In return, Dr. Krafft benefitted from having inexpensive staff run his clinic. In this school-hospital, the hospital (annex of the school) was used for training. The theoretical knowledge learned at the school could be applied immediately and enriched the experience and knowledge of the care practice.

Three schools were in a similar situation in French-speaking Switzerland at the beginning of the 20th Century: La Source in Lausanne, Le Bon secours in Geneva and the first state school in Switzerland in Freiburg. These three schools had no financial or architectural constraints with a hospital and were located outside of any hospital compound when they were founded.

After having used the space of the military hospitals in Crimea to denounce and put in order what was then "sanitary chaos", in particular using statistics and pie

21 Ironically, 128 years later, on January 26, 2019, Valérie de Gasparin's school, the *Haute école de santé "La Source"* which is part of the *Haute école spécialisée de Suisse occidentale* (HES-SO), officially inaugurated its virtual hospital at the *Palais de Beaulieu* in Lausanne (daily newspaper *24 Heures* from January 28, 2019), so that nursing students could learn their profession, which has become increasingly complex, in conditions close to reality.

charts, Florence Nightingale also decided to give training to female carer. "The Special Fund collected by subscription during the Crimean War was used. The pupils' board was paid to the hospital and they themselves received a small salary. The apprenticeship lasted one year in exchange for which the student, who received a certificate, was required to work for three years in the position to be designated by the Fund Committee". Two levels of training were considered. One level for the probationary nurse and one level to take up positions of responsibility (lady or special probationer). The latter did not receive a salary, but paid for her apprenticeship [CRO 60]. There was no equality of status between the student in the popular class and the student in the cultured class.

The third professional field of the profession, that of management or care management, began to exist with this student category and recalled the role of maid or *superintendent* and also announced the further training in executive schools which were created from 1950 onwards in Switzerland as well as in France.

NOTE.– At the age of 40, Florence Nightingale then used the ordinary hospital space to provide apprenticeships from July 9, 1860 at St Thomas Hospital in London. The apprenticeship was then dependent on "superintendents" and other general supervisors. At the Hospital-School, apprenticeship was at the service of the hospital. The school (hospital annex) enriched practice and experience with theory at the point of care.

The two women were therefore using their wealth and relationships to improve the quality of care and education. One came from the English aristocracy, improved the basic equipment of the English military hospitals and their organization, by developing hygiene, prevention and taking into account the daily life of the people treated. The other, belonging by marriage to the French nobility, by creating the first model (normal) school in the world for lay carers in order to prepare students for the practice of home care according to a liberal practice.

One (Florence Nightingale) had good knowledge and experience in the field of care and left important professional writings. The other (Valérie de Gasparin) knew the field, but through events interposed,[22] and left literary writings with values on the emancipation of women and its attention to the working class. "It is in nature, particularly in the mountains of the Jura, that Madame de Gasparin reaped her happiness. She fought for all marginalized people, of any kind. She removed the barricades between generations, understood the young, celebrated the old, their

22 At Valeyres-sous-Rances (canton of Vaud, Switzerland), Valérie de Gasparin transformed a wing of her manor house into a hospital to accommodate the sick and wounded French military internees of the Bourbaki army in 1870. "They were treated, bandaged and fed and when they finally left, they were cleaned and disinfected" [MÜT 94].

charm, their love" [SMI 92]. Victor Hugo said to Valérie de Gasparin in 1867: "You tell, you teach, you meditate, you charm. I don't have all your ideas, you know it, Madame, but I have almost the vanity that I have all your tastes (…). Fools and evil abound, alas! And keep on writing. You have a role. There are many men here below, and a woman like you consoles us. I am at your feet, Madame" [NAD 12b].

It was therefore against a backdrop of religious polemic around the symbols of charity, between the Catholic, Protestant and Anglican churches, between consecrated women and pious laity, between religious and civil institutions, between submissive and emancipated women, between women of the educated class and women of the working class, that Valérie de Gasparin faced the world to open her school. These polemics reflected the changes in society in the mid-19th Century and the emerging hospitable modernity. With a relatively similar profile and interests, but nevertheless polluted by a few latent rivalries and competition between socialites, the values that opposed the two women made them rather complementary. It is difficult to classify Valérie de Gasparin in major currents of thought. Valérie de Gasparin "escaped the definitions of her gender". She only asked "to break the mold of the type she felt trapped in". She was used to changing tone and genre without complexes in her writings. According to her literary critics, she "had a cheerful, if not downright funny virtue, and had no problem with reverence for vaudeville and rightful aims. She was at ease in her body and totally present in the moment […] in her work as in her life, she was a committed woman" [SMI 92].

The nursing profession is therefore indebted to these two committed women who opened up innovative ways for the social advancement of women and not to one woman alone. These two women enabled all classes of the population to glimpse humanistic professional perspectives in the field of care. Indeed, until now, care had been provided in the public domain either by women servants (the common people) or ordinary people (working-class women) who could not access lay care training. As for the private domain of religious Charity, it was by becoming a nun that one could have access to charitable care. From the middle of the 19th Century, training was also "to be safe for girls from good families" [SIN 08].

With Valérie de Gasparin, innovation in the 19th Century consisted of allowing those who had only learning on the job as a horizon to receive special training given in a new institution, the School. "According to her, it was excellent training and a decent salary that the sick nurses needed most of all" [MOR 14]. The most spectacular result was that a group of lay schools was established which were models. They developed throughout the world in two ways (School-Hospital or Hospital-School), first private and then public, some of which today are university faculties or higher schools of nursing. As we know, training status often determines the status of knowledge taught.

There was no longer a need to invoke the vocation, to become a nun and to withdraw from the world to be trained within the nursing discipline. Despite their different world views, Valérie de Gasparin and Florence Nightingale left behind them two prestigious institutions with almost identical aims: the Florence Nightingale School which is today part of the Royal College of London and the *Haute école de santé La Source* in Lausanne which is today one of the important university level sites of the *Haute école spécialisée de Suisse occidentale* (HES-SO). Many schools around the world have been inspired by these two models since 1860.

7

The Advent of Medical Writing

School or not, regular hospital service needed to continue. The care of the estate and its organization always needed to be ensured. The care of the group and the coordination of activities still needed to be ensured, while the need for institutional organization and functioning remained also. And it was always necessary to ensure the help given to the individual in maintaining and autonomously carrying out his daily activities. The hospital changed at a slow pace. The status of women was slowly changing as well. The care practice continued, but it was then enriched by new knowledge (natural sciences, hygiene and medicine, therapeutics). More and more people were admitted to the hospital. And as the school demanded, new trainers and care experts with good experience later became instructors in their turn.

The apprenticeships for caregiving, for example, were already effective in the hospital under the *Ancien Régime* for hospital maids. In the lay age of knowledge, it was known that "the musshafera or sick maid who had stayed a few months beyond the term for which she had requested her discharge, had to instruct the person who was to replace her" [FON 59-62]. The *musshafera* transmitted her knowledge. Among the nurse servants of God, it was in the novitiate of the religious community with the assistance of the novice mistress that the transmission of knowledge was effective. In Valérie de Gasparin's new school, the founding couple did not give classes. The management of the school was carried out by a couple of pastors: Albert Muller and his wife. Mrs. Muller managed the boarding school, and she spoke to the heart of the students and made them understand the beauty of their vocation. She helped them in moments of inner struggle. Two doctors gave the first lessons: Charles Pellis, then director of a psychiatric hospital (the Champ-de-l'Air in Lausanne from 1833 to 1845), taught hygiene and elements of physiology; Auguste Burnier gave a private lesson three times a week on the art of caring for the sick [NAD 93]. While it was probably useful to begin by giving such courses to understand the foundations of the medical knowledge that would later be delegated, they did not help much in identifying the specific knowledge required by the discipline of institutional "caring". But that was not yet the point. It was not the intention at the time to value a discipline separate from the medical profession. It was still far too early!

From this point of view, Valérie de Gasparin's English rival, Florence Nightingale, seems to have had a certain lead in the field and more up-to-date knowledge with proven experience in care and scientific research as well. Florence Nightingale was the first to write about what nursing constituted and what it did not. With the help of statistics and serious reports, hygiene and nursing were improved in terms of image and representation. Her publications, initiatives and interactions within her social network brought out of the shadows a part of nursing from the lay era of knowledge. Indeed, she was able to surround herself with influential allies to defend her cause and give hospital activity its letters of nobility.

However, Florence Nightingale "did not see the nurse as an assistant to the doctor or as a holder of medical knowledge. The less medical knowledge the general nurse had, the better, as this could hinder her health practices" [BAL 93]. This opinion was almost identical among Valérie de Gasparin's circle, where one of Gasparin's spouse's counselors, the famous[1] doctor Frédéric Recordon from Lausanne, enthusiastically exclaimed when Valérie de Gasparin presented her project to open a school: "Yes, sick nurses! A school for nurses! But… let them not get involved in medicine!" He developed his thoughts and gave his advice to Valérie de Gasparin [NAD 93].

NOTE.– At least these are words that have the merit of clarity. Whether it was Florence Nightingale in London or doctor Frédéric Recordon in Lausanne, we can guess that the foundations of the nursing discipline have little to do with medicine or biomedical knowledge. The presence of the discipline today among the humanities and social sciences is only strengthened by this. Unfortunately, scientific research, which was non-existent at the time, is struggling to homogenize the many disparate pieces of knowledge that make up the stock of knowledge useful for practicing the profession.

Fifteen years after the start of nursing training in Switzerland, the latter started to be introduced in Canada. According to McPherson, it was not until 1874 that a training program was established in Ontario at St. Catharine's General Hospital. Two nurses who had attended Florence Nightingale's school in the United Kingdom and a doctor established the first school of nursing in Canada at St. Catharines Marine and General Hospital. The school, called the Mack Training School for Nurses, offered a two-year program of practical hospital-based training. The first graduating class of

1 A street in Lausanne is named after him.

1878 included six nurses. These hospital schools, with their "hospital–school" style of learning, remained the central mechanism used by Canadian hospitals to staff sick rooms long after World War II. Quoting medical historian Rosenberg, McPherson elaborated on the economic logic of hospital schools: "Both hospitals and future nurses faced a lack of financial resources, so it was natural for both sides to barter: work for a diploma". In hospital schools, "students acquired their skills as they progressed through their learning, so that by the year they graduated, they were qualified in direct patient care and ward supervision" [MCP 05]. This situation would later also exist in Switzerland. In particular at the time when the cantons, disinterested in a national training of nurses, implicitly entrusted the Swiss Red Cross (SRC), a subsidiary company of the Federal Military Department, with the supervision of training in all the cantonal schools in the country between 1944 and 1999. "Until 1976, there was no formal legal basis for the SRC to act in the field of nursing education" [BEN 91]. Nurses and their training were then under the constant influence of military doctors and the Swiss Red Cross. The final straw! In terms of autonomy, there was still a long way to go.

Once again, we find the devil and his details. Explaining the details of the first training course at its beginnings makes it possible to not only identify the process that was beginning, but also understand how this process with its two models, "hospital–school" or "school–hospital", were able to become generalized in most nursing training courses throughout the world. The hospital–school (Florence Nightingale) in which an apprenticeship was carried out became generalized, even when a school was associated with it. The school that had a hospital for its needs (Valérie de Gasparin) remained an exception. In both cases, however, the state later recognized the training system, but sometimes forgot to officially indicate in its statistics the level of qualification obtained through certificates, certificates or diplomas issued for nursing training.

However, two major elements contributed to cultural conditioning and the generalization of the system. On the one hand, the status and role of translator of scholarly discourse played by the knowledge supervisors (instructors, trainers, teachers). On the other hand, the role played by the first instruction manuals and those who published them as vehicles for the knowledge taught. In other words, the role played by the first pedagogical actors (instructors) as knowledge supervisors and the role played by the writing of the first instruction manuals. The teacher's status (doctor) or trainer (instructor) influenced the status of knowledge. Writing, its publication and dissemination were not a power given to everyone!

The pastor couple who led La Source at the beginning had to be initiated into the knowledge taught. They attended the first classes sitting at the back of the classroom. The directors "became students themselves, in order to be able to complete the work of the teachers with their notes and supervisions" [DEG 60a]. In 1863, Pastor Antoine Raymond, pastor of the de Gasparin's place of residence, became the director of La Source and remained so until 1891. After copying the courses given by the doctors, he also wrote an anatomy and physiology textbook that was much appreciated and used in other establishments. This knowledge delegated by the physicians was then reproduced by those in positions of power who had the ability to reproduce it.

By following the first courses in 1864, the director of the *Ecole Antoine Reymond* was therefore rehearsing medical knowledge. He took notes and, in order for these notes to be used, he had them printed. The knowledge for the use by the sick nurses became legible and visible. In addition to Dr. Émile Beaugrand's book, *La médecine domestique et la pharmacie usuelle (1860)*, purchased by Valérie de Gasparin and given free of charge to her students, the students had, as early as 1866, a book written by Antoine Raymond entitled *Cours d'anatomie et de physiologie à l'usage des élèves* de *l'école normale de gardes-malades* [FRA 09][2]. Thus, in addition to his role of evangelization and preaching, which he did not completely abandon, Mr. Reymond repeated in detail all the lessons given by the medical professors. But the care workers who were in post and who, at the birth of the first schools, were still working in hospitals, wrote nothing about their practices, and yet they were already carrying great responsibilities.

Faced with the home care given by the students to various patients of all conditions, Agénor de Gasparin mentioned in his first report on the La Source school that some patients:

> They demanded long and often painful vigils, for which our students had to take turns to conserve their strength for their studies. Apart from these cases, one or two students were assigned to each patient, who had full responsibility for their care. May we say that the care given in this way at home, in houses where often nothing was prepared, where it was necessary to provide for the unexpected, seems to us to be one of the essential aspects of the education of Christian nursing sisters? There they encounter life as it is; there they find to exercise the resources of their minds and the charity of their hearts. [DEG 60a]

"Providing for the unexpected" and encountering "life as it is" is a constant in the nursing profession, whether in the age of lay knowledge in the 18th Century or in

2 Forty care practices were taught in 1867 to the students of La Source.

the age of scientific knowledge in the 21st Century. This characteristic inhabited by skills has therefore not yet disappeared today.

It should also be noted that from the end of the 18th Century, there were a few works that allowed carers or housekeepers who knew how to read to familiarize themselves with a number of writings such as books on domestic medicine for households (Buchan Guillaume[3]), those on civil medicine (Samuel Tissot[4]) or the Carrère manual (1786) that we have already mentioned for the service of the sick.

As early as 1891, the "guiding pastor" gave up his place to a doctor, a director (Charles Kraft)[5] who was very interested in having power over training in order to find suitable staff for his own private clinic, the Clinique de Beaulieu, later annexed to the school at La Source. But as his colleague and director of the Lindenhof private hospital school in Bern (Dr. Walter Sahli) said: "I have long understood that Dr. Krafft has no consideration for the general interest and has regard only for his own particular interests" [BRA 10]. Starting with 1891, male and medical domination in La Source school "will be little contested and may extend over several decades, shaping the sick-nurse and the medical profession's needs" [FRA 09]. This type of dissemination of knowledge became widespread throughout the world. This cultural dominance remained in place until such time as caregivers began to publish and gain recognition for the originality of their own thinking about care. This was not going to happen any time soon!

In spite of this, *Domus–familia–hominem* remained! The care of the estate and its organization always needed to be ensured. It was always necessary to ensure the care of the group with the establishment and maintenance of collaboration and coordination of activities, including with the medical profession, and to learn how to manage or face conflicts. And one always needed to ensure the care of people at all stages of life with the support and assistance given to daily activities within a health organization. But in addition, one needed to speak a language close to that of the hospital administration as well as that of the doctor and surgeon so that one could be

3 Buchan G., *Médecine domestique ou traité complet des moyens de se conserver en santé, de prévenir ou de guérir les maladies, par le régime et les remèdes simples*. Useful for people of all states and available to everyone. Translated from English by J.D. Duplanil, Doctor of Medicine of the Faculty of Montpellier (work in seven volumes totaling nearly 3,000 pages), 1775.

4 Tissot S., *Avis au Peuple sur sa santé,* Didot le Jeune, Libraire quai des Augustins, Paris, 1782. Republished by Quai Voltaire, Edima, Cité des sciences et de l'industrie, Paris, 1993.

5 Born in 1863 to a pharmacist father. Studied at the Faculty of Natural Sciences in Lausanne, then continued his studies at the University of Freiburg, then at the Universities of Bern and Zurich, where he obtained his state diploma in 1887 [FRA 09]. He died of a heart attack at the age of 59 on August 10, 1921.

of service to them. The nurses, who were already "specialist practitioners" before their time, continued to increase their knowledge.

Since Dr. Krafft published his course content in seven volumes[6] between 1895 and 1921, it was this content enriched by their experience that was translated and given by the instructors. The oral tradition of care was fading in the face of the medical written word. It should be noted that the title of the first treatment manuals often masked their content. In the book on *Thérapeutique à l'usage de la gardemalade* (1907), one finds notions on massages as well as on the hygiene of the sick, wills as well as the hygiene of the dead, surgical care with bandages, medicines and how to give them, injections, dressings, anesthesia, etc. The book also contains a list of the most common treatments for the sick. And of course, there was no question of talking about "nursing care"! We already find in the description of the program for the first students in 1859 in La Source, these aspects concretized by Dr. Krafft and his predecessors (Dr. Charles Pellis and Dr. Auguste Burnier). It was indeed foreseen that the doctors would give them regular lessons in hygiene, minor surgery and elementary medicine. They learned how to take blood, how to apply leeches and suction cups, how to give first aid in case of illness or accident, how to dress various wounds, how to supervise the administration of remedies and how to assist with dressings [NAD 93]. It was self-explanatory! When a sick nurse applied dressings or gave therapy, she was doing the medical profession a service, since it was the medical profession that had the privilege and the power to delegate the knowledge needed to do so. In *Thérapeutique à l'usage de la gardemalade*, not only was this a compendium of scholarly and domestic medicine, but Charles Krafft in his 1907 foreword also gives his own conception of the sick nurse as "the physician's helper":

> Should the doctor's assistants be taught the art of caring for the sick, or is it better to let the doctor explain to the sick nurse what to do in each case? The woman is born a nurse", I once heard it said, "we are the first to appreciate the special qualities that characterize the woman, but it is a complete misunderstanding of what modern medicine, surgery and obstetrics require to support such an aphorism; no, the woman is not born a nurse, she becomes one. [KRA 07]

---

6 *Le massage des contusions et des entorses* (1895), *Éthique* (1905), *Thérapeutique à l'usage de la gardemalade* (1907), *Pathologie à l'usage de la gardemalade* (1909), *Hygiène à l'usage de la gardemalade* (1911), *Physiologie à l'usage de la gardemalade* (1919), *Anatomie à l'usage de la gardemalade* (1921). Francillon [FRA 09] reminds us that "Charles Krafft imposed in his writings the term gardemalade [sick nurse] written in one word. For him, it made sense: it was not someone who looked after a sick person, in the first sense of the term, but a professional title, since it did not yet officially exist in French-speaking Europe".

After the hospital maid and the servant of God, arrived the doctor's maid. Servitude prevailed! Knowledge requirements were linked to the requirements of medicine, surgery and obstetrics. But absolutely not to the requirements of lay knowledge, that is, to what the basic triptych *Domus–familia–hominem* demanded as competencies! It was normal, the nurses did not talk about it and did not write down the requirements related to this basic triptych. However, the basic triptych was still being practiced. But above all, it continued to be silent! The totality of the works published by Krafft (and he was not the only one!) represented in fact the structure of the knowledge which accompanied, in a sometimes contrasted way, the development of the nursing profession throughout the world over the course of the 20th Century.

In 1894, supervision of the courses was then entrusted to a very good student, Sophie Maeder, who had graduated four months before and extended her apprenticeship and took on the role of class-mistress. The time had now come to make the voice of care professionals heard within the school. It was indeed the instructors who sometimes attenuated or nuanced medical knowledge by adding to it knowledge specific to hospital practice and experience. Unfortunately, Sophie Maeder had to be replaced, as she was appointed director of the infirmary in Orbe (canton of Vaud, Switzerland) in the fall of 1894, "alongside the sick women she had to care for, she was in charge of housework, linen, etc." Even in Orbe, the triptych remained. For information, in 1895, the Board of Trustees of La Source agreed to extend the duration of training to eight months [KRA 95].

As new actors in the educational field, the instructors that Valérie de Gasparin had probably heard of in her close circle, especially when she was with Mr. Guizot, did not have the mission, according to their status, to produce new knowledge in writing. That was not why they were hired. They did not publish. They had themselves learned their knowledge from medical or ecclesiastical professors who were legitimate holders of theoretical knowledge. They would add their knowledge acquired in the first textbooks, their knowledge of experience and their practical knowledge to the medical knowledge, while at the same time essentially performing a supervisory role.

The training method provided by the instructors was of the order of both representative and tutelage. The participation of students in teaching was done in accordance with knowledge models, techniques and values in force at the time. In addition to a scientific-medical discourse, a discourse that was both evangelical and paternalistic was put in place. At the start of the La Source school, this discourse developed as part of the moral education of the sick nurses. This form of teaching continued in Europe until the years 1975–1980 (!) by reproducing and imitating the mutual teaching method[7] applied in the first nursing schools. Thus, in the second lay school in French-speaking Switzerland, which was founded in 1905 under the title: "Le Bon secours, a private school for nurses for young girls and women of the educated class and an association of volunteer nurses to care for the indigent sick at home", the first employee of Marguerite Champendal, a doctor and founder of the school, was entrusted with managing the practical training of the students.

Céline Pelissier, who had no professional training, "but who had a developed social sense and organizational talent, then took the first class with the other students, organized the supervision and, later, perfected the art of massage for which she had a marked gift and exceptional hands. She was then assisted by young graduates, 'hired as instructors' for the positions of House Nurse, City Nurse and Nursery Nurse" (Bersch quoted by [NAD 93]).

With this transmission model of dominant knowledge, little research was carried out in order to constitute new knowledge that could homogenize the multiple knowledge contained in the constituent knowledge of the *Domus–familia–hominem* discipline and thus highlight the specificity of the care discipline. It was not yet the time! The knowledge resulting from the care practice and the diffusion of people's own knowledge were minor elements left in the background. Care techniques dominated. We can see then all the influence that the introduction of instructors (tutors or supervisors depending on the country) exerted in the training system and the consequences that this form of knowledge had over the years on future training and the development of knowledge. But could it be done otherwise? Nevertheless, this did not allow the nursing instructors, trainers and other nursing teachers in the nursing schools of the time to develop their own knowledge. It was still far too early for that! It was only a case of reproducing the original dominant knowledge.

---

7 This form of pedagogy launched in Madras in 1789 by Reverend Bell, taken up by the Lancaster method, a method introduced in France by Carnot in 1815, discovered the same year by the famous Freiburg pedagogue Grégoire Girard through a Lasteyrie writing, has been in force in Switzerland within the public education system since about 1850. Girard's instructors, who had themselves learned from the master, were, for the most part, merely supervisors; they were not involved in the conceptual elaboration of the text. Girard's instructor was still an assistant to the master, the master being in the case of the school for the sick, very often the doctor. It was usually the best students who were employed as instructors. Moreover, as evidenced by a report of the Committee of Nursing Experts approved by the World Health Organization in 1950, it is stated that "teaching instructors should be chosen from among the elite nurses and should be freed from the responsibilities of hospital services, so that they can devote themselves entirely to their teaching responsibilities" [NAD 93]. It was then that they would be trained in the executive schools that were set up in 1950 in both Switzerland and France.

Following the educational auxiliaries that were the instructors[8], a second consequence of the birth of schools was that of the knowledge-supporting vehicles that were the instruction manuals. Indeed, manuals were needed so that what was taught began to be standardized and that it still left some traces in the professional memory. It was then access to written knowledge that structured and supported the protodisciplinary period of knowledge. At the beginning of the 20th Century, the discipline had not yet been established, nor had the profession. The latter, characterized during this period by sociology as a semi-profession, nevertheless already represented a profession. However, the need to have written materials to learn and prepare for exams was a necessity of the time. This also had the consequence of distributing knowledge collectively within a group, contrary to what was practiced in the lay era.

Medical culture then entered the school. No hospital maids at the beginning of the school in Lausanne, for example, were there to pass on their knowledge and Valérie de Gasparin had no intention of participating directly in training.

We identified the existence of healthcare manuals as early as the 18th Century. In fact, as soon as doctors were trained at university, they had this natural tendency to publish. Between 1775 and 1878, there were 11 textbooks in France; between 1878 and 1920, 70 textbooks; between 1920 and 1960, 65 textbooks [MAG 88a].

The works of Bourneville in France and Charles Krafft in Switzerland seem to us to represent, in a general way, the future archetype of the typology of knowledge that came to mark the protodisciplinary period of the nursing discipline.

– The work of Désiré Magloire Bournevile, *Manuel pratique de la garde-malade et de l'infirmière*, 1st and 2nd editions, Bureau du Progrès médical, Paris, 1878. Written in the "for the use of…" mode, these manuals oscillate between the popularization of summary notions and the learning of precise techniques. The teachers, doctors or interns, taught too little or too much and did not seem to know which public they were addressing: did they want servants or care professionals? "In 1880, 61 lessons were planned in the municipal courses set up by Bourneville (hospital administration, anatomy, physiology, dressings, hygiene, pharmacy, care of women during childbirth). This teaching was supplemented by practical exercises under the supervision of instructors" [LER 92].

– The works of Dr. Charles Krafft of Lausanne, then director of the La Source school concern: *Le massage des contusions et des entorses* [The massaging of

8 Sometimes referred to as "*instructrices*" in French-speaking Canada.

bruises and sprains] (1895), *Éthique* [Ethics] (1905), *Thérapeutique à l'usage de la gardemalade* [Therapeutics for the sick nurse's use] (1907), *Pathologie à l'usage de la gardemalade* [Pathology for the sick nurse's use] (1909), *Hygiène à l'usage de la gardemalade* [Hygiene for the sick nurse's use] (1911), *Physiologie à l'usage de la gardemalade* [Physiology for the sick nurse's use] (1919), *Anatomie à l'usage de la gardemalade* [Anatomy for the sick nurse's use] (1921).

Other textbooks and teaching books followed in the course of the 20th Century, almost always with the same themes, certainly more in-depth, more voluminous, and often with the title "for the use of…" indicating that it was a question of knowledge delegated to carers by the one who had the power to write and publish.

With many publications, publishers rubbed their hands together!

It was then a particular process of insidious and tacit cultural domination that took place, as shown by the work carried out in educational sciences at the University of Geneva in 1999 [GHA 99].

How did knowledge begin to structure itself within the nursing discipline?

This process highlights the fact that it was almost impossible for caregivers in the period from the end of the 19th Century to the last third of the 20th Century to scientifically explain what they were doing using theoretical knowledge conceptualized and published by themselves.

7.1. The ERR process for practical knowledge

The structured written knowledge published by doctors supplanted the knowledge of some clergymen who had also begun to publish[9] on practices of charity.

9 Notably, Abbot C. Vincq who wrote in 1904 for the *Compagnie des filles de la charité de Saint-Vincent-de-Paul* his work *Manuel des hospitalières et des gardes-malades* (540 pages) or 797 pages in the joint reprint between the Abbé C. Vincq and doctor Chicandard in 1923 and 1934. The first part includes elements of anatomy and physiology (151 pages). The second part includes elementary notions of hygiene and microbiology (89 pages). The third part includes surgery and medicine (467 pages). Finally, the fourth part includes notions of pharmacy (65 pages). A few pages here and there present a few words on morality [GHA 99] but in the 1939 edition, morality disappeared. The work shows how the medical supplanted the religious [KNI 84].

	Extraction	Reduction	Reproduction
Type I	Doctors extracted notions of their discipline and published in writing recommended values of "how to do things" and "how to be"	Teaching needed to be understood and practical, eliminating any overall view, any possibility of being summarized.	The reproduction of discourse was confined to the first instructors (the best students), hence the creation of the first schools.
Type II	In turn, instructors taught the contents of medical discourse and selected medical manuals which they judged to be good for their students	Teaching did not necessarily cite the knowledge sources which were authoritative in terms of the matter and were often limited to principles (theoretical or technical) which enabled "knowledge or action"	Reproduction was faithful to knowledge, technique and value models. Elements of knowledge from experience were sometimes added to existing knowledge.
Type III	Using writing manuals by the first instructors, other instructors and teachers involved in nursing care summarized content and presented them as handouts (care techniques)	The overproduction of voluminous works resulted in their reduction to handouts. What remained enabled care techniques to be applied in institutions. No book was obligatory during training.	The teachers (novices) who did not know how to structure content reproduced this reduction. Without knowing the history of how their discipline was founded, they struggled to conceptualize and publish new knowledge.

Table 7.1. *The ERR process, synthesis [GHA 99]*

This medical knowledge did not reflect the experience of the caregivers, which was normal! It is difficult to know what they did.

The sick nurses and nurses of the 20th Century referred increasingly to medical knowledge, as well as to handouts, even instruction manuals written by instructors.

This cascade of knowledge concealed a subtle process of cultural domination in three acts that was repeated worldwide through delegated and borrowed knowledge before nurses entered university and higher education and, through their research (last third of the 20th Century), produced their own conceptual or reflexive knowledge (constructed knowledge, scholarly knowledge, care theories).

The ERR process, for Extraction, Reduction and Reproduction of Reduction (see Table 7.1), began with the presence of two pedagogical discourses in teaching.

That of the teacher, often invited or hired to give lessons on an *ad hoc* basis, and that of the instructor (monitor) or the nursing teacher, hired full time at the school to supervise the students, organize training, implement the logic of exposing the knowledge in the study plan and organizing the examinations.

The process took place chronologically according to three types.

Type I: the professor, first a doctor (late 19th Century, early 20th Century) and then later, other people with university knowledge in the humanities, for example, (1970–1980) gave the course. The doctors extracted knowledge from the courses they had received at the university[10], from their own reference books and published textbooks adapted to the students. Anatomy, physiology, therapeutics and pathology were on the curriculum. The instructors who also followed the doctors' first courses were assigned a supervision and evaluation role in accordance with the values and orientations of the dominant knowledge.

Type II: in turn, the instructors took over some of the contents of the manuals written by the doctors, extracted technical notions from them and wrote practical manuals for nurses. In the period 1935–1953, the prototype of this type of manual seems to have been that of Marie-Louise Nappée, a nursery nurse in France, who, as instructor, wrote the *Manuel pratique de l'infirmière soignante*, comprising between 400 pages in 1939 and 938 pages in 1953.

---

10 "We must confess that this manual has been written more on the basis of individual interviews and notes taken in Professor Chaussier's lessons, than on the basis of specific observations that we have been able to collect over a long period of time in the course of our daily practice." [MOR 34]

Type III: new instructors in turn extracted concepts from outdated and voluminous textbooks written by previous instructors who seemed to be the authority on the subject. They then wrote handouts, thinner and less expensive than a textbook, summarizing the technical points considered important for the creation of a nursing course. In the 1960s in French-speaking Switzerland, groups of instructors were officially set up[11] in order to reflect on the unification of nursing techniques and their teaching. The standardization of knowledge began. These think tanks were made up of instructors from schools in French-speaking Switzerland and Ticino. "Confronted with different ways of teaching care techniques, the aim of these reflection groups was to unify the techniques learned and their teaching between different schools" [GHA 99].

7.2. Nursing students and writing

Before the instructors wrote textbooks, the students were careful to copy the teachers' course content into notebooks and received application notes from the teachers in charge of supervisions[12] to keep them. This way of proceeding was provided for in Article 9 of the Regulations of the Nursing School of Freiburg in 1913 [GHA 99]. The notes taken by a student in 1929 (Mathilde Page) are emblematic of the knowledge received and represent 839 pages (!) of quality calligraphy. The eight notebooks concern:

– Dr. Reymond's science course, 77 pages of physics and 15 pages of chemistry. At the end of the book are the science questions for the June 14, 1930 exams;

– Dr. Bonifazi's anatomy course, 146 pages completed by an eight-page maternity course given by Dr. de Buman. In the anatomy notebook, there are no diagrams illustrating the text. The students represented the different parts of the human body from anatomical charts displayed on the walls of the classroom;

– Dr. Treyer's 93-page physiology course, supplemented by a 26-page diet course;

– Dr. Comte's 157-page course in medicine and therapeutics;

11 *Groupement des monitrices romandes*: *unification des techniques,* interest group of the *Association suisse des infirmières diplômées* (ASID).

12 Since they were Catholic nuns, the term "mistress" was commonly used in the environment since there were already novice mistresses in the novitiate. It was therefore not a question of instructors for the department of public education in Freiburg, even if the status of mistresses was close to that of instructors.

– Dr. de Buman's 86-page course in minor surgery. At the end of the binder are 27 questions that constitute the subject matter for the summative evaluation;

– Dr. Perier's course on healthy living and childcare, 118 pages followed by 13 pages on breastfeeding. At the end of the booklet are 26 questions from the June 14, 1930 exam and 10 questions from Dr. Treyer's course;

– Dr Clément's course on surgery and surgical treatments, 179 pages followed by 13 pages on asepsis, narcosis and disinfection of the surgical field. At the end of the booklet are three general questions for the major surgery exam with the answers that were expected in this exam;

– Courses in surgery, medicine, radiotherapy and physiology began with notions of physics, chemistry and other general knowledge required for the understanding of the discipline studied.

This type of notebook clearly shows the structure of knowledge that prevailed during the protodisciplinary period of knowledge. It was to avoid this type of note-taking, which was considered tedious, that manuals such as the Mademoiselle Nappée manual were published. From the 1950s onwards, this type of textbook tended to become expensive, heavy, mixing notions of biological sciences with medical sciences, therapeutics, morals and attitudes towards the sick. This amalgam of theory and practice was to prove inconvenient for common use in the hospital environment. The instructors of the 1950s were increasingly learning to differentiate between content that was useful in the practice of care and content that was part of the knowledge delegated by physicians. Nappée specified in its 1953 manual "that it would be up to teaching instructors to select for their students the essential notions for the State diploma, the rest being reserved for general information for professional nurses, particularly those who needed to update their knowledge, since the evolution of hospital methods had become considerable" [GHA 99].

Often, the contents presented in manuals such as Nappée's for carrying out care techniques, as well as the modalities of the latter (diagrams, photographs, drawings), very rarely correspond to the realities encountered in the field. By the time the manual was written, it was already out of date inasmuch as technological progress frequently led to changes in equipment and techniques as well as in the renewal of hospital equipment and the organization of work. In any case, students and graduate nurses had to adapt their ways of working to the equipment present and used in each establishment, as well as to the customs and habits that prevailed. From about the 1960s onwards, the care techniques contained in the textbooks were gradually replaced by handouts written by the teachers. This principle symbolically showed that only the techniques deserved to be included and promoted in training. Since the methods of training in different care schools sometimes differed greatly, school admission, the basic program, the evaluation and unification of care techniques were regulated and coordinated between the instructors of the different schools in French-speaking Switzerland. "It was in June 1957 that the instructors of the nursing schools of Sion, Fribourg, Pompaples (St-Loup), Lausanne Hospital, Le Bon Secours in Geneva and La Source in Lausanne met for the first time in order to harmonize care techniques. This group for the unification of techniques had to work hard to develop a common method for the refurbishment of beds. A technique for French-speaking Switzerland was established" [CRO 59].

As they had no scientific tradition behind them, unlike other disciples, or even more so, simply thinking that they did not have to have one, the instructors who wrote the handouts unwittingly reduced their own work by associating to their functions a writing task consisting of writing handouts that mainly contained "action" techniques, that is, for immediate social use.

Preparing a course was like writing a handout and not a didactic transposition of scientific disciplinary contents from research or the language traditions of the profession. The critical elements of knowledge and the scientific argumentation of values that accompanied it were absent from the knowledge taught. Only practical action was valued. Reflection on the meaning of action was simply not on the agenda; it remained in the realm of the implicit or the oral. The fragmentary or residual knowledge of scientific disciplines often delegated by medical professors and later by professors in the human and social sciences remained fixed in books or manuals written and published by the latter.

From there, to symbolically communicate to the students that what was theoretical or scientific was not operational, whereas practice enabled action, doing and being recognized as the one who knew how to do, it was only a step. The title of François Walter's (1992) book on the history of nursing: "*Peu lire, beaucoup voir, beaucoup faire*" is emblematic of this reality. Insidiously, theory was opposed to practice by the caregivers. Theory belonged to the whims of school, while practice was part of the seriousness of professional practice" [GHA 99]. While there were not necessarily any compulsory books recommended to students during training, in the choice of contents and the formatting of the handout, the course glossed over "the operational meaning of the contents taught, that is, the contexts, questions, demands and resources that gave rise to them, as well as the contexts, projects and uses for which they continue to be fruitful and/or problematic today" [MAT 96].

The duo of instructor and handout operated an important reductionism for knowledge when it left aside the argumentative function of language. This exclusion of the argumentative or explanatory function of language was one more handicap for nurses to assert their cultural difference. For Popper, this function of language was part of the intellectual responsibility included in "the tradition and discipline of speaking and thinking clearly: the tradition of criticism, the tradition of reason" [POP 85].

With the ERR process, the resulting representation on nursing school teachers indicates that it was not the instructors who were scientists, but physicians, sociologists, psychologists and other academics who, based on research to which they had access, were the bearers of academic theories. As non-scientists, nursing instructors and other nursing teachers also lived without discipline. Before the scientific period of knowledge, the questioning of the existence of a discipline, its foundations, its nature, and its scope was simply not yet relevant. We now move to 1970.

8

Towards Higher Education

Distributing care and offering services in organizations that were constantly growing, becoming more complex and increasingly expensive, also meant having to think about the management of the "big household" that was the hospital. There was a need to get organized! After having provided care, its organization and management needed to be. The demand was to have notions of work organization, regulation and evaluation of the application of different knowledge (who did what? Who knew what?), to manage several qualification levels, to coordinate a group or several groups of actors within the health system, to prevent and manage conflicts within public (or private) service organizations while understanding and optimizing the sources of financing specific to health organizations. We could not stop at the *Domus* part of lay knowledge. The demand was then for access to higher education (level 2b, Figure 10.1).

With vocational education in place (level 2a, Figure 10.1), there was also a need for teacher training, student recruitment and selection, training of school principals, and training in pedagogy, school management and development, taxonomy, docimology and science didactics. Having a good knowledge of national education, health policies and international education policies would be an advantage. But teaching what and publishing what? In what universe and for what audience (students, teachers, field partners)?

Bringing together professionals, creating associations, legitimizing the titles obtained, sharing knowledge, sharing innovations and publishing journals that served as a link between members were the first objective facts leading to the structuring of higher education. But not everything happened at once and at the same time. There were spaces to be conquered, especially when one was a woman and did not always share the same values within the group. Diverging views from previous dominant cultural influences created some tension and fostered controversy.

Profession first, discipline and science second. This could be the collective watchword implicitly given by society to professional organizations and the elite.

Among the vehicles of knowledge, and apart from the manuals seen above, other writings opened minds and showed healthcare professionals that not only could they group together by areas of interest or in professional associations, but that the latter could also be places of reflection through writing. A person could travel, participate in congresses, invite foreign personalities who were authorities in the field of knowledge, promote training and participate in the circulation of ideas in the group concerned. Professional journals entered the fray! Books would follow.

8.1. Women's groups

Knowledge for caring for human life, for caring for the life of the group and caring for the life of the care environment was developing. More concerned about having power over the organization of care and its teaching, women caregivers were not really present in the first women's groups. Rather, it was in relation to gender that the first voices called for better training for care managers and school principals. The profession no longer needed more female servants and Mother Superiors. In this adventure, we must not forget the new role played by the military relief organizations that were set up towards the end of the 19th Century (the Red Cross), followed a few years later by women's organizations, notably the *Société d'utilité publique des femmes suisses* (SUPFS) founded in 1888. Women began to come together to discuss their own interests[1]. The existing influences could be witnessed

1 It should also be noted that female doctors (i.e. both women and doctors) made their voices heard on women's issues in order to develop the training of female care workers, in particular: Elisabeth Blackwell, the first female doctor in the United States in 1849, friend of Florence Nightingale who opened the first nursing school in the United States in 1873; Anna Heer, a doctor in 1892 in Zurich, the first female gynecological surgeon, who opened the Zurich Nursing School (*Pflegerinnenschule*) in 1901; Anna Hamilton, the first student of the Faculty of Medicine in Marseille, graduated from the Faculty of Medicine in Montpellier and in 1900 took over the management of the Protestant Health Center of Bordeaux founded in 1865 (a Protestant city influenced by the Protestant Revival, i.e. the same system of values as those of the Gasparin couple). Nurses trained in Lausanne (La Source) were already working in the Bordeaux institution. A school for nurses has also been active in this nursing home since 1884. In order to modernize this school, from 1901, it was inspired both by La Source's school in Lausanne to modernize training in Bordeaux and by Florence Nightingale's nursing principles, and from 1902 (22 years before the French state diploma), it awarded the "garde-malade" (sick nurse) diploma [DIÉ 90].

between educated women[2] who, following the first two schools (Lausanne and London), added training models which in turn became "schools". In fact, from the moment there were exchanges, experiences abroad or the publication of news in the press, knowledge was shared and did not remain confined within the national boundaries of a country. The basic triptych of the *domus–familia–hominem* discipline remained. What was to be done, the care of the sick remained to be done at the institutional level! Care was to be given even if new training courses were created. And it was in order to give better care that training was developing. But the development of multiple training models and care also conveyed, at the beginning of the 20th Century, the confusion about roles, knowledge and competition between various protagonists.

While the model proposed and played out in Canada from about 1897 to 1945 by the VON was the most developed form of care to be provided in keeping with the traditions of language that formed the basis of the discipline and ultimately the nursing role itself, "it is physically impossible for a nurse to do heavy housework and provide adequate care to a patient at the same time" [KED 05]. We agree! But it was also possible to envisage the use of professional pairs or trinomials (one person responsible for the care project assisted by one or two auxiliaries paid by the system) to carry out all the tasks. Be care needed to be exercised, it was not a question of dividing up the work. It was not because tasks were delegated to certain professional categories that the nurse was totally relieved of them. One would thus find the role of servant and maid of the past, the nurse and her nurse's assistant of the 1960s, or the roles of *Matron* and *Superintendent* of the early 20th Century (somewhat analogous to the experience of the hospital servants of the 18th Century). The evolution of knowledge was then in continuity with previous knowledge. And research could offer food for thought. Why did nursing research not find objects and research problems oriented towards work, responsibilities and knowledge useful for solving currently uncontrolled health problems, particularly in terms of costs, organization and stakeholders in this case? Nurses have been in the field for a long time, it is up to them, or more precisely to their hierarchy, to propose today, in partnership with others, solutions to the institutional problems encountered.

---

2 Here, the case of Canadian Helen Richmond Young Reid, a renowned Montreal philanthropist, is noteworthy as a member of the first class of women admitted to McGill University in 1884. She helped the Victorian Order of Nurses (VON) to develop a high moral activity for women of the educated class that Cohen described as "the most complete aspect of the constitution of the nursing role" [COH 00]. Indeed, in this case, the basic triptych of the discipline of *domus-familia-hominem* care was very present and demonstrated its usefulness through the knowledge deployed.

But let's return to Switzerland. It was on the occasion of a congress on women's interests held in Geneva in September 1896 that Dr. Anna Heer of Zurich made proposals for the development of training and the creation of professional associations in order to develop a corporate consciousness. Having stayed in London to specialize in surgical gynecology in 1893, she was interested in the effects of good training for nurses. Aware that Florence Nightingale, as an aristocrat, insisted that nurses should be of the same social class as doctors, she argued that further professional training for nurses "went hand in hand with the creation of a Swiss organization of nursing personnel" [BRA 10]. It was therefore at the same time that a problem of class, a corporate problem, a problem of representation and a problem of training was raised.

Anna Heer, a doctor, had been the head of the *Société d'utilité publique des femmes suisses* (SUPFS) since 1901 and had been the head of the *pflegerinnenschule* of Zurich founded by the women's association (SUPFS/*Frauenverein*). She was soon to compete in her business with the activities of the Swiss Red Cross (SRC) founded in Olten on April 25, 1882. In 1893, the SRC established an education department on its own initiative and on a private basis, without any agreements with the cantons and the Confederation, with the task of promoting the training of hospital staff, the promotion of courses for Samaritans (first-aiders), the creation of uniform programs and manuals, the keeping of statistics on existing auxiliary staff and the control of professional practice [VAL 91].

On November 1899[1], the first secretary of the Swiss Red Cross, Captain Walter Sahli, took up the ideas expressed by Anna Heer in 1896, opened a Swiss Red Cross Nursing School in Bern, attached to the private hospital in Lindenhof. Anna Heer had been informed of her project in June 1898 and gave his "an assurance of the readiness of the SUPFS to collaborate closely with the SRC". A draft agreement between the SRC and the SUPFS was even welcomed in 1899. It was necessary to "encourage hesitant and fearful sick nurses who, in Bern, were extremely inexpert in creating associations" [BRA 10].

Women at that time were less emancipated in Switzerland than in the English-speaking world, and the association of the Zurich-born Anna Heer, who lived in London, and the Bernese Walter Sahli was a compromise between two different conceptions of women's autonomy. Walter Sahli was in fact committed to the implementation of training for carers, because he wanted them to be more effective in the service of the medical profession and the sick. "Anna Heer, on the other hand, while recognizing the relevance of this objective, emphasized the professional promotion and social emancipation of women" [VAL 91]. Anna Heer founded the Zurich Association of Nurses in 1909. She wrote regularly to Walter Sahli and, together with him, founded the "*Alliance Suisse des gardes-malades*" (ASGM) on November 13, 1910, of which she was the president until 1916. Walter Sahli, for his part, founded a professional journal, the first issue of which was dated December 15, 1907. The *Blätter für Krankenpflege* (sick-nurses bulletin), published by the Central Secretariat of the Swiss Red Cross in collaboration with the nursing schools of the Lindenhof Clinic in Bern (Walter Sahli) and the Frauenspital in Zurich (Anna Herr), served as a link and an ideological and professional vehicle for the Swiss nursing profession. It was an excellent means for military doctors to monitor the training of healthcare workers at the national level.

This bulletin, in military green, olive green or khaki, as one wished, with a Red Cross in the center and a legend "inter-Arma-Caritas", majestically and symbolically affirmed its membership of the Red Cross and the Army (via the Federal Military Department) and, consequently, the symbolic superiority of military-medical (Red Cross) culture over ordinary knowledge and care practices. Bilingual French–German since January 15, 1924, it was the forerunner of today's Swiss professional journal *Krankenpflege, Soins infirmiers, Cure infermieristiche.*

In the period 1910–1920, the members of the ASGM bore a number of qualifications representative of the medical specialties in practice: medical and surgical sick nurses, private home care sick nurses, obstetrics nurses, infant nurses, masseurs, nurses for the mentally ill and special nurses for those with medical illnesses. Tensions and disagreements between doctors and ASGM members concerning the practical orientations of the training polluted the associative climate. These tensions concerned, in particular, the training to be given to carers working in maternity and obstetrics and those working in psychiatry. Could they receive the same training as nurses who provided general medical or surgical care? These tensions led to the exclusion from ASGM of those working with children and the mentally ill, who would later be called maternal and child health nurses, *infirmières en hygiene maternelle et infantile* (MCH) and psychiatric nurses, *infirmières en psychiatrie* (PSY). Each medical discipline seemed to recognize its "children". But at the time, there were no specialties within the nursing discipline. They didn't even talk about discipline itself.

Infant nurses and babysitters were excluded from the ASGM at the 12th assembly of delegates on October 5, 1924. Psychiatric sick nurses and nurses were similarly excluded from the ASGM on January 22, 1925. On June 3, 1925, the *Alliance Suisse des infirmières diplômées* was re-formed, and on May 12, 1946, it was renamed the *Alliance suisse des infirmières diplômées en hygiène maternelle et infantile* (HMI)[3]. The second group of nurses came together under the name "*Alliance*

3 In 1968, this became the "*Association suisse des infirmières diplômées en Hygiène maternelle et pédiatrie*" (HMP).

suisse du personnel des soins aux malades nerveux et mentaux", which in French-speaking Switzerland became the "*Association suisse des infirmiers en psychiatrie*" in 1936. It should be noted that in the titles of the professionals and their associations, the name reflected the identities of people working in a specialized medical environment (dominant cultures) symbolized by a type of establishment. It was not a distinction related to the identity of a science or discipline specific to nursing. These different associations were merged into one at the founding meeting of the "*Association Suisse des infirmières et infirmiers*" on April 29, 1978 in Olten (Switzerland), the current (2018) name of the professional association at the national level [NAD 12b].

The care and institutional values associated with the traditional role of women, as well as their status in 19th Century hospitals, reveal tensions between the various protagonists of the modern hospital of the 20th Century. Generally speaking, in the caring tradition, household maintenance was part of the assistance to the healing process. In order to have control over the patient's overall environment, the sick nurse in Switzerland, as in Canada, needed to supervise the facilities, manage visits and control both outside noise and the noise she was likely to produce herself. She also needed to ensure the patient's moral well-being. She needed to teach the patient exercises and an appropriate diet that would ensure his physical well-being. She learned certain techniques such as how to make a bed and how to clean oneself when one was ill. Patient observation was used to evaluate the healing process and the adjustment of treatments [COH 02]. But the entirety of the service rendered by *domus–familia–hominem* was not yet globally perceived, at least not expressed. Sometimes acrimonious conflicts between different conceptions of nursing continued for several years on both sides of the Atlantic. The question of the nature of nursing or the role of language tradition within a discipline had not yet been asked. Scientific research on the subject was not yet established. It was people and their images, their status, their roles, their functions that gave rise to seeing, thinking and speaking. We wonder, but with varying degrees of understanding, about the differences between the maternal role, domestic role, household sciences, hospital sciences, medical sciences, the "nurse", the "sick nurse", differences which are most often subjective and more symbolic than scientific.

In 1908, the *administration générale de l'Assistance publique*, which issued the nursing certificate, noted for the Salpêtrière School in Paris "that the domestic staff provided for pupil service had not been hired. The pupils make it a point of honor to keep their homes clean and to prove themselves good cooks. Their self-esteem need not suffer. It is their house, it is their room that they keep clean and that is their honor. A good hospital master must first of all be a good housewife" [DIÉ 90]. This conception of the housewife nurse was castigated by Anna Hamilton, who in 1909 began a long polemic with Mr. Mesureur: "Is it true that at the Salpêtrière the students work in the school, for several hours a day, as domestic servants?" Mr.

Mesureur had his answer published in *La Garde-malade hospitalière* of 1909: "The students have, only during the first year, two periods of one month divided equally between cooking and cleaning, the heavy work being done by men of sorrow and it is not excessive for them to fully possess the difficult art of the housewife: they will need it as hospital nurses, not only to command and train the staff, but to put themselves when necessary will be the hand to the task. They will need them as hospital masters, not only to command and train the staff, but to do the work themselves when necessary. They do not think themselves dishonored by this housekeeping teaching, by this attitude of doing better than the girls on duty" (*Ibid.*). It was the employer who needed to be happy! Instead of hiring paid helpers, he made cheap use of unpaid students who were forced to do housework "for their own good". The knowledge of the lay age remained.

The religious term of *infirmier* (nurse) and its images were institutionalized without further reflection with the establishment of the French state nursing diploma. In fact, following the report submitted by Léonie Chaptal[4] in January 1921 to the *Conseil supérieur de l'assistance publique* on the "need to regulate the exercise of the nursing profession", a decree was issued on June 27, 1922 giving the nursing profession official recognition with three certificates of competence[5] allowing it "to bear the title of French State Nurse" [KNI 84]. A training program recognized by the French State standardized the teaching in the *Journal Officiel* from September 14, 1924. Disputes were not settled, however. In addition to the symbolic difference between "*garde-malade*" (sick nurse) and "infirmière" (nurse), there were also different points of view between the advocates of good theoretical training and those who favored practical, down-to-earth training. For Anna Hamilton, a *garde-malade* needed to be equal to a doctor, but in a different choice of

4 Born January 6, 1873 in Paris into a noble family, in a deeply Catholic family context, she had a brother ordained a priest in 1897. She was active in the parish works of Notre-Dame de Plaisance (about 20 works and the parish newspaper *Écho de Plaisance* served the principles of popular education and the reasoned exercise of Charity of the Catholic Church). Léonie Chaptal's grandfather was Napoleon's prime minister and officially reintroduced Catholic religious nurses into hospital establishments. "She participated in the creation of the Maison-École d'infirmières privées de Paris which was inaugurated on July 1, 1905 and became its director in June 1907" [COL 88].

5 *Brevet de capacité d'infirmière hospitalière* (hospital nurse certificate), *Brevet d'infirmière visiteuse de la tuberculose* (tuberculosis visiting nurse certificate) and *Brevet d'infirmière visiteuse de l'enfance* (children's visiting nurse certificate). These certificates characterized people and their work spaces, not knowledge. There was a sedentary "hospital" function and two "nomadic" functions, home visitors for two categories and priority public health problems: tuberculosis patients and children.

education. For Léonie Chaptal (who was not an *infirmière*), the *infirmière* needed to, on the contrary, remain in a hierarchical relationship with the doctor. Léonie Chaptal's entry level to nursing school was lower than in Anna Hamilton's school. Anna Hamilton wanted to admit students who obtained the *brevet supérieur*, a kind of higher certificate, the baccalaureate or even a diploma to her school. On the contrary, Léonie Chaptal believed that too much study was detrimental to the training of a good nurse, because, as Diebolt [DIÉ 90] reported, "Too much study can be detrimental to the development of practical skills (housekeeping or domestic science) and therefore to the practice of nursing".

In short, the differences of views and values between Léonie Chaptal and Anna Hamilton are such that the latter even complained about them to Dr Krafft in Lausanne [DIÉ 90]. The main antagonists worked in a network. It was also Léonie Chaptal who founded the *Association nationale des infirmières diplômées de l'État Français* (ANIDEF) on June 22, 1924[6]. This was an interesting takeover in terms of care, for a person who was not a nurse (in the religious sense of the term), who came from outside and who had a monopoly on knowing what skills had to be assessed to obtain a diploma that she herself did not possess!

For laymen or strangers to the professional field of institutional care, all appellations were good, provided that the services expected by the ruling class were rendered within the hospital field. *Infirmières*, nurses or *gardes-malades* were "cut from the same cloth" to use the popular expression. And so much the worse off if the professional identity was damaged!

No longer wishing to belong to associations that were exclusively headed by doctors and medical experts, the Swiss sick nurses were trying to escape their tutelage by offering to run their own associations so that they could also participate in the development of their profession. The International Council of Nurses (ICN) accepted as members only nursing associations that were run by themselves.

Thus, on June 7, 1936, the "*Association nationale des infirmières diplômées d'écoles suisses reconnues*" (ANID) was created thanks to the presence of 24 sick nurses from the *Schweizerische Pflegerinnenschule* in Zurich and a few sick nurses from La Source in Lausanne. But when one says "recognized Swiss schools", recognized by whom? In any case, not recognized by the Swiss Confederation and the cantons, since everyone seemed to be satisfied that it was a private organization such as the Swiss Red Cross (SRC) which is responsible for recognizing qualification levels and diplomas. "The SRC has gradually given itself the right to

6 Léonie Chaptal was also elected President of the International Council of Nurses (ICN) at the Montreal Congress in 1929.

regulate nursing care, occupying a legal space abandoned by the state" [BEN 91]. In 1976, the SRC again gave itself a simple "non-binding" mandate for the Confederation states to continue to supervise training and recognize diplomas. As a result, in 1936, in terms of dependence on the military doctors of the ASGM, there were no major changes since they were the ones present in both organizations (ASGM and SRC). This was still evident in 1950, when there was talk of developing non-university higher education for nursing executives. See Dr. Martz's position on university education for nurses below (see section 8.2).

Thus, the Swiss Red Cross continued to steer the organization of training through its guidelines and recognition until around 1999[7]. In fact, the latter subsidized several training institutions in exchange for providing the army with medical columns and, on the other hand, the Confederation did not consider it useful to regulate the health professions when the law on compulsory education in the arts and crafts of 1930 was established. There was even a law announcing the Vocational Training Act, which excluded nurses from its scope of application until 1999. The Swiss Confederation thus left this prerogative to the cantons, which relied on the lead taken by the SRC and military doctors in this field [NAD 93, BRA 09]. It was quite practical!

In this way, let us not forget the Federal Decree of June 25, 1903 on "voluntary assistance to the sick and wounded in time of war" of which Walter Sahli was the author and which associated the Confederation with nursing schools. Every nursing school that received the annual federal subsidy of CHF 20,000 was obliged to mobilize its nurses (students and graduates) in the event of conflict. Through this federal decree, a real obligation to serve was also introduced for a specific category of women, namely nurses. "Being admitted to school implied *ipso facto* a duty to serve in the event of war in one of the training courses organized by the Red Cross, the number of which was determined by the schools themselves. The schools therefore decided which nurses were to be enlisted" [VAL 91].

On July 21, 1937, Swiss nurses were admitted to the International Council of Nurses. Nurses being a hasty translation of the term "*infirmière*" whose linguistic origins we have seen above. Here, then, were the Swiss healthcare organizations that

7 In the meantime, military doctors gradually withdrew from their "default interference" in the nursing field and new associations were formed, including the *Association suisse des infirmières diplômées* (ASID) on December 3, 1944, which became the *Association suisse des infirmières et infirmiers* (ASI) on April 29, 1978. Thus, all categories of nurses, who still had associations separated by various medical orientations (general care in medicine and surgery, psychiatry, maternal hygiene and pediatrics), then had the same association of professional nurses. This was a move away from medical power. It was now up to the nurses to direct their own orientations.

were confronted with at least three different names in terms of identity[8]. *Infirmières*, *gardes-malades* and nurses posed translation problems. These terms were not synonymous and did not have the same etymology and linguistic history. This gave rise to different symbolic representations.

The 40-year relationship between the *Société d'utilité publique des femmes suisses* (SUPFS), the Swiss Red Cross (SRC) and the *Association suisse des gardes-malades* (ASGM) explains how the SRC played a role in the development of the profession's third field of practice, that of management and higher nursing education in Switzerland and France. The creation of executive schools[9] for teachers, school directors and directors of nursing services in the 1950s complemented the nursing training institutions. The nursing discipline did not yet exist and therefore had no place in the Swiss university environment.

8.2. Non-university higher education structures

Non-university postgraduate education in the field of nursing in Switzerland led to the implementation of the third field of practice of the nursing profession, that is, the practice of nursing management in healthcare settings, including the practice of educational management (degree 2b, Figure 10.1). This was a logic of regulation and knowledge management as well as knowledge teaching. It was not a logic of knowledge production and research. This training influenced France and its colonies, but differed in time and space from the North American and other English-speaking models. The aims were more or less the same: to train head nurses and school principals for the organization of care and training and instructors for teaching.

The idea of higher education for head nurses was already mentioned on June 15, 1921 in the *Blätter für Krankenpflege*, no. 6. Then, in 1931, Lydia Leemann, Doctor of Arts and Director of the *Schweizerische Pflegerinnenschule* in Zurich (the school

8 *Krankenswester* in use until 2002 among the German-speaking Swiss nurses can be added. As of 2002, *Pflegefachfrau* or *Pflegefachmann*. Female carers or male carers do not really say in terms of identity what kind of skills or knowledge these professionals had. And there were many "female carers" at different levels.

9 The word "executive" is regularly used by the Red Cross and the military to refer to those who have received special training to supervise medical servicemen and Samaritans in their relief activities for the wounded. In the 1950s, for example, Nursing Sisters did their "Red Cross executive course" at the Chanet barracks in Neuchâtel. In the 1970s and 1980s, in Switzerland, a head nurse or a nursing teacher wore a blue badge with two gold edgings on her white hospital gown to clearly indicate her status as an executive.

founded by Anna Heer) expressed the wish, at the meeting of the central committee of the *alliance suisse des gardes-malades* on October 10, 1931, "that courses for managerial positions should be set up". It was only from October 11 to 23, 1943 that the first course for executive nurses was organized at the La Source school in Lausanne by the *Association nationale des infirmières diplômées d'écoles suisses reconnues* [VAL 91].

On April 27, 1948, Monika Wuest, then president of the *Association suisse des infirmières diplômées* (ASID), wrote to Lieutenant-Colonel Hans Martz "asking him to do everything possible to be able to found a Swiss school for nurses with managerial functions as soon as possible" [BRA 10]. In May 1948, the Swiss Red Cross decided at its General Assembly to initiate a project for a higher school. Dr. Hans Martz prepared three proposals for the location, one in Bern, one in Geneva and one in Zurich. As early as 1945, there had already been proposals from the *Bon secours* nursing school in Geneva, which was familiar with the training given in North America. The school was ready to take over this training on the model of the university schools in North America. The Geneva school had already written in March 1946 to Hans Martz and Monica Wuest to persuade them to open this school in Geneva, but the Geneva proposal was rejected by the medical lieutenant colonel Hans Martz because he was opposed to imitating North American schools. Although they did not yet have the right to vote at both cantonal and federal levels[10], Swiss female nurses did not need a university education, even if it was to become a director of care or a teacher in their discipline (which was not yet the case).

In his presentation to the central committee of the SRC on December 29, 1948, Hans Martz stated that the Swiss university should not imitate foreign models. "Schools in other countries do not correspond in any way to the cultural, political, religious and linguistic realities of our country". Of course, the medical profession and politicians did not understand why nurses should be given a higher education. Monica Wuest, president of ASID and future director of the executive school, said that the school "should not, as in some other countries, aspire to a university education either. We must not scare away the existing staff". The students who graduated from the school remained modest executives and were discreetly employed[11] [VAL 91]. It is difficult to contradict the man who was sought to create a higher school, especially when he was both a doctor and a senior officer and, moreover, the head of the organization that oversaw the normative development of nursing

10 At the federal level, women's suffrage was introduced on February 7, 1971 after having been accepted in a vote by 65.7% of voters.

11 This modesty was also to be found in France on November 14, 1958 when the public authorities created the *Certificat d'aptitude aux fonctions de monitrice* (CAFIM) and the *Certificat d'aptitude aux fonctions de surveillante* (CAFIS).

education[12]. This eternal discretion imposed on female nurses (sometimes with their consent) by male doctors consistently prevented nurses (particularly in France) from progressing in their roles other than by becoming a nurse or health executive. This continued to be the case until around 2010.

In order to demonstrate the desired discretion, the *école supérieure de la Croix-Rouge suisse de Zurich* in its early days modestly positioned itself as a "training school for nurses". It opened its doors on October 23, 1950 and kept the same status from 1950 to 1971. ASID President Monika Wuest was the director of the Zurich Executive School.

The composition of the School Council provides us with particular information about the compromise realized and all the groups or associations wishing to share their power, presence and visibility behind this private school (of course, we must not forget anyone!):

– Dr. Hans Martz, Medical Officer, Chairman of the School Council;

– Lydia Leemann, Doctor of Arts, former Director of the Zurich Nursing School (Vice President);

– Helen Martz, Headmistress of the Lindenhof School in Bern, Dr. Martz's sister;

– Jakob Heusser, State Councillor, Director of Health Affairs of the Canton of Zurich;

– Dr. Hugo Remund, Lieutenant Colonel, Chief of Staff of the Swiss Red Cross;

– Adèle Evelyn Rau, Director of the *école de l'Hôpital cantonal de Lausanne*, represented the lay nursing staff;

– *Schwester* Josi Von Segesser, Director of the *école de l'Hôpital cantonal d'Aarau*, represented the Catholic nursing sisters of Switzerland;

– Sister Marguerite van Vloten, Director of the Nursing School of the Deaconess Institution in Riehen, represented the Protestant nursing sisters [VAL 91].

In order to give an idea of the number of people claiming to be nurses, we can find a figure of 11,500 nurses in Switzerland in 1939, calculated by Anna Hoffmann,

12 "The language of authority only ever governs with the collaboration of those it governs, that is to say, with the assistance of social mechanisms capable of producing that complicity, based on ignorance, which is the principle of all authority" [BOU 82].

then president of the *Alliance suisse des gardes-malades*[13]. According to Lydia Leemann, this corporate grouping was divided into:

- 550 nuns from 21 Catholic orders in 50 hospitals;
- 1,600 deaconesses from 10 houses in 106 hospitals;
- 1,100 nurses from 13 schools in 64 hospitals;
- 280 self-taught nurses with ASGM certificates in 154 hospitals.

To these should be added maternal and child health nurses, called *infirmières d'hygiène maternelle et infantile* (HMI)s, approximately 540, and nurses and psychiatric nurses (number unknown) [CRO 42]. There was a whole mosaic of professionals to consider and there were many issues of power and property related to the history of the groups involved. Each group struggled to position itself, but there was not yet the kind of unifying knowledge that could be found in a specific discipline.

Thirty-six years after the School of Graduate Nurses of McGill University in Montreal[14], the French-speaking branch of the Swiss Red Cross School of Nursing, named "*École supérieure d'enseignement infirmier*" in 1971, opened its doors in Lausanne on October 22, 1956 under the title: "*Croix-Rouge suisse, école supérieure d'infirmières*". Its first director, Mireille Baechtold, had received a scholarship from the World Health Organization (WHO) to spend a year of study in Boston to prepare for her duties [VAL 91]. The program of the first course for head nurses in 1950 at the *école supérieure de Zurich*, which lasted 392 hours over four months, revealed new knowledge in the internal structure of what was taught.

In the main branches, as was normal, there were notions related to the stated aims[15] of the course (instructors and head nurses), notions on the care environment (hospitals, law, insurance, architecture, hygiene and prophylaxis, medical and surgical novelties), notions on professional issues (ethics, rhetoric, reports and statistics,

13 Until 1999, the profession and professional titles in Switzerland were not legally recognized and protected by the State.

14 Who in 1920 offered a certificate in teaching and supervision of care [COH 02].

15 "Whether it is known or unknown, whether it is cared for or neglected, whether it is managed within an institution or by an isolated person, the act of teaching articulates variables that are always the same, even if their respective contents vary across space and are constantly evolving over time" [AVA 91]. These variables, always three in number, whatever the country concerned by a training course, are the aims of the training, the internal structure of what is taught (logic of knowledge exposure) and the representation of the subject.

dietetics[16]) and various categories for a further development in general culture (education, physics, chemistry, French, English), as well as exchanges with the management and the outside world. With regard to the third component of any teaching activity, that which concerned the representation of the subject, the SRC specified that in order to be allowed to take part in the courses, candidates to the higher school "must be particularly gifted and possess sufficient maturity of mind. They must have a good general education, hold a diploma recognized by the Swiss Red Cross, have at least two years' experience after graduation in either a school or a hospital, be at least 28 years old and be recommended by the school or hospital management" [NAD 83].

The logic of exposing knowledge (the program) revealed the following subjects:

– pedagogy (48 hours);

– applied psychology and personnel management (48 hours);

– general instruction (32 hours);

– exercise at the conference and discussions (rhetoric) (32 hours);

– hospital organization (24 hours);

– hygiene and prophylaxis service (24 hours);

– new surgical and medical therapeutics (24 hours);

–patient care ethics (16 hours);

– law and civic education (16 hours);

– methodology (16 hours);

– free time schedule (seminars) (16 hours);

– miscellaneous (English, typing, lectures, visits, exchanges) (16 hours);

– physical–chemical introduction (8 hours);

– the insurance system (8 hours);

– interior construction of a hospital (reading of plans) (8 hours);

– reports and statistics (8 hours);

– commercial arithmetic and budget (8 hours);

16 At that time, a head nurse was responsible for ordering from the hospital kitchen the diets prescribed by the doctor. Let us recall that diet medicine also marked the beginning of the systematic medical checkup.

– professional issues (8 hours);

– history of patient care (8 hours);

– dietetics (8 hours);

– French (for German speakers) (8 hours);

– correspondence (4 hours);

– relationship with the authorities (4 hours).

Abroad, particularly in North America, nurses could pursue university studies as early as 1899. But just because you went to university didn't mean the discipline existed. It had yet to be created! For example, Adelaide Nutting, a nurse graduate of the first class of the Johns Hopkins Hospital School of Nursing (1890), was a leading figure in the nursing profession in the United States. A pioneer in many fields, she initiated with Mrs. Robb the first course open to nurses at Teacher's College (part of the Educational Sciences Department of Columbia University in New York) in 1899. It was for Linda Richards' course in hospital economics [COL 94]. Nothing could be more normal! "Hospital Economics" at the time, meant "Home Economics" because we have seen it, taking care of the household, of the house, taking care of the life of the estate (*Domus*), represented the first body of autonomous practical knowledge that structured the discipline for centuries. The fact that hygiene was subsequently added onto this body of knowledge showed that the traditions of language were respected and left traces, which was normal, to say the least. Knowledge, regardless of status, was passed on from generation to generation. And in this adventure, we recall that nurses were above all not "cleaning ladies" even if housekeeping schools and nursing schools were put on an equal footing[17], that is, at the elementary professional level in several countries! Community awareness of the role of hygiene in large living communities such as hospitals was a common concern as soon as these "Houses" (*maisons*) evolved, grew and developed.

In Canada, it was from the public health nurses that one can begin to glimpse higher education in nursing through *the Association des gardes-malades enregistrées de la province de Québec* (AGMEPQ) in 1920. Supported by major international organizations such as the Red Cross and by pan-Canadian organizations such as The Canadian Nurses Association, they called for the establishment of university education for nurses. They were successful after World

17 Generally speaking, from the elementary professional level up to 1940 for Canada [COH 02]. ISCED 3c or 35 for Switzerland, according to the nomenclature of the International Standard Classification of Education (CITE/ISCED), 2011 or secondary level I before 1999.

War I: "The Red Cross funded public health nursing courses at English-speaking universities, including the Universities of British Columbia, Toronto, Alberta and Dalhousie". It should be noted in passing that there were also nurses in Canada as well as in Switzerland and that the Red Cross was also active in nursing education in North America. "The School of Graduate Nurses at McGill University in Montreal trained qualified nurses for teaching and administrative positions in nursing schools in Canada. It was then heavily subsidized by the Red Cross. For the first time in Quebec, it offered a public health nursing course for nurses". As for the *Institut Marguerite d'Youville* (IMY) of the Université de Montréal, it was in 1923 that the first advanced courses for nurses were offered. Hospital administration, nursing education and dietetics (also part of the curriculum of the Swiss Red Cross Nursing School in 1950) were specialties in the first professional development program offered by the *Institut Marguerite d'Youville* in the Franco-Catholic sector [COH 02]. But the discipline still did not exist! Certainly, "the elite of nurses in Quebec, composed of members of the Franco-Catholic and Anglo-Protestant secular religious communities, aspired to the establishment of a higher education in nursing to train, initially, qualified nurses in the field of administration, teaching and public health" [COH 00]. But not yet to train researchers involved in the production of new knowledge for a specific discipline.

It is therefore understandable why Dr. Martz (who held a leading position at the Swiss Red Cross) and Dr. Wuest (former president of ASID) were ordered in Switzerland to ensure that higher education in Switzerland "being not in a position, as in some other countries, to aspire to a university education". Conditioned since 1910 by the discourse of influential doctors within the SRC, Swiss nurses and nurses were subject to a class *linguistic habitus*[18] by not being able to access training in the same way as abroad. This did not mean that the training abroad was better; it was the status of the latter that was the issue! There remained a kind of voluntary servitude in terms of knowledge! At the semi-professional stage, nurses were more interested in completing the ongoing process of professionalization. In order for this process to be complete, the fourth field of practice, scientific research, that is, that which was part of the logic of producing autonomous knowledge and its recognition, was lacking. As already mentioned, the profession indeed needed to succeed in producing "specific knowledge that was not the lower or residual level of a dominant knowledge. This knowledge needed to be recognized by the elite of other professions, the public and governments. Moreover, this knowledge needed to be transmitted to the highest level of the educational system" [JOB 85].

18 "The linguistic habitus is the product of the social conditions of discourse. It is what we have acquired, but which has been consistently embodied in the body in the form of permanent dispositions that makes us reproduce the social conditions of our own production, but in a relatively unpredictable way" [BOU 84].

NOTE.– It is important to understand the issues involved in this construction/production/use of knowledge so that the profession is no longer exclusively dependent on knowledge other than that which it is capable of producing. “Knowledge and training represent a major issue in any professionalization process” [COH 02]. With the successive creation of all their schools, nurses are well placed to talk about it.

In the venture to set up higher education and executive schools (level 2b, ISCED 5, Figure 10.1), the main focus was on training head nurses and teachers. Not everything involved developing the discipline. However, since public education in Switzerland was a prerogative of the cantons, the subject was dealt with in a private setting, that of the Red Cross. Not in the training structures of the Swiss Confederation or those of the French national education system. In Switzerland, as in France, the state could recognize diplomas, but it did not invest much in the construction of educational structures or directly in research and the funding of teachers. Who was interested in nursing? The questioning was too premature and there was probably a lack of experts on the subject!

The idea of the Swiss Red Cross was taken up in France also on October 1, 1951, when the French Red Cross executive school opened in Paris (ISCED level 5, see Figure 10.1). The national “Red Crosses” communicated and exchanged information with each other. Prior to this date, one became a supervisor without any special training after eight years of service. Other schools followed, notably in 1954, the *école de cadres de l’Union nationale des congrégations religieuses d’action hospitalières et sociales* (UCSS), then in 1956, the *école de cadres de l’Assistance publique* (AP) in Paris. Then, following the decree of November 14, 1958 on the certificate of aptitude for instructors and supervisors, other schools were successively opened, executive schools in Lyon, Marseille, Bordeaux, Strasbourg, Toulouse and Reims.

We have not yet reached the scientific period of the discipline. Even if we speak of “household sciences” or nursing as “arts and sciences”, the knowledge needed for nursing was not yet homogeneous and seen as scientific. Will it ever be? The knowledge available helps to do what needs to be done. The long tradition of the language of care continued, but no one thought of structuring this knowledge carried by women caregivers. The 20th Century saw new training structures being put in place, but did not provide much more information on the knowledge used in care than we have already mentioned. Rather, it revealed the struggles of those who had the power to do so, for example, to participate in controversies over women’s place in care and to control the women’s organizations that were being formed. Training and school were good playgrounds because who controlled training and instruction manuals also controlled the autonomy of thought, the logic of action and the powers given to the actors.

8.3. Towards university schools and scientific research

Over a period of about 40 years, nursing education changed its status on both sides of the Atlantic. Quebec nurses, for example, who entered university around 1960 and were admitted to the Professional Code in 1973, and more particularly the professors and researchers in the nursing faculties, raised the question of the content and knowledge that made up the sciences they were trying to develop. For whom was this knowledge? What more did the scientific knowledge developed at the university bring in comparison to the knowledge taught at the higher level (college education in Quebec or graduate schools in Switzerland)? In addition, the name given to the various Canadian faculties in French-speaking regions was the subject of debate in Montreal. As early as 1967, despite the fact that "the word nursing represented a North American reality that could not be translated by French terms", a physician proposed that "faculty of nursing" be Gallicized as "*école des sciences infirmières*" (school of nursing). In 1977, and without any other form of epistemological or linguistic reflection, the subject was back on the table. After relatively heated debates, however, it was decided to Gallicize the term nursing[19] by "*sciences infirmières*" (nursing sciences) [COH 02]. A strange decision! No attempt was made to demonstrate how nursing could be a science, but it was decided that it could legitimately be one. Without perceiving it at the time, this decision would pose major problems for 21st Century professors when it comes to nursing faculties defining the nature, scope or identity of their own discipline. If, to be a nurse, you have to enter a school of nursing, there are obviously nursing sciences to be taught!

NOTE.– It is well known that "discipline is the main strength of the faculties which, in turn, make it reign" [DEB 00]. The notion of discipline "is irremediably associated with the development of the university, of which it is an organizing principle" [FAB 13].

Under the "insistent recommendations" of the WHO and with a Swiss consultant (Marjorie Duvillard), who was the Swiss director of the nursing school of Bon secours in Geneva and to whom we owe the idea of training nurses at a university level, a school for university nursing executives (in partnership with the University of Lyon II) for school or nursing department directors, opened its doors in Lyon on October 21, 1965[20]. This came to be the *École internationale d'enseignement infirmier supérieur* (EIEIS, the International School of Nursing University Education in Lyon). From the beginning, the Ministry of Public Health was

19 Let us recall that Florence Nightingale never conceptualized or gave a meaning to the term nursing. "I use the word nursing for want of a better one", Nightingale wrote in the prologue to her *Notes on Nursing* [ROU 08].

20 For more details on the beginnings of this school, see Michel Poisson's article [POI 12].

represented by the management of the *Hospices civils de Lyon* (HCL, May 30, 1961) which closed the school in 1995 (after 34 years of existence). In 1965, for the Director of Health Services at the WHO Regional Office for Europe in Copenhagen, "it is essential to prepare nurses for leadership positions in various specialized areas of nursing, to train them to perform administrative functions and to organize and direct nursing education, as well as to participate in research in the field of nursing". But what does nursing consist of?

The French Minister of Public Health and Population at the time confirmed the intention in three points: "(1) This school will train nursing school directors, it will also train heads of nursing departments in healthcare institutions; (2) it is a university school: students will be given a diploma established by the University of Lyon; (3) this school will also be a research center and this research will be very useful for all other nursing schools" [POI 12]. The aims are clear! But in spite of everything, it is the Minister of Health who was speaking. It was not the Minister of National Education or Research, who would have been more concerned with higher professional training. "Higher education", "university degree" and indication of a "research center" began to situate the linguistic event for a period to come, that of the scientific period of knowledge. But we are not there yet, even if language preceded action!

It was in 1961 that the future director and deputy director of the Lyon EIEIS Nicole Mennesson and Huguette Bachelot, both WHO fellows, met at the airport on their way to Quebec. From August 1961 to October 1962, they prepared for the bachelor's degree in nursing at the *Institut Marguerite d'Youville* (IMY) of the University of Montreal. In a letter signed by the two of them and addressed in May 1962 to the Director General of Public Health, they wrote: "We are pleased to announce that we have both obtained the Bachelor of Science in Nursing from the University of Montreal and that we are going to begin a study trip across Canada and the United States. Huguette Bachelot, for her part, even received a very great distinction, along with the Bishop's congratulations" [POI 12]. For four years, they prepared for the creation of the EIEIS until its opening on September 6, 1965 under the leadership and in the company of Marjorie Duvillard, missionary for the WHO from November 15, 1962 to January 30, 1964. With substantial financial resources made available by WHO, including an airplane at their disposal for all their travels, the two founders of the Lyon EIEIS went to visit the Higher Schools of North America (United States and Canada). This took them to Quebec City, Ottawa, Toronto, Winnipeg, Edmonton, Vancouver, Detroit, Seattle, San Francisco, Iowa City, Washington and New York [POI 12]. Their visits impressed Huguette Bachelot, who discovered that nurses in the United States had a much more independent vision of nursing than in France, where "French nurses had only one dream, which was to scratch the surface of medicine[21]" [POI 12]. It was also during this period that a network was gradually established between Lyon (Rhône-Alpes region), Geneva (French-speaking[22] Switzerland) and Quebec with the aim of "moving nursing care away from a pseudo-medical education towards what nursing care really is" [POI 12].

The first directors of the EIEIS were assisted by female teachers who also had received a university education. Thus, Catherine Mordacq, in her turn deputy director of EIEIS with a WHO scholarship, studied at Teachers College, Colombia University New York, and obtained a Bachelor of Arts in 1963, a Master of Sciences in 1965 and a doctorate in educational sciences in 1980. Marie-Françoise Collière, with dual training as a nurse and social worker, a certificate as an instructor at the executive school of the *Institut Catholique de la rue de Vanves* in Paris, obtained a Master of Science, Teaching Public Health Nursing from Wayne State University in Detroit in 1965 and a *Diplôme d'Etudes Approfondies* (DEA, M. Phil equivalent) in the History of Civilization at the Université de Paris VII. She died in Lyon on January 27, 2005 after having worked from 1964 to 1994, one year before the final closure of the EIEIS, and was posthumously awarded an honorary doctorate by the University of Las Palmas in Spain in 2005. Finally, Elisabeth Stussi, a former student of the *École de cadres de Rhône-Alpes* and instructor at the *École d'infirmière de Strasbourg*, was hired as a "trainee instructor" at the EIEIS in Lyon while waiting for a WHO grant to complete her training in the United States. After a one-year stay in Detroit, at Wayne State University, she obtained a special certificate in nursing education administration. She "left EIEIS in 1979 for the WHO Europe office in Copenhagen. The school disappeared. It became a department of the Hospices civils de Lyon, DIEIS" [POI 12]. Why was a school of this scale not more protected by the public administration, which remained prisoner of the word "executive" for health personnel? Given the skills deployed by the teaching team, there were probably the beginnings of a French nursing faculty at the university in Lyon.

---

21 What seems to be the case today, moreover, can sometimes be found in the remarks made about so-called advanced practices [TAI 18].

22 The director of the *Haute école de santé de Fribourg*, Jean-Claude Jaquet, who knew Marjorie Duvillard very well, also graduated from EIEIS in 1976. And in 1994, the *école d'infirmières de Fribourg* under his direction became (regardless of what the Swiss Red Cross thought) the first nursing school in Switzerland to legally position basic nursing training (nursing diploma level II) at the higher professional level (ES or ISCED 5) for the canton of Freiburg. The basic training of a nurse then reached the level of executive education in French-speaking Switzerland (see Figure 10.1). Evidence of the achievement of this higher professional level for nurses is evident in the statistical yearbooks of training courses in the State of Freiburg for the period 1994–1999.

Speaking several languages, trained abroad, DIEIS nursing teachers remained instructors. And "why not teachers?!" Mordacq was already outraged in a professional journal (nurse-teacher) in 1977. It is fortunate that they did not have a doctorate in nursing sciences, because they would still be instructors, if necessary acting as supervisors if they were in a hospital establishment. In fact, the French government seemed incapable of developing its nursing schools, which still fell under the Ministry of Health. And the national education did not feel concerned about higher education in nursing. There was no status provided for nursing professors with a doctorate in France. This was promising. With the signing of the Bologna agreements on the European Higher Education and Research Area in 1999, the university environment could certainly be tinkered with!

In 1945, as we have seen, Marjorie Duvillard, then director of the nursing school of Bon Secours in Geneva, wanted to promulgate a university curriculum for the training of nurses. But the project never saw the light of day. However, it was another nurse-director of the school, Rosette Poletti, who returned from the United States with a doctorate in 1975, who approached the Department of Public Education of the Canton of Geneva to develop a university program for graduate nurses. But "as no faculty seemed interested in hosting this course, even at the postgraduate level, the university attached this course to the Faculty of Psychology and Educational Sciences" [BRA 10]. Nursing seemed to be an oddity and was not by far universally accepted, especially among the few sociologists who taught in nursing schools. You never know when nursing is overshadowing its expertise. And since there were no such faculties, funding for this course was not assured. From 1976 to 1992, this first Swiss experience of a two-hour weekly university course, while it was indeed a challenge, nonetheless allowed students to raise the question of university education, the knowledge required to teach at university and the future of nursing promotion in the country.

It was then at the University of Geneva that from February 7 to 9, 1980 the "first French-speaking conference on nursing theories" was held. This major event, with 600 participants from several countries, symbolically gave a strong message to the nurses of the country and to the population of Geneva, with the banner displayed on the front of the university, that conceptual models in nursing sciences and theories of nursing care existed in North America and that the latter could be presented in a university setting. Rosette Poletti, while recalling the main characteristics of any six-point care theory, explained in her opening lecture at the three-day congress that "university nursing education in Europe was taking a long time to be structured", that "the nursing profession was on the move" and that nurses no longer had to "accept to be medical auxiliaries and assistants forever" [ACT 80]. They must have been concerned with building up knowledge to feed their discipline. But the discourse about the latter was above all "an operation of domination before being a structure for the production of knowledge" [FAB 13].

8.4. Europe and the *Hautes écoles spécialisées* (HES)

As early as 1992, with a view to Switzerland's possible accession to the European Economic Area (EEA), the question of universities of applied sciences, called *Hautes écoles spécialisées* (HES) was addressed for professions that were still not regulated by the Confederation. This was the case for the nursing profession. In 1994, there was a conference, the *Conférence des offices cantonaux de formation professionnelle de Suisse romande et du Tessin* (CRFP), which decided to create a single HES for Western Switzerland. In 1995, the Federal Assembly passed the Federal Law on these schools. In order to comply with the Bologna agreements on the European Higher Education Area, the Swiss constitution was also amended in 1999. Existing non-university higher vocational education and training needed to be upgraded to university level (ISCED 6 bachelor's degree). This was another level of education which had now been reached 49 years after the opposition of Lieutenant-Colonel Hans Martz. Finally, here were the nurses entering university-level training (degree 2c, Figure 10.1). The *Haute école spécialisée de Suisse occidentale* (HES-SO), also known as the University of Applied Sciences, was founded in 1998, and in 2002, it was integrated into the nursing program in the health sector, as well as in the social, music and visual arts fields. HES-SO mainly covers the French-speaking part of Switzerland. With almost 21,000 students in 2018, the HES-SO is the largest HES in Switzerland. Its various study courses and research are divided into six fields of study: Design and Visual Arts, Economics and Services, Engineering and Architecture, Music and Performing Arts and Health and Social Work. In 2016, healthcare professionals accounted for 3,657 students or 17.6% of the student group. Of these 3,657 students, 2,382 (65.13%) were enrolled in the Bachelor of Science in Nursing program and 36 (0.98%) in the Master of Science in Nursing[23] program. The higher the academic levels of education, the smaller the number of students. Indeed, not all nurses aspire to become professors or researchers. Research, the production of new knowledge, scientific language and publications will only concern a minority of them.

From 2006, the Confederation introduced the three-year bachelor studies at the tertiary level. The Bachelor of Science in nursing provides access to a two-year master education (ISCED 7) which is also a gateway to a doctorate in nursing (ISCED 8). This access to a university education could be followed from 2000 at the *Institut des sciences infirmières de l'Université de Bâle* and from fall 2008 at the *Institut universitaire de formation et de recherche en soins* (IUFRS) as part of the Faculty of Medicine and Biology of the Université de Lausanne [BRA 10]. At the beginning of this university training, Céline Goulet (Nurse PhD, Montreal) and

23 More information available at: https://www.hes-so.ch.

Diane Morin (Nurse PhD, Quebec City), both Quebec nurses with a PhD in nursing, were in charge of the studies. We can thus see that the Swiss-Quebec nursing links already active in France at the birth of the EIEIS in 1962 were also continuing to be strengthened in Switzerland. With its six domains and its network of higher education institutions, the HES-SO plays an important role in the socio-economic and cultural development of the seven cantons of Western Switzerland and positions itself as a recognized player in the Swiss and international higher education landscape.

Having schools at university level is good, but the normative aspects of science and research also come with them. Research is one of the main tasks of universities and universities of applied sciences [24]. For example, the reference document of the Swiss Conference of Universities of Applied Sciences on research of September 21, 2005 states that these universities "do not limit themselves to research and development in well-established and proven fields of knowledge, but seek and discover future-oriented areas of applied research. They carry out basic research when this is necessary to achieve the goals set for applied research" [KFH 05]. But how many school principals understand the message of the moment and how many nursing faculty members are in a position to practice basic research in their field? The environment allows knowledge to be generated, but nurses are not getting the message. It is difficult to produce new knowledge without reference to the context that authorizes it!

Indeed, when one does applied research and asks the question "what do I apply?", it is indeed theoretical elements related to the discipline concerned and stemming from basic research that must be carried out in applied research. The scientific frame of reference used in research generally reflects the research discipline concerned. Researchers need to be aware of the functioning of the research and its environment, including guidelines for funding and recognition of research work. For example, a reference to the Frascati Manual (OECD)[25] is unavoidable. Inevitable also are the funding application forms that the independent nursing researcher writes with the agreement of his/her academic management and in which any research project must be argued according to a protocol and international

24 "The law makes research a basic task of the universities of applied sciences. The supervisory authorities must therefore create better organizational conditions to facilitate its implementation and to promote the development of R&D (...) training and research in the health sector should be completely rethought" [CSS 10].

25 Document for use by governments, scientific means and incentive agencies, and research statistical offices. See the *Manuel de Frascati,* Proposed Standard Practice for Surveys of Research and Experimental Development. OECD, Paris, 2002.

scientific standards. In addition, researchers must not ignore the issues behind research activities conducted at universities. If society makes a financial commitment to scientific research, it expects in return a production of new knowledge by the discipline concerned. This is also the basis for the recognition of nursing sciences. When evaluating and accrediting universities, the Swiss Science Council points out that "if the evaluation shows that research is of negligible importance at a university due to the nature of the institution, consideration should be given to reclassification in another category (e.g. university of applied sciences)" [CSS 10][26]. With access to university education and funding for the production of new knowledge, that is, funding for scientific research, the protodisciplinary period of the nursing discipline is coming to an end.

Then comes the scientific period of knowledge. This requires us to consider the evolution of knowledge and to question the science and theoretical proposals that can feed a discipline. In what way are nursing sciences, nursing? In what way are nursing sciences, sciences? Is access to transdisciplinarity an outcome that would make it possible to avoid thinking about the nature of the discipline itself? We do not think so. Although benefits can be expected from working in partnership, power sharing among researchers often puts them in competition rather than synergy. In science, people willingly exchange their scientific output for recognition. Even if the aim of the scientific institution remains that of extending knowledge, it is nevertheless known that "scientists tend to produce knowledge on their own in order to benefit[27] from recognition and to accelerate their personal progress, not that of the institution, nor that of knowledge. They produce knowledge in order to gain recognition. Conversely, the institution grants them recognition in order to obtain knowledge" [VIN 95].

26 The Swiss Science Council (SSC) is the advisory body to the Federal Council on matters relating to science, university, research and innovation policy. As an independent advisory body of the Federal Council, the SSC takes a long-term view of Switzerland's education, research and innovation system. For more information on this mission, see: http://www.swir.ch.

27 Even in the case of collective research or publications, it is usually the first author who is recognized as the lead author.

9

A Return to Image: The Shaping of Knowledge

The protodisciplinary period of knowledge saw the creation of the first nursing schools and the entry into training of female caregivers. Two renowned women from the aristocracy, who were neither nurses nor caregivers and had no qualifications in the field in which they were involved one year apart, innovated and gave the initial impetus to the training by proposing to set up an education for female caregivers. Coming from French-speaking Switzerland and Great Britain, the models were quickly imitated: apprenticeships with supervision in a hospital environment, on the one hand, and on the other hand, new spaces of speech called "schools" were created. This practically led to the implementation of the second field of activity of the nursing profession, that of training with its logic of exposure and transmission of knowledge.

As a reminder, the first field of practice was that of the practice of care in the lay era, based on the logic of application and use of knowledge. Whether this knowledge was experiential knowledge, tacit knowledge or local knowledge, it was necessary in any case for caring for the estate, caring of group life and caring for human beings. Was training necessary or not? Were they credible people or not? No matter what knowledge was used, it needed to be applied and used in a way that made it useful for something. It was imperative to keep the hospital running even if the conditions of exercise were not what we would expect today. And the nurses today, by the way, continue to make the system work.

With the practice of training on the job, a second field of practice emerged. First, basic training, then non-university higher vocational training (e.g. executive schools) and, finally, university training played a decisive role in the development of the profession (see levels 2a, 2b and 2c, Figure 10.1). This second field of practice even played the main role in the whole process of future professionalization worldwide.

The historical role played by schools was rarely emphasized when discussing the discipline of nursing or nursing science. Regardless of the type of school, basic or higher education, the values held by the founders of this new field or the initial orientations, it was necessary in any case to define beforehand, as for all educational institutions, the aims of training, the representation that one made of those trained and the logic of exposure of the knowledge that one wanted to see applied. This logic of exposure of knowledge and the way of exposing this knowledge to students were decisive factors. The study of knowledge, its production and transmission were essential. At the beginning of the 20th Century, the first professors (doctors and sometimes clergymen) played an important role in the orientation and level of knowledge delegated. These first professors "by default" in a way, because there was no one from the healthcare sector to give the courses, were to determine the orientation of the training by themselves. Their auxiliaries, such as instructors and supervisory staff in the hospital environment, played a role in ensuring the logical application and use of knowledge. But the first instructors, by their status, could not teach what they wanted to teach and the first instruction manuals structured the knowledge to be memorized. This is how books, as vehicles for the dissemination of knowledge, would also condition the nursing culture.

9.1. Duplication of reduced knowledge

At the beginning of the creation of schools, the important thing was that the training was effective, not necessarily that it was the best, but that it at least participated in changing the status of the female caregiver and provided the benefits that society had a right to expect.

The arrival of instructors and the writing of textbooks did, however, have incalculable epistemological consequences for years to come. Of course, women were allowed to train. They were given access to knowledge, but this knowledge remained in tatters, unrelated to other knowledge and to the history of knowledge and language traditions. A manual here, a manual there! The protodisciplinary era was marked in particular by the proliferation of books and manuals teaching care techniques. These manuals were useful for sharing the knowledge delegated by those who wrote them, but did not contribute in any way to the development of the nursing discipline.

Among the vehicles of knowledge in use in the 20th Century within the French-speaking world, let us briefly mention: Molignier A., *Pathologie médicale à l'usage des infirmières*, Douin, Paris, 1979; Carillon R., *Anatomie et physiologie à l'usage des infirmières*, Douin, Paris, 1969; Bernard P., *Manuel de l'infirmier en psychiatrie*, Masson, Paris, 1974; Lacombe M., *Précis d'anatomie et de physiologie pour les infirmières*, Lamarre-Poinat, Paris, 2009; Mercier J. and Clogne R., *Manuel de pharmacologie à l'usage des élèves infirmières*, Poinat, Paris, 1963; Lacombe M., *Dictionnaire médical à l'usage des IDE* (Infirmière Diplomée d'Etat), Lamarre, Paris, 2009; and Harel-Bireaud H., *Manuel de psychologie à l'usage des soignants*. The expression "for the use of" explicitly shows that knowledge was delegated to a subordinate group that did not have the power to publish its own knowledge. There were few works written and published by nurses "for the use of the medical profession". Those that did publish were the delight of medical publishers. For example, the knowledge in anatomy and physiology delegated to nurses by Dr. Lacombe and published by Lamare in Paris was into its 31st edition in 2016 (!). It should also be pointed out that during the protodisciplinary period of the discipline, neither discipline nor nursing science was yet spoken of. These notions were coming to the scientific period of the discipline which saw the nursing faculties and the HES developing.

Unable to conceptualize the meaning to be given to lay practices and knowledge and reproducing in the long term dominant values contained in textbooks and their derivatives such as handouts, the instructor remains alienated from the training system for which she was invented. As Pierre Bourdieu points out, "the school institution is the only one to hold completely, by virtue of its own function, the power to select and train those to whom it entrusts the task of perpetuating it, and is thus in the most favorable position by definition to impose the norms of its self-perpetuation, if only by using its power to reinterpret external norms" [BOU 70].

With the help of handouts, the instructors unknowingly took over from the doctors in order to maintain their students in the cultural *habitus* induced by the previous textbooks, thereby demonstrating the composition of the professional experience which seemed to be permanently embodied in the form of permanent dispositions. By limiting the exposure of their knowledge to care techniques and ensuring their proper practical application in the field, the instructors tried to reproduce "the objective logic of the conditions, but by making it undergo a transformation". The transformation in question took place at the training level and consisted of going from a book, sometimes voluminous[1], to a collection of typed sheets. By transforming previous care manuals, by extracting knowledge from written works into a mosaic of common or borrowed ideas, the instructors reproduced the social conditions of their own production, "but in a relatively unpredictable way, in such a way that one could not simply and mechanically move from knowledge of the conditions of production to knowledge of the products"

1 Brunner and Suddarth's 1979 1,314-page textbook, *Traité de soins infirmiers en médecine et chirurgie*, Éditions du renouveau pédagogique, Ottawa, may represent the archetypal work in this category.

[BOU 84]. The production of handouts perpetuated the myth of the name-centered nurse. That is, the nurse who practiced care techniques in a medical-hospital environment without asking the question of the nature of the knowledge taught, until recently. The types of care taught were those of the digestive or cardiovascular system, those of psychiatry or pediatrics, those of the person suffering from urinary tract disorders or those of the person with respiratory insufficiency, etc. In short, it was by dividing medicine into systems or specialties that knowledge was exposed. Thus, according to Dessautels quoted by Mathy, "the creation of myths and the learning of half-truths are sources of alienation, because they deprive individuals and groups of the possibility of objectively and critically apprehending their environment, acting on it and orienting their development" [MAT 96]. With the textbooks reduced to handouts:

> Patient care became technique, then technical care. Knowledge remained in tatters, unconnected to other knowledge. Thus, the technical role became know-how, while the moral role was replaced by know-how. The two did not meet; they remain dissociated. Both of them could be learnt from the nurses' manuals. From the model nurse, we moved on to the model for nurses without even realizing it. All this was indicative of the unease in which caregivers found themselves in order to reappropriate care knowledge. The consequences were reflected in the analysis of workloads, insufficient staffing, the limitation of an economic reading that stopped at costs without taking into account the economic impact. [COL 96]

The first schools for women caregivers were established and instructional materials were written as a model of what to teach. Just as the Native Americans were not asked to present their views, first Christianized, then driven off their land and finally settled on reserves in the midst of advancing scientific–technological cultures, neither were female caregivers asked as early as 1850 to present the ancient historical foundations of their art or knowledge. They were simply unable to do so. It was another class of women who took the initiative and the power of the word! Faced with cultural dispossession and the imposition of legitimate language (by textbooks), "nurses could not understand the role of history in understanding the issues of current scientific struggles" [GHA 99].

We then discover, with regard to the foundations of knowledge related to the nursing discipline, that the unconscious led to lay knowledge being forgotten, *domus–famila–hominem* and their history. The first constitutive elements of the discipline in terms of knowledge were not always really taken into account. It is as if the discipline and its actors could not or did not know how to get anything out of it! Not taken up at the beginning of the protodisciplinary period of knowledge, these constitutive elements were concealed even though it was imperative (and unconsciously) necessary to continue to apply them in the practice of care and its organization on a daily basis. These elements of knowledge related to basic care that was often devalued and delegated to nursing auxiliaries or orderlies. The word "basic" was not perceived as basic knowledge of the discipline was still yet to appear. In general, virtual knowledge went beyond the actors who carried it. "The unconscious of a discipline is its history; the unconscious is the hidden, forgotten social conditions of production: the product separated from its social conditions of production changes its meaning and exerts an ideological effect. Knowing what one does when one does science – which is a simple definition of epistemology – presupposes that one knows how the problems, tools, methods and concepts that one uses have been historically made" [BOU 84].

9.2. The problematic identity of knowledge

In the protodisciplinary era, there was indeed knowledge that was taught, knowledge that was published, knowledge that was delegated and knowledge that was borrowed from all kinds of disciplines. But since caregivers were not allowed to do science, they produced mainly textbooks, but not books. They were excluded from access to the argumentative function of language. Then, later on, they learned through the unspoken words of their training institutions that they should be wary of science and the development of scientific thinking, which, according to Popper, was composed of "language, problem formulation, the emergence of new problem situations, competing theories, reciprocal criticism through arguments: all these means are indispensable for scientific development" [POP 94]. In accordance with the customs of those who held authoritative discourse and who were accustomed to giving a symbolic value to the written word in the same way as the values carried by their class habitus, the teachers of the time reproduced the social conditions of their own production. This in no way advanced basic research for the conceptualization of knowledge.

As mentioned in Marrakech during the 4th SIDIIEF World Congress in 2009, the so-called "nursing" profession is not paramedical. The history of its knowledge shows that this is by no means its essence. It is even mainly "para-nothing of all" according to the malicious assertion defended by the director of a Swiss university. Why is it always positioned as an "auxiliary profession" or as "para-something"? Just because female care workers from the servant and working classes were prevented by voluntary servitude from accessing education in the 18th Century does not mean that the specificity and complexity of their task should be ignored today, interpreting it only from a medical paradigm. It is therefore easier to understand the "*ni bonnes, ni nonnes, ni connes*" (literally, neither good, nor nuns, nor dumb) shouted in the streets of Paris during the nursing demonstrations in France in the fall of 1991. But then what are nurses? We would like to know!

Contrary to what many textbooks and some books written by doctors with the famous formula "for nurses" suggest, the nurse today has no more a parareligious, paramedical or paramilitary tradition than the little African had of Gallic ancestors with blue eyes and blond hair, as the school textbooks distributed by the colonial powers claimed. It was the predominance or attraction of medical knowledge delegated to nurses at the beginning of the 20th Century through textbooks that led to the symbolic belief that the nurse was, as mentioned in a circular dated October 28, 1902 from Émile Combe, Minister of the Interior and Religious Affairs, addressed to the prefects in France, "the disciplined but intelligent colleague of the doctor and the surgeon"[2]. Thus, at the beginning of the 20th Century, in all French departments, a strong image dominated. We may finally wonder what secondary benefits nurses derive from persevering to situate their spaces of speech, reflection and work behind this "awful word, paramedical" denounced in France by the psychoanalyst Michel Renault in 1991 [MOR 91]. Cut off from the history of their knowledge and conveying certain class *habitus*, some of them make a point of participating in the influence of medical science, sometimes to the detriment of the visibility of their own discipline. What advantage can be gained from these symbolic representations that persist and punctuate the process of professionalization?

The extraction, reduction and reproduction of the reduction of knowledge brought about by the ERR process is a three-step process of cultural domination that must necessarily be integrated in order to better circumvent it. This pernicious cycle highlighted at the University of Geneva in 1999 will continue unbeknownst to teachers and their training institutions. Reflection on the very existence of a discipline will not take place. The very origins, nature and scope of this discipline will go unnoticed, as it is anhistorical and buried in the collective "guilty" unconscious of teachers who cannot produce anything other than the reproduction of their own conditioning.

Attempts were made to gather or synthesize the knowledge of discipleship at the time when nurses were beginning to enter higher education. But between domestic sciences, household sciences, hospital sciences, knowledge for caring for human beings (*ad-hominem*), knowledge related to the role of women, medical scientific knowledge, the knowledge of servants and the knowledge of nursing executives, what place does knowledge have within the discipline? In Europe, in 1950, there was still no mention of discipline, scientific research, science, theories of care or conceptual models. The very foundations of the discipline as well as any reference to our

2 *Journal officiel français* from October 30, 1902, p. 7. 043. Circular of October 28, 1902, addressed to prefects, relating to the application of the law of July 15, 1893 on free medical assistance and the creation of nursing schools.

language traditions or to the foundations of experiential knowledge concerning the triptych of care (*domus–familia–hominem*) were also neither perceived nor mentioned. The English heroine Florence Nightingale was quoted over and over again, and it was hoped that a discipline would grow "out of the ground". As scientific research and the epistemology of science were not yet on the agenda to question existing knowledge or contribute to the development of the discipline, it was impossible for nurses to demonstrate the rationality of their own interventions in the system. At the end of the protodisciplinary period and even at the beginning of the scientific period of knowledge, society did not in any way ask all nurses to produce or conceptualize knowledge and make it known. One only has to look at the employment contract or their job description to be convinced of this.

When knowledge needed to be incorporated into higher education, existing university structures often had problems with the identity and nature of the discipline. In which discipline did they want to study? Between the bachelor of hospital sciences, the bachelor of housekeeping sciences and the bachelor of nursing sciences, the authorities of the University of Montreal and the gray sisters of the IMY (Institut Marguerite d'Youville) seemed to have some problems of understanding when, after many hesitations, it was necessary to register training courses in the academic world [COH 02]. What were these so-called "nursing" sciences composed of? As we have seen, the Catholic nun was a "nurse" who had to deal with smells, worm-filled wounds and the powers of darkness. So she was not the one who today is trained in a nursing school or in a nursing faculty. What representative image is created when we refer to the etymology of the term "hell" of nursing? Is it possible to preserve, without damaging the identity of the discipline, a term full of theological symbolic connotations, even mythological if we go back to the third millennium to scientifically represent the so-called "nursing" thought?

The problem of the identity of the discipline remains, even when it is possible to train at the doctoral level in nursing sciences, as is the case at the Université de Lausanne, for example (*Institut universitaire de formation et de recherche en soins* or IUFRS). What autonomy does a university institute have in the field of knowledge when it depends on a faculty other than that of the discipline supposedly leading to a doctorate in nursing? As mentioned in Montreal, creating an autonomous faculty in nursing seems to be "contrary to the very objectives of higher education to elevate to the dignity of a faculty schools which, although it is sometimes necessary to establish them on a university campus, must remain under the dependence of the faculties directly involved in maintaining them" [COH 02]. Should the knowledge produced by scientific research be limited to the dominant faculty interested in the maintenance of nurses in the university, or should it participate in the development and strengthening of the discipline in question? Who benefits from scientific production? Society or the discipline? And why not both? "It is impossible to deal with the disciplinary issue today without linking it to the political dimension of scientific activity" [FAB 13].

Around 1975, university courses in nursing faculties across North America became stronger around the American nursing literature. Faculty teaching was based on the work of care theorists, "particularly those of Peplau, Abdellah, Orlando, Wiendenbach, Hall, Henderson, Levine, Rogers, Orem, King, Neuman, Roy, Watson and Parse. Other work has focused on the need to draw on the science in nursing, particularly that of Schlotfeldt, Ellis, Johnson and Leininger to name a few. Others have proposed guides or frameworks for developing scientific theories, including Dickoff and James, Ellis, Johnson, Suppe, Allen, Chinn, Parse, Fawcett, Kim and Roy" [DAL 15]. Some of these theorists were already mentioned in the work of Rosette Poletti in Switzerland, whose aim in 1978 was to introduce nurses to the nursing discipline with its theories and concepts [POL 78].

Does scientific research produce new knowledge, write yes! But in what places, with what means, using which media and for what audience? Writing is not always extracting or reproducing, but scientifically producing one or more works that would be original by improving existing knowledge and respecting the standard of scientific production. In this case, we must keep the historical linguistic capital, the one that is interesting for the profession, the discipline and society, as well as, and fortunately, the one that today is still as applied and in the process of being developed. With its different scientific approaches and references and its different conceptual models, the nursing discipline, bounded, on the one hand, by the biomedical sciences and, on the other hand, by the social sciences, is now entering the scientific period of knowledge and the reflections it will give rise to.

PART 3

Scientific Knowledge

10

Nursing Sciences?

The scientific period of the discipline began with nurses' accessing university and the scientific language held there. It involves access to the discourse of professors, the reading and publication of scientific articles and access to different types of research and their methodologies. This moment is quite contrasted from one country to another. In terms of language, the word "science" and its components (epistemology of science, scientific research, scientific knowledge, scientific approach, nursing, scientific congresses, etc.) are beginning to be perceived, desired, used, heard and understood. They are perceived as being of some use for the development and recognition of the nursing profession and its knowledge. It is a period during which human beings acquire a little more power, emancipate themselves from the dominant cultures, read, start to gather and have access to articles on science, professional journals, newsletters and scientific journals, which allow the exchange of experience, especially at the international level with congresses. After the basic vocational training, the need for professional development or higher education is perceived. It is also possible for the elite to move up the social ladder by means of an elevator effect.

After a short period in non-university higher education schools (executive schools especially in Europe), the first step is for nurses to gain access to university studies, and then the development of specific programs in nursing sciences, the development of scientific research and the dissemination of its results, the conceptualization of the first care theories, the creation of doctoral programs in nursing sciences and, finally, the epistemological reflection on the status of nursing sciences and the identity of the discipline that is emerging. Of course, we must name the spaces of science and give a name to the new faculties. We can then envisage access to writing, access to higher education or even access to academic training, to a position as a university professor and to scientific research and its promotion (scientific journals, congresses) up to the doctorate in nursing or even the post-doctorate.

NOTE.– Just because nurses go to university does not mean that the discipline springs spontaneously from the academic world. Access to university does not immediately contribute to the identification of the discipline. Disciplinary knowledge remains to be identified, constructed, produced and homogenized, in particular through the worldwide implementation of basic scientific research, its problems and the recognition and publication of its research results.

10.1. Profession first, discipline and science second!

From the semi-professional stage that prevailed in the 1970s and 1980s to the professional stage, nurses reach the end of the professionalization process with access to university studies, scientific research and the production of their own knowledge. The four practical fields of activity, and therefore of the profession, are in place. But before accessing scientific research and the epistemology of science, before benefiting from research subsidies by official bodies providing incentives and support for research, it was necessary to position oneself as a profession both legally and academically. It is at the heart of the universities that the scientific steering bodies prescribe in a normative way the conditions for the production of knowledge and access to funding. Universities and higher education institutions, particularly doctoral schools, for example, are indeed places where knowledge is produced, disseminated, valorized and thus recognized as a discipline. The status of schools in general often determines the status of knowledge.

Profession first, discipline and science second. This was the implicit motto launched on several continents. Historically, the nursing profession has determined the nursing discipline, not the other way around. The two generally accepted components of the nursing discipline, "the nursing profession" and "nursing science", are not to be separated. It is within the profession that the discipline was born, not the other way around. It is even mainly within educational institutions (the second field of practice) that the level of knowledge is distinguished. This requires a training structure with at least three levels (ISCED 4, 5, 6) for training to convey the discourse on nursing (Figure 10.1). It also requires justification of the professor's status (and the salary that goes with it) in the various nursing faculties and universities.

At a time when the creation of university programs was being considered and the nature of the discipline was not really defined, the question pertaining to the status of the training given in hospital schools arose in the Canadian province of Quebec.

NOTE.– It is not really the nature or the status of the discipline (sciences?) that is debated for the classification of training courses, but a parallel reflection, the harmonization of studies (structures) between different countries.

At the heart of the economic, professional and academic issues, the *Ordre des infirmières et infirmiers du Québec* (OIIQ) decided in 1977 that initial nursing training would be done in a college of general and professional education, called a *collège d'enseignement général et professionnel* (CEGEP) [COH 02]. The CEGEP is a public college-level educational institution that offers technical and pre-university training. Pre-university site-specific programs last two years (four sessions) and lead to university. Technical programs generally last three years (six sessions) and lead to the labor market and some university programs. In Switzerland, the same applies, but with some nuances.

In French-speaking Switzerland, from 1999, it was decided that 100% of nurses would be trained at the bachelor level (ISCED 6) at the regional level with the possibility of continuing their studies at university at master (ISCED 7) and doctorate (ISCED 8) levels in nursing. In German-speaking Switzerland, about 90% of nurses are trained at tertiary education level (ISCED 5) and about 5–10% obtain a bachelor's degree at a HES and can continue their studies at university at master and doctorate levels. Very often, the implicit purpose of non-university higher education (ES school) is to respond to acute personnel problems in the short term or for economic reasons. If we have the same professional title and, in addition, the same discipline (nursing), why is there a difference in salary and no difference in professional practice[1] between a nurse trained at ISCED 5 (ES school) and a nurse trained at ISCED 6 (bachelor's degree)? Admittedly, it is often the status of training and knowledge that determines different salary conditions. A university teacher is in principle better paid than a teacher in an ISCED 5 school. But the absence of a difference in the conditions of professional practice within the same subject area is simply an aberration. If a nurse at ES level can do the work of a HES nurse and vice versa, why maintain a lower level of knowledge and two salary scales within the same discipline? Should we then only value the higher level in terms of skills for the proper functioning of the health system? This aberration, which can lead to role conflicts, is quite simply likely to make the best trained nurses turn away from a professional and scientific career. Moreover, it does not contribute to the

1 The federal law of September 30, 2016, on the health professions in Switzerland (not yet in force at the time of writing) states that "authorization to practice a health profession under one's own professional responsibility is granted if the applicant holds the diploma for nurses: Bachelor of Science HES/HEU in nursing or nursing diploma ES" (article 12). Moreover, the Master of Science HES in osteopathy is mentioned in this law, whereas the *Master of Science HES* in nursing sciences, which has existed since 2009 in Lausanne, is not mentioned [CON 16]. Presumably, the politician and his consultants do not know where to situate nursing and what to do with master's and doctoral degrees in nursing to make it consistent with the Bologna agreements on higher education and research.

identification and strengthening of discipline. Can we find doctors at ES level and others at university level? No. Are there sociologists, psychologists or PhDs at ES level and others at university level? No, there are not. Then what is the problem? A dependence on representations of the past both in politics and nursing? It is simply a return to the 1990s when in Switzerland there was a nursing diploma (ISCED 4) of level I (former nurse assistants) and a nursing diploma (ISCED 5) of level II (former general, psychiatric or pediatric nurses) within the same profession. In 1988, the Swiss Red Cross even proposed to train nurses at levels I, II and III, level III being a university level of education. By creating nursing sub-categories, it is felt that they should be integrated at a later stage in the higher levels of training when knowledge is evaluated. In the 1990s, however, in Switzerland, there was still no mention of discipline. And the debate is not over yet! Just look at what is being said on social networks in 2019 when the French-speaking cantons (Bernese Jura and Valais) are trying to reintroduce a level of education at the birth of HES, the ES level of education for nurses. We were just coming out of the old representations linked to the division of medical work set up in the protodisciplinary era of knowledge. Admittedly, the requirements are higher for access to ISCED 6 and access to more complex scientific knowledge. However, the Swiss federal law of 2016 on the health professions does not mention "scientific skills" for nurses. In this law, they are only entitled to have "general competences" with "as a priority,[2] patient-oriented practical training" and "to apply new scientific knowledge in the exercise of their profession" (Article 3.2.b) [CON 16]. They have been doing this for a long time without waiting for this new federal law. Therefore, there is nothing very new on this subject at the legislative level.

However, there are also different representations of the image of the nurse in the political world. These differences could explain the difference in image between French- and German-speaking Switzerland. For some people, the bachelor-level HES nurse would be an executive; for others, she is the basic professional expected. We just forget that we are changing paradigm with the advent of university-level training and the globalization of training structures. This is a societal problem. There is a break with the old historical divisions of labor related to medical specialties (general care, psychiatry, maternal and pediatric hygiene). With university-level training, we are moving to the level of a representation of the international academic divisions of higher education (undergraduate or bachelor's degree, graduate or master's degree and postgraduate or doctoral degree) applied to disciplines, particularly with the establishment of the European Higher Education and Research

2 This avoids taking an interest in anything other than patients (in other words: staying in your place). In the history of her knowledge, the nurse has always had knowledge that allows her to do more than just "being patient-centered".

Area and the Bologna agreements. In French-speaking Switzerland, and contrary to what happens in neighboring countries, particularly in France, for example, nurses are not placed in any university faculty. We simply create specialized university structures (HES) for them, which correspond to their actual field of competence and knowledge.

The basic level of the university typology in nursing is the bachelor's degree. Why then, with a basic academic degree, is a managerial position envisaged? And if a HES degree is seen as a degree carried by management, what about the master's and doctoral degrees within the same discipline? "Super-executives"? Probably not. What also happens to nursing specialists in management and organization trained as executives in the third historical field of professional practice? Why continue to think about "divisions of labor" when we are confronted with an international division of knowledge and academic higher education within a discipline?

NOTE.– A discipline is neither ES, HES, nor CEGEP. It is simply developed and taught at the highest level of the education system. This is the case for the majority of university disciplines, including nursing. As Kleinpetter points out, quoting Edgar Morin (1994), "a discipline naturally tends towards autonomy, through the delimitation of its frontiers, the language it forms, the techniques it is led to develop or use, and possibly, through its own theories" [KLE 13].

Yes, in several countries, the discipline exists and is taught at the undergraduate (bachelor) level as well as at the graduate (master) and postgraduate (doctorate) levels! These are international divisions of higher education. This is not at all the same in terms of language as the local and practical divisions of medical work developed during the 20th Century. Why do these problematic distinctions exist within nursing and not in the medical sciences? Strangely enough, when there is a shortage of doctors or when the costs of healthcare are unbearable, it is rarely proposed to develop a medical education in a higher school (ES) or college (GÉGEP) to cope with the shortage! Is it still to be seen, in terms of language, as a voluntary servitude, historical sequelae or *habitus* of nurses in terms of knowledge?

It was also in university training institutions, particularly in North America, that people began to talk about "nursing sciences". Historically, care was first practiced. We did not yet talk about discipline. Then care had to be taught in schools designed for that purpose. There was still no talk of discipline. Then, we had to organize, coordinate, regulate and supervise nursing work. There was still no discipline. We were talking about nursing executives, health executives, head nurses, directors of care, school principals and *superintendents*. It is with access to scientific research in the university environment and the theoretical development of knowledge in doctoral schools that the discipline began to take off. Comparisons between academic disciplines became possible. "In the United States, there were four doctoral programs in 1960, 30 in 1984, 48 in 1989 and 75 in 2000. There were 106 doctoral programs in 2006 and 133 programs in 2014 with more than 5,000 people enrolled in the different programs." [DAL 15]

"Disciplines depend on each other and on the actions of their members. Between these actors, more or less complex games, tensions and negotiations produce, stabilize and transform the divisions. The knowledge taught then becomes an indication of the institution and social recognition of the discipline." [VIN 00] The taught knowledge that divides those who care, those who teach and those who lead, will then lead to a questioning of the content of teaching. The language about the discipline only appeared within the fourth field of practice, that of research, once the process of professionalization was in its terminal phase. It was the research practices of theorists in the fourth field of practice of the profession that gave birth to the discipline, even though the foundations of lay knowledge date back to well before the Nightingale era. "A discipline does not exist in itself: it presents itself as a vast network of exchanges of people, notions and flows of matter, but it is part of a wider network of reticulations that presupposes ever unstable modes of articulation. (...) Competition between disciplines is the rule and there can be no disciplinary peace. The mapping of knowledge does not have a perennial character." [FAB 13]

Just because the foundations of lay knowledge existed and have been applied for a long time did not automatically make it an academic discipline and then books. There is still something to be written about what we know, and not just anywhere! The first theorists asked themselves questions about existing practices and thought about giving them a meaning through writing. This was something that women caregivers could not do in the 18th Century, for example. Before publishing, most women theorists held different statuses within the profession. They gained experience and a certain amount of power, if only the power of authority. And "the language of authority only ever governs with the collaboration of those it governs, that is to say, with the assistance of social mechanisms capable of producing that complicity, based on ignorance, which is the principle of all authority" [BOU 82]. It is the same for a nursing professor or researcher today. He has had to climb the ladder of knowledge acquisition, often as far as the doctorate, before being able to talk about it. You do not become a doctor in a discipline on the first try. You cannot conceptualize and synthesize all the knowledge that exists in one day either. Objective knowledge is gradually discovered, built up and written down in stages. Nor is it because nurses value the reflective aspect of their work that the production of new knowledge is legitimized.

The disciplinary meta-paradigm, philosophies, conceptual models, theories, came into being because we were able to bring our reflexivity to bear on our practices and make it known using the structures available. This reflexivity developed within the fourth and final field of practice (that of research) which emerged around 1950–1960 behind the American theorists and researchers at the university level. It was thus within the university that the discourse on the discipline began. This fourth field of practice is that of the practice of scientific research in an academic environment, the practice of writing, the practice of publishing and disseminating knowledge, the knowledge of the third world. The latter is the world of objective contents of thought, the world of critical arguments, the state of discussions and the content of journals, books and libraries. The world of books as the third world in particular "originated as a product of human activity. Scientific knowledge belongs to the third world, to the world of objective theories, objective problems and objective arguments" [POP 94]. Who writes? In what place? Who publishes care theories? Who is inspired by science? Who disseminates these reflections? Who reads the reflections on display, especially when they are mainly displayed in English in the French-speaking world? And the development of knowledge within the nursing discipline started from its own writings[3]. In nursing, as in other sciences, knowledge production often consists "in improving existing knowledge and changing it in the hope of getting closer to the truth" [POP 94].

Generally speaking, at the university level, and especially at the postgraduate level, new knowledge is generated through research. A thesis must be an original production. Publications also contribute to the recognition of the knowledge produced. At the CEGEP or ES school, we expose the knowledge to be applied. The school is not mandated to produce scientific knowledge. We do not look at things through the same glasses. Training at the CEGEP or ES school leads to the job market. University training, under certain conditions, also leads to another job market, that of science, that of professors, researchers and senior managers. It is research and the production of new knowledge or innovation that becomes the issue of valorization of a discipline. Once the doctorate is in hand, it is possible to be an independent professor or researcher (in any case not an instructor or trainer). Let us avoid mixing up both the actors of the same profession and their logics of action. All the actors of the profession are nurses. But not all nurses, however noble their motivations, are involved in research, management or teaching. The practice of care

3 For example, a famous publication by Virginia Henderson, then Research Assistant at the School of Nursing, Yale University, New Haven, Connecticut, USA, *The Nature of Nursing: a Definition and Its Implications for Practice, Research, and Education*, Macmillan, New York, 1966. The International Council of Nurses (ICN) widely disseminated this writing as early as 1960. The French-language version "*Principes fondamentaux des soins infirmiers*" was published by the *Association des infirmières et infirmiers de la province de Québec* with the permission of ICN. This relatively modest work of 49 pages for the first edition and 62 pages for the eighth printing in 1977 were part of the general professional works distributed in the French-speaking world to nursing school students.

financed by social insurance and health insurance funds is not the practice of research financed by the state bodies responsible for higher education and scientific research or by funding agencies such as the Swiss National Science Foundation (SNSF) or specialized foundations, for example. The practice of research has a status. It is primarily linked to universities. One day we will have to accept and become our different statuses within the same profession.

It was only when the discipline began to assert itself as such in the university that comparison with other sciences was possible. Moreover, a researcher who explains that he or she produces scientific knowledge with funds from a scientific agency of means, such as the *Fonds national suisse de la recherche scientifique*, for example, must also be able to justify that his or her discipline is in financial need of funds distributed by scientific agencies in order to develop. The discipline then appears. And it is generally within the universities themselves (sometimes in partnership with a field of application), where researchers and other theorists in the profession live and work, that conceptual models in nursing, theories, guides for professional development, etc., are produced and evaluated for their relevance.

Together with scientific research, this is the fourth practical field of the profession: that of the production and dissemination of scientific knowledge. Research must find some solutions to the problems encountered in daily life and maintain, increase or update the theoretical or practical knowledge available. We know that the four practical fields have been established according to an identical and irrefutable chronology throughout the world (see Figure 10.1). These fields of practice have not necessarily developed at the same time around the world, but always in the same order. 1) we heal; 2) we teach; 3) we manage; 4) we research. How do we research how to heal? We seek how and what to teach? We are looking for how to organize, coordinate and evaluate applied knowledge? Finally, we look for how to search, where and what to search for in order to develop knowledge and discipline to make it more efficient? These are some of the questions that the elite and the actors (leaders) of the profession have asked themselves over time and space in order to develop their discipline.

Within the same profession, there are not only care practices or so-called “nursing” practices. There is not only “the” practice, whether it is reflective or contributory to the knowledge production process. In the same profession, there are also professors’ practices, managers’ practices and researchers’ practices. The weight of training structures on research is enormous for the recognition of a discipline in relation to other fields of practice. Moreover, training structures have developed chronologically into three levels of varying complexity, vocational education, non-university higher vocational education and university higher education (see Figure 10.1). Many researchers are doctoral-level experts and all of them feed the discipline with their new knowledge. However, this is not necessarily expressed[4]. What good are all these practices if they are not talked about? Why should it only be care practices that take center stage? Can't society also benefit from the knowledge produced by research in other professional fields?

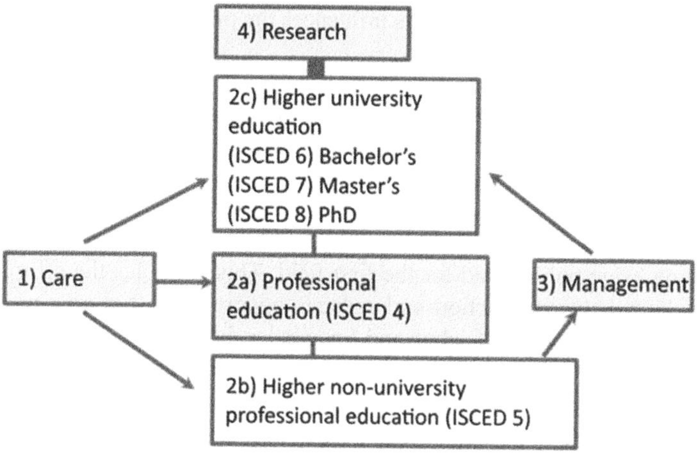

Figure 10.1. *Chronology of the emergence of the four practical fields of occupation and levels of education according to the ISCED*[5]

Furthermore, not all nurses are necessarily interested in becoming a pro-scientist or researcher in their scientific field. And even with regard to researchers, the *Conférence suisse des hautes écoles spécialisées* in its 2005 reference document on research draws the attention of those involved in scientific research, including in the field of health, to the fact that "it should not be forgotten that it is usually a few creative personalities who really succeed in advancing research in a given field" [KFH 05]. This applies to all disciplines.

Knowledge must then be produced and disseminated in the four professional fields through basic, applied or clinical research. The fourth field of practice, that of

4 It is not only a question here of making people feel that scientific knowledge from research is superior to other forms of knowledge. Scientific knowledge is quite simply produced and funded by other institutions whose role is to support knowledge production, innovation and increase the reach of a discipline.

5 International Standard Classification of Education (ISCED).

research, works for all other fields of practice[6] of the profession and not only for the field of care practice. There is not always a need to also seek knowledge or new functions in disciplines related to nursing. The practice of scientific research also follows a particular logic of construction, evaluation, dissemination and recognition of the knowledge produced. The production of knowledge also takes place within specific structures. The context always influences the production of knowledge.

Moreover, as we have seen, the nurse has been at the heart of the daily care system (cultural intermediary) for centuries. It is she who ensures the daily organization at the operational level. Caregivers have never been enclosed in an exclusive and hermetic caregiver/cared for bubble. We cannot, on the one hand, claim that the profession has been chronologically involved in four fields of activity, as shown in Figure 10.1 and, on the other hand, present research as serving to produce knowledge only in and for the first field. This crumbles the efforts and the process of knowledge production and reduces opportunities for intra-professional collaboration. The division of labor and knowledge lurks and the overall vision is altered! The profession has needed to develop four knowledge fields chronologically in order to build up. Each field can sometimes contain several levels of training. This is not for nothing!

NOTE.– The three practical fields that historically precede the field of research are therefore mainly concerned with scientific research and its results. How can we take better care of them? How to better teach how to take care of it? How to better organize, coordinate and finance care? And even better, how can fundamental research be better developed in order to build knowledge useful to the profession as a whole and to society? These are questions to which the discipline should at least provide some answers.

Then come the epistemological questions. How is knowledge constructed and developed, what knowledge should be taught? What is the origin, nature and scope of the knowledge taught? In what way is nursing part of the sciences or are they nursing? What are the places and role of research in the production and recognition of knowledge? What new knowledge modifies, enriches or complements previous knowledge? How does the knowledge produced circulate? How can it be useful both for the discovery and enrichment of the discipline and its knowledge and for the

6 A practice is not just a technical or relational application in a given environment. As already mentioned, it is also, as a reminder, "a human action controlled and guided by symbolic elements included in a cultural system (knowledge, values, ideologies)". The practice, even if only that contained in the four disciplinary fields of the discipline, "is then a consequence of the translation and understanding of values into norms of action" [NAD 93].

functioning of health organizations (administration, schools, hospitals, social insurance)? It is a question of ensuring the quality of the knowledge available, of ensuring professional succession and of ensuring the organization and safety of care and, why not, the financing of the services provided.

The construction of knowledge and theories, their conceptual elaboration, their dissemination and their social recognition represent the last stage of the professionalization process. Within the framework of this process of professionalization and for the autonomy of knowledge, we have seen that it is necessary to produce knowledge at the highest level of the academic system. This has now become a possibility. But be careful not to be attached at the university level to just any faculty. Because disciplinary confusion lurks. With the multiplication of schools, the second practical field, that of training, has had to be reinforced (several levels of training). It has been necessary to envisage the training of teachers who cannot indefinitely confine themselves to a permanent role as repeaters of knowledge. After graduating from higher education, they may one day have to not only transmit knowledge, but in turn be teachers who produce their own knowledge, publish it or use it for application. They will have to have access to research, to its financing, to its valorization and to its recognition. In turn, knowledge producers use their research results by sharing them (conferences), disseminating them (professional and scientific journals) and publishing them (books). This knowledge must certainly be of interest to students and colleagues, as well as to society, first at a local level before the international level. This society often finances through various incentive schemes or the salaries it pays to members of academic institutions what it thinks is useful for them to operate or make decisions within the health system.

Nursing care theories and conceptual models of nursing were the first forms of knowledge of nursing care conceptualized from scientific research as early as the 1950s. This knowledge is part of the discipline. Indeed, as early as the 1970s, various theorists trained in the United States made known the main theories and methods of nursing itself. The aim was to break with the pre-eminence of the old conception of the paramedical nurse, assistant to the doctor, and thus to isolate those aspects of practice which do not fall within the scope of medical prescription in order to elaborate, clarify and specify their autonomy of thought in order to exercise their professional role within the health system. The emancipatory function of knowledge emerged. "The discussion of the process of care becomes the subject of many debates that both legitimize and constitute the new nursing sciences as an academic discipline." [COH 02] After the "fad" or craze for "care plans" and "philosophies of care" came in language "nursing diagnoses", "basic evidence" as in medicine, "evidence-based" (EBN[7]) and "advanced nursing practices". But since the discipline is not only about care, how did an English epidemiologist (Archie Cochrane), for reasons of economy and rationalization of care, lead nurses to join the evidence movement as early as 1972, when this epidemiologist was completely alien to the foundations and orientations of the discipline? Why, in turn, do nurses who do research follow such a reductive movement for economic reasons because healthcare resources are likely to be limited according to the economic-managerial desires of the great neo-liberal narrative?

In the university environment and based on epistemological reflections, especially in doctoral school, nursing sciences must compare themselves to other sciences (not imitate them) and define as precisely as possible the object of the discipline. Otherwise, confusion lurks! This is how "clinicians" or "practitioners" were born in the 21st Century, as if practicing nurses were not. There is an attempt to expand the scope of practice at a time when there is difficulty in recognizing the standard benefits already available to many categories of beneficiaries, as well as the nature of the discipline.

Confusion is still clearly perceptible when the director of a university institute that is nevertheless authorized to award masters and doctorates in nursing sciences specifies, probably on the basis of Article 124 bis of the Vaud law on public health that came into force in November 2017, that specialized nurse practitioners "will be able to assume medical responsibilities. They will be competent and authorized to make medical diagnoses and perform medical acts. They will provide treatment-oriented care and will have the right to prescribe and monitor medication and to make adjustments in medication". Thus, by allowing the physician "to free up time to concentrate where his or her added value is most significant", the nurse practitioner specialist "will be an answer to the looming physician shortage in the future" [TAI 18]. Of course! Moreover, the delegation and supervision of knowledge by the medical profession is often a source of profit and comes at a cost. According to the *Institut canadien de recherche et d'information socio-économiques* (IRIS), even if this way of accounting for the delegation and supervision of knowledge by the medical profession was only temporary until 2019, the fact remains that this activity can be costed economically. And with the nursing shortage that has been looming for some time now, who is taking care of it? The various care assistants trained by nurses? This is what happens when we do not distinguish, in terms of knowledge and language, the medical discipline from the nursing discipline, and the natural sciences from the human sciences. And it is nothing exceptional to hear this kind of

7 Evidence-based nursing as the best combination of knowledge from scientific research related to problems of care.

argument, especially when we discover that there are "medical deserts" in several countries that need to be filled. The shortage of general practitioners must be addressed. Since when have nurses been legally mandated to relieve the doctor of his or her responsibilities in a discipline that is not theirs? "To make a profession with professional autonomy in a specific field evolve towards the acquisition of knowledge of another profession is a way of deconstructing its foundations. It is also an insidious way of turning away from an in-depth reflection on the nursing knowledge specific to the discipline and developing research programs related to the development of this knowledge." [DEL 19a]

Not only are nurses unable to provide for their own professional replacements, but they are also seeking to take on new roles and alleviate the medical shortage. In using their skills to address the medical shortage, they are not spending enough time advocating for the recognition of their own discipline (Figures 10.4 and 10.7). Nursing thinking may simply be confiscated by medical thinking [DEL 19b]! While the Federal Health Insurance Act of 18 March 1994 (LAMal) and its implementing ordinance of September 29, 1995,[8] require a medical prescription or a medical mandate to provide care that is the basis of the nursing discipline (independent function of the professional role of type CS1–CS3), the Vaud Health Act that came into force in November 2017 allows nurses to assume more medical responsibilities of type CS2 (medically delegated function of the professional role). This highly contrasted political discourse on care is perhaps also only a reflection of the internal contradictions carried by the nursing elite during the long historical adventure of its knowledge.

That nurses are already simply assuming the orientations of their own discipline and their responsibilities, which are much greater than what the future Swiss federal law on the health professions says in legal terms [CON 16]. They also have to fight their own shortages. In France, for example, "there is a lack of a real university structure in nursing, capable of producing its own knowledge to guide the actions of the profession to support the overall health of the population. France is showing its inability to provide leadership in the development of the French-speaking nursing discipline for many years to come" [DEL 19a]. Until proven otherwise, nursing research continues to build on its methods and defines itself precisely as "a systematic investigation designed to improve knowledge on issues of importance to the nursing discipline" [LOI 07]. "Disciplinary societies are human societies made up of those who adhere to disciplines, initially defined as subsets of a universe of knowledge that they are constantly building, reshaping and adapting to." [AUB 13]

---

8 Article 7: definition of care: benefits include examinations, treatments and care carried out according to the assessment of care required on medical prescription or medical mandate by nurses.

The discipline that comes from the care activity certainly exists. But does this discipline concern nursing? Is this a crazy question? Linguistically speaking, we may doubt the existence of the nursing discipline, as Collière already expressed it in 1996 [COL 96]. And the etymology of the word "*enfermier*" as we saw in section 3.3 reinforces the doubt and tells us about the values the term conveys. *Enfer* (hell) is not the conceptual field of the discipline, nor is the eschatological promise of the nun or the demonic etiology of diseases. So, if the discipline cannot be nursing, can it not envisage another identity? Is this forbidden? Is it taboo to ask the question? Among the important questions for the discipline, that of the foundations of knowledge is particularly stimulating. We know with Nicole Rousseau, Professor Emeritus of the Faculty of Nursing at Laval University in Quebec City, that as we approach the 21st Century:

> The nursing profession is in crisis and does not seem to be able to rely on legislation or its theorists to get out of it. (…) The first attempts to conceptualize nursing should have been inspired by this tradition or at least developed from the daily practice of autonomous nursing, i.e., from the interventions that nurses make when they do something other than fill medical prescriptions. (…) The early theorists of care did not draw on the books and practices of the women's nursing tradition. Without explicitly saying so, they viewed nursing as a field of study built on knowledge drawn from a variety of disciplines rather than as a specific discipline drawn from language traditions. The professionalization of care should have led to self-nomination, but neither access to professional status nor access to university education has yet succeeded in restoring to women caregivers the independence they have lost over the centuries. [ROU 97]

We may indeed wonder whether nursing science has an interest in being dominated by theoretical orientations coming first and foremost from medicine and sometimes from psychology or sociology, and whether we are really dealing in these conditions with "nursing science". Nursing science by state or by nature? What nursing is this science? Apparently, few nursing researchers have worked on the theme raised by Rousseau! Rather, it is the headlong rush that dominates! Philosophers who emphasize the role of history and language traditions as the ultimate source of knowledge (Popper, Foucault, etc.) are also not really taken seriously.

How can we talk about the knowledge that underpins our discipline if existing and pre-existing knowledge is obscured, forgotten or systematically devalued? Without really knowing how care existed before Florence Nightingale, fashion phenomena replaced language traditions and knowledge. Florence Nightingale was inspired by the religious vocation and the message seemed to apply automatically to lay educated women. But at the time, the aim was to spare everyone, lay and religious alike. If knowledge is not to be fragmented and keep its unity, if research is not to be dispersed according to the orientations of funding agencies or the major fields of research decreed by the State[9], it is in our interest to refer to existing knowledge in our language traditions before borrowing elsewhere what we would like to replace at home. Some knowledge has been handed down through the centuries and is even timeless. Before doing applied research on all kinds of problems or interdisciplinary research, we need to assess where the limits of our own discipline lie and where we are in the production and cohesion of our knowledge. But basic nursing research is not necessarily the "teacup" of our university faculties.

Certainly, society has been transformed. We must now learn to use computers, data banks, digital languages useful in the age of cost accounting for services delivered within the health system and "take care of computers". Medical computing will not say otherwise! But the little sheets of paper kept by hospital governors and used to feed hospital accounts in the lay age of knowledge in the 18th Century have certainly given way to computerized management of the quality of care and other computerized care records. This is not to say that the skills required for the "complex practice of information management" or the "practice of information gathering"[10] have disappeared! There is still language to be translated, held, shared and understood. And nurses have never had enough time to spend with patients. They have always spent time doing something else!

With the emergence of critical research on the nursing discipline, the epistemological status of the knowledge mobilized to teach care can be analyzed and knowledge useful to the organization and coordination of care activity within the health system can be criticized. We can also criticize the practice of scientific research or the so-called "clinical" research, particularly when it involves a human clinic related to the human life process. There is a wide range of approaches to the criticism of knowledge or the analysis of the epistemological status of our different types of knowledge. Certainly, "research activities make it possible to refine existing theories and to contribute, on the basis of new knowledge, to the development of other

9 Who often continues to see nurses through symbolic representations of the function or what is said about them.

10 These two important practices are part of the cultural intermediary model, which is the first conceptual model in nursing in French-speaking Europe. They are briefly described on pages 86 and 87 in the modeling of nursing activity published in 2013 [NAD 13]. See also section 10.2.5 of this book.

theories that will guide action or change in nursing practices" [DUC 02]. But what links can be made, for example, between our pre-Nightingale language traditions and nursing diagnoses, the evidence-based movement (EBM) or advanced nursing practices (ANP)? These links appear in Figure 10.2, but they are not constant. Rousseau concluded: "Nurses would benefit from being aware of the historical roots of their profession and using them to better define the type of services they can provide to society" [ROU 97]. This is precisely the singular theme of our work! The historical roots of the profession show that the service rendered to society by nurses is much broader than what is said.

10.2. Historical constants of the discipline

As in many fields of knowledge, contemporary knowledge builds on previous knowledge. There are historical constants that span the centuries. Recognizing them allows us to apply or develop them and avoids inventing new roles. Long before Florence Nightingale, what we knew how to do was already transmitted to us by elders. The nursing knowledge of a period often integrates that of previous periods in order to keep it alive [PÉP 08]. What do we do with this ancient knowledge that is still alive today? The aristocratic knowledge of the "mistress or housekeeper" mobilized by Florence Nightingale is certainly useful for organizing the space and time of care and promoting hygiene, but it is neither the first nor the only one to structure the discipline. In order to rediscover and valorize the constants of knowledge held in the space and time of language, we will then borrow some reflexive knowledge from the philosophy of science to recall that "it is tradition that obviously represents the most important source, in quality as well as in quantity, for our knowledge" [POP 85].

Therefore, if we ask ourselves about the difficult relationship between nursing knowledge and the discipline of the same name, we cannot escape the analysis of our language traditions. Philosophy of languages is therefore well placed to give us avenues of analysis since we are interested in these traditions and the first statements of "caregiving". Philosophy then becomes a reflexive science to examine existing knowledge. The first languages that appeared to take care at the institutional level and in the public sphere[11] are manifested by what Foucault calls a discursive

11 We deliberately leave aside the language of the practical Charity of the Church already conceptualized around the term "hell" (hell, the shut-ins, the powers of darkness, the Church's practice of exorcism, the works of mercy (7 bodily and 7 spiritual), the therapeutic effects of holy oil or holy water, etc.). These aspects of the practice of care seem to us to belong more to medieval theology and to the history of the Church, than to the caring knowledge of the magistrates, maids and hospital servants who preceded us.

practice. As far as we are concerned, this is the discursive practice of the maids, servants and sick nurses of the lay era. Discursive practice "is a set of anonymous, historical rules, always determined in time and space, which have defined, in a given period and for a given social, economic, geographical or linguistic area, the conditions for the exercise of the enunciative function" [FOU 69]. That is, the one that accompanies us when we enter into a relationship. And precisely, the relationship with the human being as the first act of care places our discipline in the human sciences with an extension to the communication sciences.

What was said in the first lay hospitals to welcome suffering humans already required skills to carry out this enunciative function. The positivity of a discourse characterizes its unity through time. This form of positivity (and the conditions for the exercise of the enunciative function) "defines a field where formal identities, thematic continuities, translations of concepts, and polemical games can possibly unfold. Thus, positivity plays the role of what could be called a historical *a priori as a* reality for utterances" [FOU 69]. It is not a question of knowing who is telling the truth, who is reasoning rigorously, who best conforms to his own postulates if any. Before being able to criticize a piece of knowledge or a theory, we must begin to identify the statement, its sources, its archives.

We find in the hospital archives an incredible amount of statements that can account for the knowledge to care. A series of signs will become enunciated, as long as it has a specific relationship to "something else" that concerns itself. It should also be noted that the enunciating function "cannot be exercised without the existence of an associated domain" [FOU 69]. No statement on institutional and professional care without the constitution of the hospital domain. Within the Domain (*Domus*), the House, the Hospital, the care statement "always has margins populated by other statements". The associated domain "forms a complex framework". See the energetic metaphor of the weaver's shuttle (end of Chapter 10). The statement is "part of a series or set, playing a role in the midst of others". For example, the language of caregivers played its own role in the midst of other languages. This is still the case today! These other languages coexist within the health system (other health professions, the medical profession, the administrative body, partners outside the hospital, hotel services, technical services, computer services, etc.). This is why we refer to "cultural intermediaries" in our nursing conceptual model [NAD 13]. The identity of a statement, and this is the case with the caregiver statement, is still subject to a "set of conditions and limitations: those imposed by all the other statements in the middle of which it appears, by the domain in which it can be used or applied, by the role or functions it has to play" [FOU 69]. Nursing science did you say?

Yes, provided that "science is located in a field of knowledge and plays a role in it. A role that varies according to the different discursive formations and that changes with their mutations" [FOU 79]. But there is no "nursing" science if what constitutes this science is only composed of borrowed knowledge such as anatomy, physiology, physiopathology, pharmacology or applied therapeutics. This was the case as we have seen in the protodisciplinary period of knowledge. Why would this science be qualified as nursing if the applied knowledge is the same as that which other trades, particularly in the health field, can also call upon (specialized educators, medical assistants, medical secretaries, physiotherapists, nursing aides, occupational therapists, etc.)? Nursing science cannot therefore be just "nursing" because it is a nurse who applies it. The argument does not hold. To use a simple example, a nurse who cares for a child in the pediatric ward of a hospital and who claims to be a nurse sees her claim disappear if it is a mother or an early childhood educator who is caring for that child. There is a risk that the language may simply be "maternal care" or "educational care". In addition to the confrontation with the original meaning of the word "nurse", whose limits we have already explained, care, like science, cannot be "nursing" by state or nature [NAD 14]. On the other hand, they are nurses by myth.

It was not enough to transform the word "nursing" into "nursing sciences" as early as 1978, as suggested in Montreal [COH 02], for nurses to be able to present the origin, nature, coherence and rationality of their knowledge. However, it is true that the literature often shows that knowledge about caring is of course conceived as a practice, and also as an art, a discipline or a science. The latter presents states of development and methods without necessarily reaching the state of science seen as an ideal. There is knowledge. Discipline as well. Science why not, provided that there is a certain homogenization and objective relation of the knowledge produced that goes beyond common sense.

In the nursing discipline, discursive practice "can form groups of objects, sets of utterances, sets of concepts, series of theoretical choices", which shows that the threshold of positivity described by Foucault seems to have been crossed (discourse becomes individualized, takes on its autonomy, is transformed). The discourse on care detaches itself and gives rise to practices as concrete actions and social functionings. This is a first stage. We can even claim to have reached a second stage, which is the epistemologization threshold described by Foucault (the statements are divided up, put forward standards of verification and coherence, propose models and theories). Nevertheless, there are a number of conceptual models and concepts that inhabit the language space of the discipline today. But it seems that the discipline as a scientific discipline has not yet reached the two upper stages described by Foucault, which are the threshold of scientificity and the threshold of formalization [FOU 69]. We can even wonder what this brings and if it is useful to reach these last two thresholds? We do not think so. Compared to the state of knowledge of the lay age, reaching the threshold of positivity and the threshold of epistemologization of contemporary knowledge over a period of less than 200 years already seems to be an important step forward for our discipline in the constitution of a knowledge of relative autonomy.

Therefore, let us rediscover this field of knowledge and "this set of elements, regularly formed by discursive practice and which are indispensable to the constitution of a science, although they are not necessarily intended to give rise to it, we can call it knowledge. Knowledge is what we can talk about in a discursive practice that is thus specified, it is also the field of coordination of statements where concepts appear, are defined, applied and transformed" [FOU 69]. As evoked in the age of lay knowledge, caregiving utterances "are a slow accumulation of the past and a silent sedimentation of things said". It is the breadth of caregiving statements that needs to be measured. Hence, we have tried to find the first statements of care, their typology and the silent sedimentation of things said, behind the knowledge, at least those that could be accessible to us. There is still a lot of historical research to be done on this side.

NOTE.– From where do the statements start, "how far and how often they are repeated, through what channels they are diffused, in what groups they circulate; what general horizon they draw for the thought of men, what limits they impose on it, and how, in characterizing an epoch, they make it possible to distinguish it from others?" [FOU 69]. From where do the caring statements come from?

The positivity of a discourse characterizes its unity and coherence over time. As we have seen, time in the nursing discipline was not the environment of the 19th Century. We repeat ourselves. Discipline does not come "from the ground" and not everything started with Florence Nightingale! Let us be serious! Over the centuries, the statements of caring increased in scope and were the subject of a structuring process in several stages. Knowledge accumulated as society transformed. Is it possible to find the discursive practices of the nursing discipline? Is it possible to find a coherent structure of knowledge and to recompose the different layers of sedimentation in the history of knowledge of the discipline of nursing? Wouldn't there be in the case of the nursing discipline, a device that makes it possible to put in relation complex relationships between the discursive and the institutions that shape the practices?

What then is the knowledge that can transcend space, time, habits, postulates, speculations, beliefs, myths, convictions, reflexes, fashion phenomena, faith or prejudices and that inhabits the third world, notably that of traces, writings and books, described by Popper? What elements of knowledge remain and remain in place despite the transformation of society and the hospital system? What knowledge has survived over the centuries since the tradition of language established itself as a source of knowledge? How has so-called "nursing" knowledge been constituted?

It is then discovered that the various layers of knowledge are piled on top of each other like a sedimentation process affecting elements of knowledge according to the times, the development of society and health systems (see Figure 10.7). The history of nursing knowledge "is its constant questioning and its astonishing capacity to integrate change" [COH 02].

10.2.1. *Domus–familia–(ad)hominem*

Among the very ancient knowledge that crossed the centuries, there is the basic triptych of ancient knowledge on which the discipline is historically grounded. There is nothing very dogmatic about this. There may be a layer of knowledge that preceded this period, but we do not have the means to verify it. It is simply a matter of giving back to the traces of our ancient knowledge the place it deserves. Starting from the lay era, we have gone as far as we can go. Taking care of life with the triptych of the age of lay knowledge (*Domus–familia–homo, homines* or *ad-hominem*) is always present in the background of the nurse's daily activity today (see Figure 10.2). It is this knowledge base that forms the foundation of the nursing discipline.

The knowledge in Figure 10.2 represents the oldest group of knowledge for which some evidence can still be found today. It is knowledge that enables basic care to exist. Observing the living environment, organizing the care space, observing the people being cared for, sharing our languages, putting people in contact with each other, anticipating our actions, sharing our knowledge within the group, taking care of ourselves, others, space, helping to survive and helping with the activities of daily life are still practices that we observe today. Ensuring the functioning of the hospital in the 18th Century, ensuring the functioning of the care unit or service is the same in the 21st Century. But the hospital and society have changed. This triptych of the care activity, as it is sometimes believed, does not depend on a mandate or medical prescriptions.

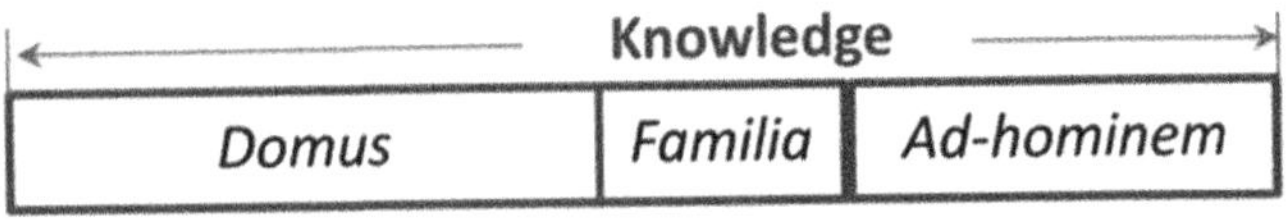

Figure 10.2. *Foundations of the care discipline. First foundation of knowledge of the lay age. A basic structure*

But it seems that it is completely absent from healthcare costs, even though it has been the subject of intergenerational transmission of knowledge since the hospital has been in existence. Taking care of the life of the estate, taking care of the life of the group and taking care of the life of humans can hardly be done without establishing links between society, its institutions, their financing, their operation and the inhabitants of the hospital or care services. This is also what we refer to as relational practices or life and health mediations in the context of modeling nursing activity [NAD 13].

It should also be noted that, in the transmission of knowledge of this era, it is always the oldest or most experienced who pass on their experiences and knowledge to the youngest, whether in the field of care or later in educational institutions. There has been no radical change in the knowledge of care despite the evolution of the hospital or the constraints it has undergone (budget saving programs, for example). There are no major breaks in knowledge. There is therefore an increase in the costs and constraints involved. In the 1970s, large sections of knowledge, know-how or skills derived from the basic triptych of lay knowledge were still perceptible.

Today, the care environment is still made up of structures, human and social relations linked to daily institutional life (existing structures, living environment, human status). According to the pragmatic philosophy, we can even say that the environment is the means that gives the care environment its own institutional characteristics. Lay knowledge is therefore already expressed "through a language that conveys cultural categories, social representations, moral notions and is structured according to the history and culture of the group from which it originates" [DAL 08b].

Before being "a female vocation", especially within religious congregations and the practical charity of the Church, caring was an ordinary domestic activity stemming from knowledge of experience transmitted by peers. This specific knowledge for taking care of the estate, the group and the human being resembled what is sometimes called today primary nursing and represents the basic[12] knowledge of the discipline.

The knowledge for taking care of the life of the estate is still in place, but has been transformed. It is no longer up to the nurses to do everything, for example, doing the laundry or cleaning in the hospital. But they continue to welcome the people

12 Who gave the terms "basic care". Let us not forget the origin of the language. Basic care is that which underlies the basic knowledge of the discipline and not the basic care of more complex technical care. Devalued over time, this specific knowledge is often delegated by nurses to their trained auxiliaries. In this delegation of knowledge, the responsibility of the nurse remains full. She can take back at any time what she has delegated. This is also a general characteristic of all delegated knowledge.

being cared for, trainee students, new staff, trainee doctors and employees from outside the department. They also strategically monitor the environmental conditions, the state of the equipment, the logistics and stock management of the care unit and facilitate intra- or extra-institutional communication.

The knowledge that allows us to take care of the life of the group remains and has even been strengthened. There is more knowledge today about group life, group work, collaboration, conflict prevention, coordination and group phenomena than in the age of lay knowledge.

The knowledge that allows us to take care of human life remains. With the contribution of the human sciences, they have also developed. Today, many care theories propose care concepts, while a great deal of objective knowledge mentions the precautions to be taken, for example, in order to individualize care. The time when the nursing process and the care plans made by nurses made it possible to develop intervention strategies is not yet too far away. Discipline and science are making their appearance. The nursing process is supposed to better convey (support) the body of knowledge specific to the nursing discipline ("reference scheme" in Adam's case) and to explain the nature of the discipline around it. "There will be a nursing science when the nursing discipline has defined its own body of knowledge." In the title nursing process, "process is taken in the sense of development and progress, designates a systematic way of proceeding, a scientific method, a methodological approach, a dynamic process" [ADA 83].

10.2.2. *Three cultural and linguistic systems*

As we have already seen, from the end of the 18th Century until about the middle of the 20th Century, the rules of action of the lay carer accompanied the carers in their passage from "domestic servant" in the service of the institution and of the sick, to this new position of servant and auxiliary to the doctor. The language specific to the triptych *Domus–familia–hominem*, included in particular the function of institutionalization (*Domus*), which first prescribed in writing what caregivers needed to do to make the environment as healthy as possible and to ensure that newcomers to the institution adapted to the institutional norms. Similarly, the caregiving function (*familia*, *hominem*), associated with the institutionalization function, did not fade away. With the arrival of medical knowledge in the hospital and the delegation of the required knowledge, a fourth function (medico-delivery function) was added to the previous ones in terms of skills. It was in a way the beginning of so-called "advanced" practices.

The arrival of medical culture in the hospital towards the end of the 18th Century (CS2 in Figure 10.4) did not eliminate the traditional tasks to be performed. Human care, group care and estate care not only remained, but were reinforced. In an insidious and progressive way, the development of scientific medicine and technological progress only added complexity to the already existing complex. Similarly, the new architecture or technological advance of a hospital was never insignificant for the development of new skills, new knowledge and the proliferation of multiple languages (technical, information technology, digital).

It was then within three major cultural systems that the caregiver was now called upon to evolve. During the protodisciplinary period of knowledge, a second layer of knowledge was added on top of the first. The "Home" of the 18th Century became a hospital with a complexity that made it a cultural institutional system. By cultural system (CS), we mean a configuration of knowledge, values, ideologies and practices shared and transmitted by the members of a given "society". A cultural system contains differentiated and particularized values and norms, all of which require cultural references, knowledge, in order to have meaning and legitimacy [NAD 93]. In the hospital setting, we distinguish, until the 2000s, three groups, three cultural systems that imposed themselves through writing according to a distinct chronology over the long term. Each cultural group provided information that triggered the reflexivity of the caregivers, who in turn translated this information into action and words (CS4).

The institutional culture remained the first culture to prescribe or incite in writing logics of action (*Domus* or CS1). *Domus* became CS1 as the first written prescriptive culture. The institution had to work! And in the first instance, it was the nurses who made it work. The hospital developed, so did the institutional culture. The medical culture, the second to prescribe standards of action in writing (CS2), imposed itself, erased or put nursing knowledge in the background. The nursing culture (CS3), which was the third to make its logic of action explicit, finally put in writing, as early as the 1950s, about part of its professional reflexive action standards (*familia-hominem*, CS3) [NAD 13]. This was the beginning of care theories. These three cultural systems, which became stronger in the protodisciplinary era of the discipline, took over from lay knowledge, but integrated it into the CS3 cultural system (see Figure 10.3). These cultural systems accompanied the protodisciplinary period of the discipline throughout its development. Let us not forget that a cultural system "ensures, within a given society, the solidarities existing between its past and present" [DEB 00].

The practices *hominem* and *familia* were grouped together in CS3 (see Figure 10.3), because it was the carers as "cultural intermediaries" between all the interlocutors involved in care institutions who were confronted daily, in time and space, at the interface with the multiple languages held by the collaborators (the group). It was also necessary to welcome and make room for the medical knowledge that was gradually invading the hospital space. This was the beginning of the colloquiums at the start of work.

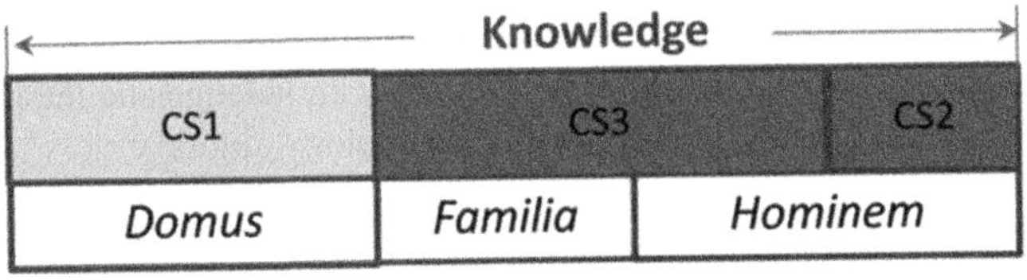

Figure 10.3. *Appearance of cultural systems (CS) in terms of knowledge in the modern hospital of the 20th Century. In Switzerland, in the 1980s, employees in the administrative services wore gray badges by name, nurses wore blue badges and the medical staff wore red badges. For a color version of the figure, see www.iste.co.uk/nadot/nursing.zip*

The *Domus* category of languages (CS1) reminds us that it is always the institution that shapes practices, and this has been the case since the birth of the hospital (see Figure 10.3). This began with the establishment of an employment contract, recognition of the diploma obtained and job descriptions that already indicated in a general way what was expected at the institutional level in terms of knowledge and skills among nurses. Hospital hygiene standards require, for example, that caregivers dress or wash their hands in a certain way when they enter the ward. The languages at the heart of which nurses work are then true cultural systems and are loaded with values, ideologies and knowledge that are not always explicit and increasingly complex.

At the foundation of a hospital, the prescriptive culture implicitly delegated by the institution behind the first cultural system (CS1) allowed the caregiver as a "housekeeper" to serve the institution by enabling it to function (see Figure 10.4). In this logic, not only were caregivers "not exclusively serving" the institution, but also they were "primarily serving" the healthcare system. Moreover, the management of institutions of respectable size generally had only a relative and deferred idea of what was going on discreetly around the clock in this specific work space that was a care service. These languages, if they were indeed used to provide services to the people being cared for and their families, were also and above all used to make the institution work. It had to work, if possible smoothly! If the nurses did not recognize this, they were not surprised that others were trying to take their place by, for example, putting coordinators on every system floor. Rising costs were a given!

In the prescriptive culture gradually delegated to them by the medical profession in the 19th Century (medical culture and language) through the second cultural system (CS2), caregivers were also doing the latter a service, because whoever had the legitimate power to delegate knowledge (anatomo-physiology, pathology, applied therapeutics, pharmacology, etc.) expected in return a correct and safe practical application of that knowledge (see Figure 10.4). However, in this "double agent" function shaped by the medical profession since the 19th Century: "informing agent" for doctors and "applying agent" for prescriptions, the carers were not, however, mandated to relieve the medical profession of its responsibilities, even if through new delegated knowledge, advanced practices or clinical evaluation, as can be seen today. As already mentioned, there were not only medical deserts, but there were also nursing deserts to be inhabited. With the arrival of medical knowledge, the knowledge and time devoted to *Domus* and *hominem* or CS1, CS3 practices were somewhat reduced in favor of the service rendered to the medical profession. The nurse then in turn delegated part of her knowledge to the auxiliaries she trained in practice and at school.

In their own reflexive culture and in interaction with the caretakers and their surroundings, the third cultural system is still evident today (CS3). This nurse/patient/entourage interaction is the last one to transform experience into knowledge through the play of writing, but it is also the second in terms of actual practice to enter into activity (during the profane period). Knowledge continues to exist, to develop, to become more complex. As we have seen, it was only from the 1950s onwards that nurses effectively began to produce the first care theories and the development of knowledge specific to the discipline (see Figure 10.4).

Care theories (Peplau, Abdellah, Orlando, Hall, Henderson, Levine, Roy, Watson, Parse, etc.) are part of the CS3 type of care culture. As with other works, Johnson, Allen, Chinn, Fawcett, Kim, Leninger, etc. are also part of the CS3 care culture. Other moderate-spectrum theories or theories of practice or theories specific to professional situations are also found under the CS3 culture. Intervention plans are then developed in conjunction with the arrival of care theories. Always between people, between things, between ills, always in the "in-between", the CS4 type of reflective culture is a combination of existing knowledge. Between man, his miseries and his life context, the reflexive combination of knowledge for taking care of the human being, taking care of the group or taking care of the estate, between CS1, CS2, CS3, means that the knowledge known as "nursing" in the scientific period of the discipline is simply the socio-constructivist and interactionist environmental result (see Figure 10.4) of the various historical elements of knowledge and their multiple combinations [NAD 13].

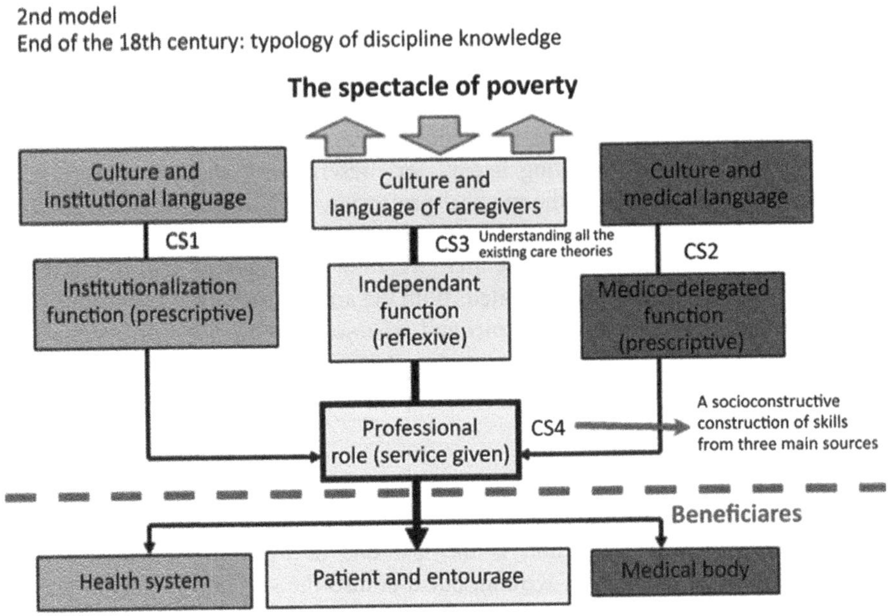

Figure 10.4. *Three cultural groups have guided healthcare action since the end of the 18th Century. For a color version of the figure, see www.iste.co.uk/nadot/nursing.zip*

COMMENT ON FIGURE 10.4.– *Recipients of services are: representatives of the hospital administration (CS1, institution), the medical profession (CS2) and the people cared for and their families (CS3). Cultural system 3 also includes all the existing care theories and various conceptual models (source: according to the Fonds national suisse de la recherche scientifique [NAD 02b, NAD 13]).*

10.2.3. *Medium, mediation, cultural intermediary*

The basic triptych coupled with the cultural systems thus formed as elements of knowledge, an institutional environment (milieu, medium), an objective of helping life through mediation (care) and a human posture among humans are then detached from the basic triptych.

With medium, health mediation and cultural mediation, a third layer of knowledge was added to the two previous layers. Three elements out of four of what North American researchers consider to be the focus of nursing knowledge (environment, care and the person) are present [PÉP 17]. These elements are important in thinking about the identity of the discipline (see Figure 12.1). With the spectacle of poverty that nurses have been facing for centuries, they were called upon as "cultural intermediaries" to develop implicitly towards the end of the 20th Century, by reflexivity, a fourth culture (CS4), an original synthesis using their own knowledge derived from experience and research, which then acted between the institutional culture and the medical culture (Figure 10.5).

This original synthesis and coordination of knowledge was in any case linked to the construction of a message (language) in the organization, to help survive by being placed as a cultural intermediary in the system. In (the organization), to (help survive or care), as (cultural intermediary), determined a "principle of DPC linkage" that is part of the constant fundamental elements of the cultural intermediary model [NAD 13]. A bit like in cooking (mayonnaise or sauces), it was necessary to find a formula for linking knowledge to make it more homogeneous and to avoid its dispersion in space and time. The identity of the discipline could take shape (see Figure 12.1). You do not do a bit of everything, anything and nothing special when you have a structured discipline. The languages held in the environment, to help people live, but as a cultural intermediary, then linked all the knowledge and interventions planned, organized or practiced by nurses and their assistants. In the language that placed the nurse in the position of cultural intermediary (way of occupying the field and the function) and that permanently related to the dynamic environment in which she was, the nurse must manage in terms of reflexivity a space of speech and action with variable geometry between three value systems that were not in synergy (CS4)[13].

In this intermediary posture, there were above all human actors, constantly negotiating with the environment, faces, places and power in general. It was from the institutional environment (milieu, medium) that it was possible to set objectives for helping people to live through health mediation and in a cultural intermediary posture. This posture of cultural intermediary generated a fourth culture (CS4) as a socio-constructivist and interactionist environmental result. The combination of institutional, medical and social language traditions is indicative of what was said, seen, done, represented, interpreted and manifested in the totality of languages exchanged with the individuals receiving the nurse's services. It took place in the environment, that is, the work medium and its characteristics. It thus became a

13 Cultural intermediary between culture and hierarchical institutional prescriptive language (cultural system 1), between culture and hierarchical medical prescriptive language (cultural system 2) and between the culture and language of the people being treated and their environment (CS3). It is on the basis of interactions with the latter that the culture and reflexive language of carers (according to a constructivist interactionist approach) belonging to their function independent (CS3) of the professional role (conceptual models and care theories according to the modalities of the CS3 + CS4 cultural system) have been developed.

"milieu", in the sense of "that which encompassed" and therefore a constructed structure. Medium and mediation are made for each other. In fact, the nurse as a professional working for the health system constantly draws information from the organization and its occupants and transforms it from her knowledge into action and speech. The service provided through cultural mediation is carried out at the perceived signal or at the request of the beneficiaries of the service. It is located at the customer interface in the front office. "The multiplicity of requests for services and their complexity generate a need to manage information flows with priority choices." [NAD 12b] This singular posture requires varied and in-depth skills to make information and perceived signals intelligible and credible. It should also be noted that it is not only humans who fill the hospital space and who make signals or give information. Walls and objects also emit signals. Whether it is the electronic alarm on a monitoring device, the internal signage of a large hospital or the wall clock on the ward. It is not much talked about in care theories.

Constrained and willing to live with humans that were struggling, the caregiver (nurse or health mediologist[14]) was confronted with the uncertainty of their reactions, behaviors, motivations for living or dying, or desires. This is still the case today. However, in addition to the people being treated and their family and friends, the nurse health mediologist still has to maintain working relationships with a number of people who benefit from his or her services. This is the case with the representatives of the medical, technical and administrative hierarchies.

The emotional space is strong enough and the sharing of time important enough for the nurse to legitimately and scientifically have something to say on the subject. Today, as a specialist in the coordination and synthesis of the multiple languages (CS4) that surround her in the institutions in which she works, the nurse spends a large part of her time developing the ability to do something with these perceived, heard, decoded and processed languages [NAD 12b]. This would be enough to justify her training in an academic setting today. To convince ourselves of the number of potential interlocutors likely to interact with the nurse, we need to only sit as an observer in the entrance hall of a large hospital at the time of visits or outpatient consultations. The number of people passing by, their attitudes, clothing, skin color, ages, interactions, gestures, signs of their role within the institution, facial expressions, objects they hold in their hands, etc., present as many messages about their state of health or their current concerns as they are almost revealing in terms of the services they are expected to provide.

It is from these languages, from the meaning given to them and from the writing that makes them exist that the healthcare discipline is constituted through its different models. For information to be transmitted, the message must find its

14 A term that is proposed to replace the word "nurse", see [NAD 13].

vehicle or channel, its environment and recipients who share something of the same code [NAD 13]. As Foucault reminds us, "knowledge is what can be spoken about in a discursive practice that is thereby specified" [FOU 69]. Thus, knowledge exists only from the relationship between language and actions in the field of a given social practice.

Nurses work in the tertiary sector, the service sector. This human activity, mostly of an informational nature, has today a heterogeneous clientele composed of people with different statuses who all benefit, in a differentiated manner, from near or far, from the services provided by the nursing profession. It is worth repeating that a healthcare institution is not only inhabited by patients. This also applies to a non-hospital structure. And since "the major element of service management is the existence of the client in the system" [BAN 99], it can be said that in a service provision it is always the beneficiaries of the service who provide the verbal or non-verbal information useful for the design and production of the service.

Becoming aware of this fact then changes many things. A new layer of knowledge is superimposed on the previous two. This information comes from everywhere: from the environment (medium), from the establishment of health or life mediations and from the cultural intermediary posture occupied in space and time (Figure 10.5). The context becomes a mediating state of the practice of caring. The client, whoever the nurse may be, a representative of the CS1 organization, a representative of the CS2 medical profession, or a representative of the CS2 medical profession, the persons being cared for and their CS3 entourage "always have two non-exclusive statuses; the client may be a target or a resource" of the services provided [BAN 99]. As already mentioned, it is of course not only patients who can be the target or resource of the services provided by nurses. This is true on a daily basis.

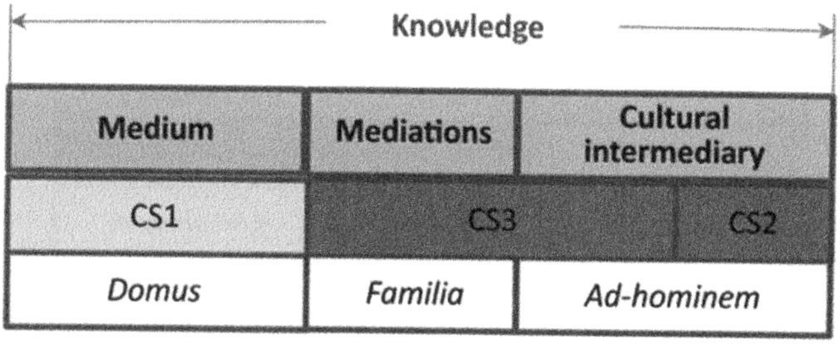

Figure 10.5. *The three MEDs: in terms of knowledge, nurses draw from the environment the information necessary to establish health mediation with a view to helping the people being cared for to live while occupying in space and time a traditional cultural intermediary position. The three MEDs can contribute to the construction of the scientific identity of the discipline. For a color version of the figure, see www.iste.co.uk/nadot/nursing.zip*

10.2.4. *Concepts of the nursing disciplinary metaparadigm*

These concepts emerged in the United States with the analysis of the knowledge produced by the discipline. There are four of them, and they represent the focus of the nursing discipline because of the work carried out in nursing. "The nursing metaparadigm is the most abstract component of the nursing structure. Personal concepts, those concerning the environment, health and care and the propositions that link them are used to delineate the field of nursing knowledge (Figure 10.6). The dialogue about the current composition of the metaparadigm remains open and possible changes to its composition are possible." [PRO 02] With the discovery of our language traditions, the composition of the metaparadigm remains, but requires some clarification of its outlines.

In the light of the three stages of knowledge of the discipline, we can say that the environment is not just any environment. It is exclusively an institutional one. In the environment as a space of speech, we can speak about… the goal to be achieved. The care it enables providing in order to help to survive. We then speak in order to take care… of humanity. And indeed in practice, we take care of humanity by focusing our attention on it. This same humanity, rather than being a philosophical form whose outlines we would seek to define, is above all a sociological humanity[15]. Indeed, the nurse's interlocutors are numerous and are above all inhabited by statuses, roles and functions (in short, powers). Let us think of health executives, doctors with their hierarchy, representatives of administrative services, etc. These will influence the relational dynamics of professional activity. It is all these human beings who benefit from the services of cultural intermediate nurses.

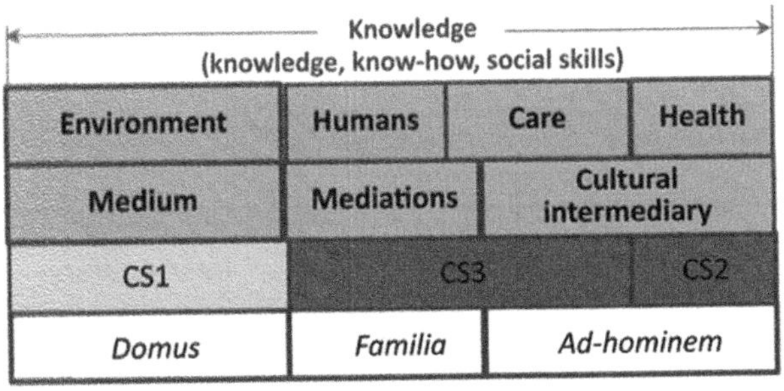

Figure 10.6. *Conceptual references are developing. North American female metatheorists in nursing bring new elements that are compatible with language traditions. The environment, humanity, care and health can also by their combination show another facet of the nursing discipline. For a color version of the figure, see www.iste.co.uk/nadot/nursing.zip*

15 Generally speaking, if we want to find different conceptions of humanity, we can consult the philosophical writings on the subject.

Humanity is therefore the target of attention, but this attention can only exist because we occupy a space representing the heart of the institutional system. It is a cultural intermediary position that nurses occupy. And the attention paid to humans is not necessarily the same if the humans are being cared for, their relatives, a doctor, an ambulance driver, a police officer, a representative of the administration and a representative of the technical or general services. As for health, the last central concept of the American metaparadigm, it must be said that everyone is talking about it… but nobody can touch it! You cannot photograph health that remains intangible. Moreover, it was only towards the end of the 18th Century that attention was paid to structures and practices conducive to the development of public health. For our part, we define health as a person's ability to lead a life with or without assistance, despite adverse conditions.

10.2.5. *Fourteen groups of practices*

By analyzing the four previous layers of knowledge applied by nurses with reference to the basic triptych of the discipline, the cultural systems present, the cultural intermediary posture, the CS4 type reflexivity and the central concepts of the nursing discipline, we can highlight several groups of practices. These practices have the characteristic of being timeless and, therefore, of being able to survive even through the centuries, but in varying proportions and qualities. Contexts change and become more complex, but the practices remain. It is one thing to have care theories, conceptual models and knowledge. Measuring their application through practices is another. A new layer of practices is then added to the knowledge already at work (Figure 10.7). This is the fifth layer of knowledge that our language traditions convey.

These 14 groups of practices apply worldwide. This does not mean that before this stage of reflection there were no practices. We have spoken about practices and knowledge of the lay age. But what is original is that we can perceive (and retain) with these 14 groups of practices (and therefore of knowledge, skills, values and ideologies), a complete typology of knowledge that has crossed space and time in five successive layers (Figure 10.7). Knowledge has come down to us and structures the discipline over the long term. Even if it can always continue to develop, fundamental knowledge persists:

– the first layer of knowledge present in the language marks the foundations of the discipline. It covers the lay period up to the beginning of the 20th Century;

– the second layer of knowledge, which is superimposed on the first, dates from around the end of the 18th Century and is still visible today. The knowledge is that which allows the posture of cultural intermediary;

– the third layer in turn encompasses the second layer. It comes into being the moment when the identity of the discipline raises questions;

– the fourth layer of knowledge at the end of the 20th Century refers to the four paradigmatic concepts of the discipline according to North American female metatheorists;

– the fifth layer of knowledge accompanies the practices still in use today. The knowledge at work in the last four interlocking layers still accompanies today's reflexive practices as the care context has changed. The body of knowledge carried by the discipline over the long term is also visible in another form in Figure 13.1 of the book.

The discipline can be inscribed at the heart of these five layers of knowledge brought successively in space and time. It is these five layers that should be preserved, brought together and made more homogeneous to form the foundations of the discipline (Figure 10.7). Care theories, for example, are derived from some of these practices, experiences or languages. The nursing discipline has a historical foundation of knowledge that should not be forgotten.

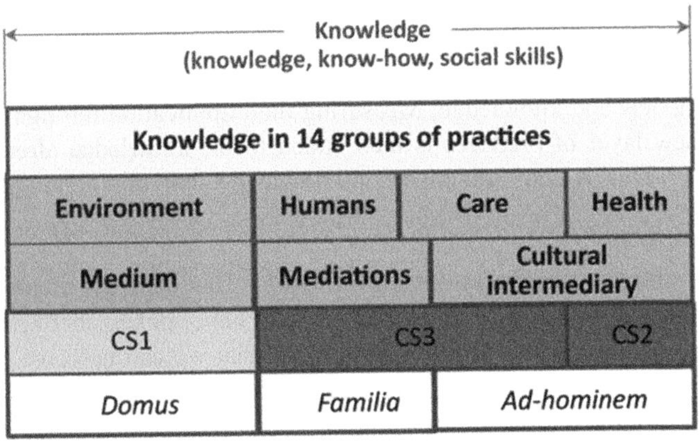

Figure 10.7. *Behind the concepts developed by the discipline, we can identify 14 groups of timeless practices that can be recalled. With this fifth stage of discourse in the discipline (yellow), the totality of the long-term thinking patterns and knowledge mobilized in the discipline at the global level are apparent. For a color version of the figure, see www.iste.co.uk/nadot/nursing.zip*

With this fifth level of knowledge, it is then possible to establish a typology of the knowledge carried by 14 groups of practices within the discipline. They reflect the norms of action resulting from the standardization of language and contemporary lay care practices. These 14 groups of practices cannot be dissociated from each other and form a whole that can be found in the reflective knowledge of the CS4 type. The knowledge required by these practice groups is in addition to the knowledge that makes up the disciplinary matrix (occupation repository) and constitutes the epistemological unit (health environment/health mediation/cultural intermediary associated with CS1, CS2 and CS3) of the care discipline. It is complicated, but it is also 300 years of knowledge that add up. It is all of this knowledge that makes up the ordinary practices of the nursing discipline, which should be valued and recognized both legislatively and economically. This cultural intermediary position occupies the heart of healthcare institutions and represents the oldest and nowadays most important part of an institution's budget. These practices have already been the subject of several publications since 2002, notably [NAD 03a, NAD 13]. As a reminder, we summarize below the characteristics of these 14 groups of practices (and therefore, knowledge groups) that accompany the conceptual model in nursing sciences known as the "cultural intermediary model". A practice can have several modes of expression, which is why we refer to practice "groups". It should be noted that these characteristics were defined by validation exercises as part of an international scientific research project, with the collaboration of forty nurses representing different care settings in French-speaking Switzerland between the *Haute école de santé de Fribourg* and a nursing faculty in Quebec (Canada) [NAD 02b].

A) Complex information management practice: the set of activities that simultaneously collect, store, analyze, redistribute, disseminate and perform special processing of information in order to transform it into action or words. The knowledge that makes up this type of reflexive practice and the time required to implement this type of practice is impressive. This information management can be induced, delegated or on the caregiver's own initiative. The complexity of this practice is due to the mixture of information from the three cultures and the heterogeneous values they carry. This practice is sometimes shrouded in noise, uncertainty, imprecision, powerlessness and questioning. Its complexity and magnitude result from the mixing of the data to be processed as well as the explanations given to the implicit and tacit expressions (CS4). After processing (transformation into acts or words), the transmission of information in turn requires linguistic and cultural skills so that the meaning of the message is not too far removed from the reference system of the person for whom the message is intended. This type of practice requires the caregiver's attention, great observation skills and is a matter of experience as well as knowledge. The first actions delegated to the caregivers started from the institutional writing (regulations, job descriptions, books of sanctions, protocols, etc.) and were based on the institutional rules and regulations), then medical orders and finally, writings and research in so-called "nursing" sciences. The redistribution and dissemination of the information that makes up this practice also presupposes mastery of the means of communication for transmission.

B) Information-gathering practice: set of activities aimed at gathering information (by listening, on demand, by observing digital screens or light signals or by research) and which the nurse needs to act. This practice requires the caregiver to consult multiple sources (telephone, office automation, documentary, computerized, scientific, technical, human, verbal or non-verbal, sound, olfactory, esthetic, etc.). It is important to know where to look for the information you need.

C) Management and coordination practice: there is also a group of practices initially called "order and discipline" in the age of lay knowledge. We will call it "management and coordination practice" in the protodisciplinary era of the discipline. All the activities that affect the management of time, space and movement necessary for the management of personnel and the organization of work, as well as the management of people present in the institution in order to avoid chaos (including management of the people being cared for and their visits). It requires both language coordination and social control. This practice also implies a control of the culture delegated by the carers to the staff who assist them in their functions.

D) Regulatory practice: set of activities aimed at preventing or managing human conflicts and dysfunctions in the organization. Serving to maintain the balance in the nurse's activity between production energy (care activity) and recovery energy. Without taking this practice into account, institutional dysfunctions and increased risks may occur. In addition to supervision and the processes of reassurance or conflict management, this practice includes various breaks and possible moments of relaxation (which never are) to cope with the tensions and constraints of professional practice. Preserves the productive power of the services provided. Without taking this regulatory practice into account, there is a predominantly emotional overload that wears out the care staff and may lead them to resign or become demotivated. It is therefore vital to the harmonious functioning of a healthcare institution. Without energy for regulation and recovery, we cannot hope to have energy for production.

E) Travel practice: set of activities that allows nurses to bring together various interlocutors and spaces, which would not exist without their intermediary. This practice is used to transmit information or objects from one place to another (a bed, for example) or to support a person on the move. This movement connects the different spaces of an institution and the people who live there, or even unites the institution with the city or living environment of the person being cared for. It also includes discharges from the ward with or without the person being cared for and is dependent on the topographical and architectural structures of a hospital (single block or pavilion structure).

F) Hotel practice: set of activities based on the domestic, family or household economy according to the characteristics of the persons being cared for and the hotel equipment or general services of the hospital (distribution of meals, repair of beds). It also includes a logistical practice (often delegated) combined with an assistance practice.

G) Collective hygiene practice: all the activities and principles that revolve around the prevention of hospital nosocomial infections, disinfection or professional protection of people. They are part of hospital hygiene or disinfection standards in establishments or at home. Practice is often delegated by nurses to their auxiliaries or to the general services of institutions. This does not prevent the nurse from occasionally participating in this activity.

H) Replenishment and storage practice: a set of logistical activities to support and sustain the production of services related to the care activity. Tidying practices also contribute to the closure of a care activity (practice L), including inventories, stock replenishment and economic accounting of materials used (linen, equipment, documents, forms, medicines, appliances and miscellaneous substances). This practice requires skills in distinguishing objects and their use or the conditions of conservation, storage (strategic locations of certain equipment) and supply.

I) Disposal practice: all activities aimed at eliminating used or defective objects and bodily organic waste (urine, stools, vomit, blood, spit, etc.) and assuming air purifying practices. Sometimes associated with practice G or practice J. It is not the most spectacular or most sought-after of the practices, but it remains essential to the development of life and the harmonious functioning of institutions. It requires that the experience of odor or deodorant practices be assumed. Often delegated by the nurse to her auxiliaries, it nevertheless requires certain skills to assume the daily routine and was already present in the professional culture at the time of lay knowledge.

J) Assistance practice: set of activities aimed at helping actors involved in one or other of the three cultural systems. It is an old activity that has become more complex in proportion to the increase in knowledge, the technological development of the hospital, society and the number of actors involved in health institutions. However, it is possible to distinguish each system benefiting from this practice: helping a colleague, which is a natural part of the teamwork used in the environment, cooperation and coordination of the activity (CS1); helping the medical profession (CS2), for interventions that require "multi-handed" skills (catheter insertion, lumbar puncture, adjustment of an assistance or control device, restraining a patient during a medical visit, etc.) and helping care recipients with daily living activities (DALs) and promoting independence. This practice was already part of lay practices. Helping people who lacked "goods, strength, health" as it was once called (CS3). We can also help them sometimes with the development of some care techniques. This help to live in spite of the adverse conditions that affect it has given rise to an activity that is not always valued and that the legislator sometimes calls "basic care". We find these DALs in Virginia Henderson's care theory, for example. This assistance also applies to the loved ones and family of the person being cared for, affected by the unfortunate or happy conditions (improvement of a state of health, birth) and how ordinary and sometimes unforeseen these things are.

K) Professional practice of the relationship: basic informational practice related to the institutional dynamics, its purposes and health mediations. It includes all verbal or non-verbal activities related to the things of life and to the promotion of autonomy, security and support. This practice includes structuring or reassuring presence, health mediation, touch, the helping relationship, active (empathic) listening, disease or accident prevention, end-of-life accompaniment and information given to the person being cared for (and to his or her family and friends), so that he or she is better informed, warned, oriented, trained to take charge of himself or herself and to become more autonomous. As the first care act, this entry into a relationship, whether verbal or non-verbal (touching, for example), is the oldest within the care discipline and assistance practices and requires the coordination of multiple linguistic codes. Often associated with practice J, it also participates in the orientation of the person being cared for in the spatio-temporal, statutory and institutional context of service provision.

L) Technological practice of care: set of activities delegated by the medical profession (CS2) and aimed at the application of the medical prescription (applicator agent). It includes the preparation of care, its execution (care techniques), its evaluation and its closure. This activity is probably the best known, the most idealized, the most dramatic and the most discussed. Sometimes referred to as a "paramedical" or "medico delegated" function, it institutes the carer in a prescribed activity and in the role of a delegated "double agent", shaped by the biomedical culture: an agent collecting data for medical analysis and an agent implementing medical prescriptions. As the "data collector" role is included in practice B (information collection), we will only consider here the role of "applying agent", the prescriptions. This is the "care technique" part of the past! This activity depends on the technology required by the therapies. It often requires the use of appropriate materials, devices or technical aids (parenteral, oral, rectal, vaginal, bladder, ENT (ear, nose and throat), ear, respiratory, skin), dressings, wound care, computer-assisted or non-computer-assisted means of investigation. This group of practices is the basis of a hospital's medical IT system and is also the main source of funding for health insurance funds in Switzerland and is used to compile hospital productivity indicators of the "SwissDRG" type (in France, homogeneous groups of patients).

This CS2-type practice has been progressively delegated to nurses since the birth of the Clinic and sometimes later improved by their care.

M) Training practice: this refers to all the activities enabling the profession to ensure and reinforce the transmission of professional and scientific culture (values, ideologies, knowledge) by welcoming and supporting students in training, for new staff regardless of their status or to demonstrate, evaluate and exhibit knowledge with a view to developing skills. These activities are the initiative and exclusive responsibility of the carers in their scientific disciplinary field. Practiced in the care territory, this also enables collaboration with partner universities in the training of students, to participate in scientific research or to present the profession during information and recruitment campaigns. It should be noted, however, that this practice is a serious service rendered to institutions and the health system (CS1) in order to reduce the shortage of highly qualified professionals. This practice is directly proportional to the number of trainees to be welcomed, supported or assessed. In principle, it is not financed by the costs borne by health insurers.

N) Inactivity practice: paradoxical "floating or hesitant" practice (we wait on something that does not come) including all the values or events paralyzing the action (loss of time by technical, human or institutional dysfunction, disorganization or disinformation).

NOTE.– All of the above practices can be memorized, measured and are often timeless. They can thus cross the centuries without being dependent on events or changes. It is possible to enrich their description, to find new modalities and to continue to develop knowledge about these practices through research.

The intensity deployed by the 14 practice groups changes according to the information that energizes the service provision. The measures of care activity for each of the 14 practice groups can be plotted on the axes of a "radar" diagram (Figure 10.8). In this way, we have, as it were, the ever-changing surface of the discursivity required by the discipline to provide care to everyone. The healing activity is never stabilized. Nothing is frozen. It remains dependent on the language of the recipients of the service and the thinking skills of the caregivers. Schematically, it is of the order of perpetual movement and mobility. It does not always allow itself to be enclosed in protocols and routines presented as reassuring, insofar as, *a priori*, we never know the nature of the message (verbal or non-verbal) that implements the service provision, nor its intensity, nor the moment when it will be delivered. It is the management of the unforeseen on a daily basis.

More importantly in terms of perspective, instead of indicating the frequency of occurrence of practices, we could indicate for each practice the sources of the information that triggers the service activity itself. These sources are multiple and of varying density. Since it is always the recipients of the service that deliver the verbal or non-verbal information useful for the design and reflective production of the service (CS4 type), it is these informative elements and sources of language delivered by the recipients of the service (CS1, CS2, CS3) that must be taken into account to identify the workload. The source of information that triggers service delivery is more important than the frequency of responses given. Let us not forget that the care environment provides a lot of signals and sources of information (colloquia, memorandums, protocols, informational data, charts, alarms, various noises, etc.).

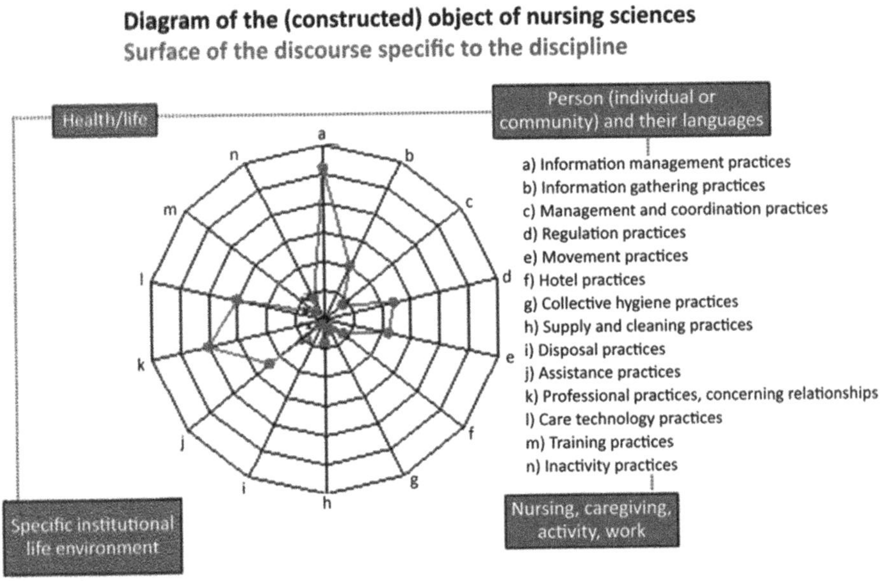

Figure 10.8. *Dynamic surface of knowledge arranged according to language traditions and the discipline's own perspective [NAD 13]. For a color version of the figure, see www.iste.co.uk/nadot/nursing.zip*

In Figure 10.8, the theoretical territory of knowledge presented in the conceptual cultural intermediary model then determines the reflective language surface of the discipline (to be colored red from the center). It is the totality of this surface that represents the daily activity accompanied by the knowledge required for caregiving. Like an oscilloscope, this surface is always in motion. Everything is moving all the time. We can, of course, conduct research on one of the many axes of the diagram, but in this case, it would be to specify the modalities of action or the specificity of the axis in question. It can also be seen that this radar diagram of the distribution of our knowledge can be at the heart of the four concepts of the nursing metaparadigm (in red on the diagram) according to the North American tradition.

Because of the knowledge they mobilize, nurses occupy a strategic place in the healthcare system. They are not always aware of this because of the proliferation of statuses that exist. They are at the heart of contradictions, have to deal with organizational shortcomings, receive complaints, grievances and questions. "They are the ones who perceive the inconsistencies or shortcomings of actions, measure their acceptability to patients and families, and make up for the shortcomings in daily life." [GRO 99] As Michèle Lacoste [LAC 01] points out, work, particularly in the provision of services, is in any case always a language considered to be "a vector of strategies, power relations, professional identities and cultural models". The constant construction of action induces speech, exchange, coordination and cooperation. The complexity of the work requires the convergence of the activities of several agents, several teams and several services. To do this, it is necessary to resort to communication: information flows (oral, written, computer, telephone, etc.), circulation of written documents, interactions, especially interactions that fix errors. "The information available is neither totally explicit nor completely unambiguous: it presupposes relying on tacit knowledge, but it must be checked with others in case of doubt, and differences in interpretation must be dealt with and the consequences repaired" [LAC 01]. The nurse's reflexive activity does not depend exclusively on the medical activity of an establishment; it is built on the moment and step by step through interpretations of the context and the intentions of others. As a result, it is difficult to codify this activity in advance with a view to determining a lump sum for financing by the health insurance funds, for example.

With a professional activity summarized in 14 groups of practices and five layers of knowledge by stratification, skills appear that are not within everyone's reach and that are not to be put into all hands. In fact, the discipline with its cultural intermediary model brings together ideas that have been developed in the field of institutional care since its inception (Figure 10.7). The unspoken emerges. The discipline is rarely mentioned in the profession's legislation. For example, in Switzerland, the federal law of September 30, 2016, on the health professions in Switzerland refers to "general competences", the discipline of nursing is not named, and the university-level study program "Bachelor of Nursing" is required to modestly offer "patient-oriented practical training as a priority" [CON 16]. In any case, "scientific competence" is not expected. In addition to "general competences", other competences are mentioned, such as "social and personal competences" and "specific professional" competences, which are still to be determined "with the cooperation of the universities concerned". As the discipline is not mentioned in this law of 2016, we are witnessing controversies and polemics in Switzerland between nurses of the ES level and nurses of the HES level. On the one hand, the good ones, on the other hand the best! But a discipline has no use for these distinctions, which determine more the levels of training and school structures than a body of knowledge. When talking about nurses, be careful not to mix a school structure, a student profile with a disciplinary body of knowledge.

In the absence of greater clarity as to the discipline taught and to illustrate this by a phenomenon of semantic innovation, let us try to introduce the metaphor which in science, participates in the setting of the plot and thus brings together the productive imagination and schematism. The role of the metaphor, this important source of lexical enrichment, figure of speech, symbolically speaking, associates the cultural intermediary with technically and socially determined sets.

The first metaphor (emotional metaphor) that we could propose for professional dynamics is that the nurse is like the "healthcare system hard drive" on which everything she saw, sees, says, hears and does is stored. Coupled with a photoelectric cell that captures and processes the manifestation of emotions from a human clinic, this hard drive contains the history of the connections and dynamics of all the information to be decoded and transformed into action and speech [NAD 12b]. If we spin this metaphor, we will say that it is important to avoid overloading the hard disk and to save it frequently, because when it is full, serious malfunctions may be programmed! This first metaphor came from the highlighting of "informational practice" in the framework of a scientific research conducted in 2002[16].

With the emergence of the posture of cultural intermediary, we proposed a second metaphor (cognitive metaphor): that of a hospital nursing department as a "control and referral tower for data traffic". Of course, it is not the airport's sky that is controlled, but the flow, use and coordination of the data transmitted, to satisfy demands, ensure safety and make the health system and its institutions function as well as possible. It is these flows of information that would be likely to provide load indicators for staffing levels if efficiency is to be achieved. This is information (verbal or non-verbal) provided by the recipients of services. But a hard disk does not move by itself, nor does a hospital nursing department! With the realization that in the space and time of the care environment, it is movement that makes the connection. We will then seek to find out who is moving within institutions to establish relational links or maintain the social link. These links made in particular by nurses are made in the "between" (the environment), between people and objects, through the technocultural mediation which then exists thanks to this "in/for/like" linking formula which accompanies the three MEDs of Figures 10.5 and 12.1 and which makes it possible to propose a third metaphorical statement.

16 Combination of "information management" practice, "information gathering practice", "management and coordination practice", "professional relationship practice" and "regulatory practice" (in 2002 represented between 57% and 72% of a nurse's workday) [NAD 02a, NAD 13].

It is the “inactive”[17] metaphor of the weaver’s shuttle. In the space and time of care, the framework of the loom is the institutional framework. The reed is used for CS1-type control. It is then the movement which makes the link, the nurses run everywhere! Between the weft wound on a shuttle and the warp threads of the weaving machine (the many beneficiaries of the nurse’s services), there is the shuttle that carries the weft (the nurse’s knowledge). This is the most mobile and independent part of the loom. A static shuttle is useless! The fabric is the result of the activity of the shuttle and the meeting of the warp, the weft and the movement of the shuttle. Therefore, the fabric, which can be of variable quality, not only corresponds to the improvement of the health status of a given society as a result of the activity of a nurse but also represents the optimal functioning of a care institution (environment and various interlocutors). A competent nurse also refers to her ability to move through the system [NAD 13].

17 The notion of enaction (Francisco Varela) is a way of conceiving cognition that focuses on how human organisms and minds organize themselves in interaction with the environment according to our CS4-type reflexive logic.

11

The Construction of the Discipline

The history of the discipline, of nursing knowledge or of nursing sciences then confronts us with problems that may give rise to a desire on the part of the researcher to "discover satisfactory explanations for everything that surprises us and seems to require an explanation" [POP 94]. Why have the knowledge traditions that structure the discipline in the long term not yet been able to claim a real epistemological status of nursing [NAD 93]? We are talking about the real scientific status, because the current status of nursing sciences, we recall, was born of a somewhat hasty decision imposed on nurses around 1977 to translate nursing as nursing sciences without having demonstrated that we were well ahead of sciences deserving in their specificity to be called "nursing". The lack of collective memory and the linguistic difficulties of translation complicated the situation. What equivalence of meaning is there between nursing and *infirmière* (from *enfer*, hell, the powers of darkness)? There is none! An almost impossible translation that has the capacity of presenting a discipline behind some stereotypes and abuse of language. As a reminder, it was a Canadian physician in the 1970s who proposed to Gallicize "nursing faculty" by "*École des sciences infirmières*" (school of nursing) [COH 02]. "The criteria that specify a discipline are difficult to determine abstractly. Today, the only coherent definition of a discipline is that which bears that name in scientific institutions" [LEV 13]. It is not surprising that the discussion of the nursing discipline is most prevalent in nursing faculties, doctoral schools, and scientific conferences.

With all the layers of knowledge that have been assembled and laid over the long term since the first knowledge group was created (Figure 10.7), it becomes possible to glimpse a logic of knowledge construction specific to our discipline. But this knowledge is not just any knowledge. We started with the foundations (basic principles) and laid the different bricks of knowledge on these foundations. This knowledge did not come out of nowhere and did not wait for the arrival of Florence Nightingale to begin to exist. To quote an old idea in the philosophy of science, we know that "if there has been no question, there can be no scientific knowledge. Nothing can be taken for granted. Nothing is given. Everything is constructed. Above all, one must know how to pose problems. Including in basic research. And no matter what one says, in scientific life, problems do not arise by themselves" [LAC 83]. Our language traditions presented in this book have been defined "after several intermediate stages, by means of considerations related, at the very least, to spatio-temporal localization, because a non-local theory cannot be considered scientific in the strict sense of the term: we know – and act – only locally" [THO 83]. These intermediate steps are represented by the layers of knowledge already mentioned in Figure 10.7, and we know from Popper that "knowledge cannot start from nothing – from a *tabula rasa*, nor yet from observation. The advances of knowledge consist, mainly, in the modification of earlier knowledge" [POP 85]. This was demonstrated in the previous chapter. By construction of the discipline, we are talking here about basic research carried out in the university environment. If there is no basic research, it is difficult to do applied research within one's one's own discipline.

To go further and try to analyze the situation, we also had to escape the framework of contemporary care theories (often deductive theories), carry out a reframing operation and escape this normal science which "never aims to shed light on phenomena of a new kind". In general, normal science is "directed towards the articulation of phenomena and theories that the paradigm already provides" [KUH 96]. This is a bit like what is happening today when it is proclaimed that one of the areas of interest in nursing science is the "human-university-health process" [PÉP 17]. This is not false, but probably incomplete! To find out more, we need to return to the traditions of language, set aside Florence Nightingale for a moment and change the paradigm.

In order to approach the fundamental scientific construction of our knowledge, and on the basis of the revisited history of this knowledge, we must consider healthcare practice in a different class from that which, for "modernity", consists of giving it meaning and values, a "nursing" orientation that only takes into account "practical training focused on patients" [CON 16], health, the sick and their families and friends. As we have seen, a nurse does much more than just look after patients. If the totality of services provided by nurses is not taken into account, it is staffing, safety of care and overwork in the name of efficiency and cost-effectiveness that will suffer quantitatively and qualitatively. Research from the perspective of the nursing discipline should include in its results not only the benefits to the person being cared for (CS3), but also the nature or impact of the service provided to the medical profession (CS2) and the contribution of new knowledge to the organization (CS1). For most of the time, it is these three groups of people who benefit together, but in different proportions, from the services provided. In almost all professional situations, and to put it simply, we would say that today we have a person (or a group) to take care of, but it is the patient of a doctor in connection with social funding and it is also a person admitted according to particular procedures within an organization that must continue to function. The nurse with her reflexive language traditions is at the heart of these action perspectives.

Of course, any theory is likely to improve as long as we know that it is presented "tentatively for testing". It progresses by eliminating errors, but not by increasing truths and, in this case, we can hope that by the incessant questioning caused by "the ignorance and uncertainty produced by knowledge" [POP 85], the theories and concepts carried by the nursing discipline will become increasingly reliable. The advantage of this vision of things is that, from the moment we perceive the other possible class membership, we cannot easily return to the trap and anguish of our old vision of reality or previous representations. By this very fact, we can then conduct our reflection according to a scientific method made up of "daring conjectures and ingenious and rigorous attempts to refute them" [POP 94]. This method then modestly allows science to be nothing other than consciousness brought to its highest point of clarity and uses, as a rule of the game, the respect of data, on the one hand, and obedience to criteria of coherence, on the other hand.

Nursing science (for us, health mediology[1]) can then be seen as a scientific title, since the research undertaken to increase knowledge reveals a thought process which has "as its starting point and ultimate goal the formulation of ever more fundamental and fertile problems, giving rise to other, as yet unpublished problems" [POP 85]. "Knowledge can only be called scientific if it has been published and thus subjected to peer review. It is also through publication that knowledge can be used or further refined when it gives rise to another study" [DEB 10]. The healthcare discipline develops its knowledge from practice and does not consist of prior knowledge, from which the latter would simply deduce its approaches. Nor is the discipline the place where annexationist disciplines are practiced or taught and is not, in its constitutional logic, an applied science in terms of conceptualizing the function independent of the professional role and the theories serving this function [NAD 93].

1 New identity reference system resulting from basic research proposed to nursing sciences since 1992. This identity for the discipline takes into account the traditions of language and knowledge interacting over the long term in an institutional setting (*domus*, hospital, medium, environment, institution), the dynamics of health mediation (care, help survive, service provision) and the position of cultural intermediary occupied in the field by nurses (CS1, CS2, CS3, CS4; see Figures 10.5–10.8). Health mediology firstly "refers to the study of the institutional postures of cultural intermediaries between three cultural systems that are nurses within the health system and the symbolic powers of languages at work in health institutions" [PÉP 17]. For a more detailed discussion of this concept, see [NAD 13].

At the end of the protodisciplinary period of knowledge and once the profession had been constituted with its four fields of practice, we probably moved too quickly towards heterogeneous applied research (problem-solving, action research, moderate spectrum theories, theories specific to care situations, etc.) to the detriment of our own fundamental research and its cohesion serving to position and increase knowledge for our discipline. That is, increasing knowledge by improving or replacing previous knowledge. Without basic research, one has little to apply as a researcher. At the beginning of the scientific period of knowledge, everyone was in a hurry to see themselves "doing scientific research". From the final dissertation to the scientific report of the funded research, everyone aspired to acquire methodologies useful to the scientific process. It was necessary to set to work and, if possible, to embrace the benefits of science. It was a time when we also had "carte blanche" to do "black research" in order to produce "gray knowledge" [NAD 07]. Much of the new knowledge or concepts that emerged from this era also consisted of little reference to the existing fundamental conceptualizations of nursing. But could it be otherwise, especially within the French-speaking world?

Having favored applied or clinical research[2] to the detriment of basic research, we now find ourselves with an abundance of "nursing research", which we symbolize by balls of different colors lost in space and time (Figure 11.1). It is becoming difficult to grasp the nature or scientific identity of the discipline. The problem of the visibility of nursing for society and politics is not far away.

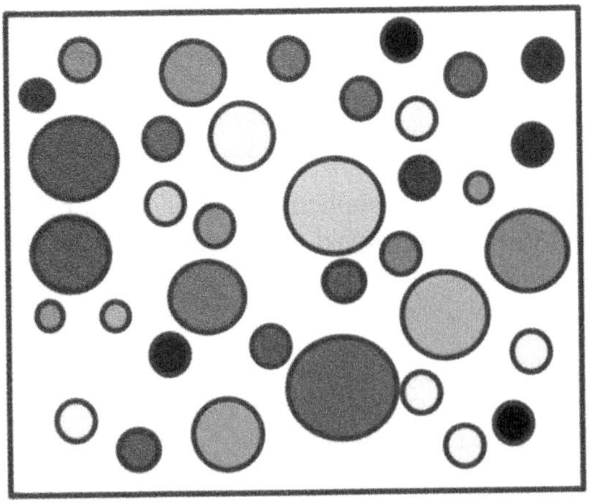

Figure 11.1. *The different "floating" multicolored knowledge within the nursing discipline today ("cut under the microscope"). For a color version of the figure, see www.iste.co.uk/nadot/nursing.zip*

2 Which clinic are we talking about, biomedical clinic or human clinic?

If we look at the state of knowledge produced worldwide, we are struck by the heterogeneity of schools of thought, the great diversity of methodologies deployed, the heterogeneity of the status of researchers, the variety of values displayed, the multiplicity of ideologies carried by the published texts, the fragmentation of research results presented at conferences or similar sessions at congresses, for example (Figure 11.1). Ultimately, in the face of this proliferation of applied research and disparate sources of funding, there is also a great imbalance between basic research and applied or application-oriented research. Beyond the fact that this research is led by nurses with a PhD in nursing, what links them in terms of disciplinary identity? Too much applied research is killing basic research. Producing scientific knowledge is not always producing "a little bit of everything, anything and nothing special" in terms of knowledge [ADA 79]. This knowledge must be able to be grounded to a basis that serves as a foundation. The knowledge represented in Figure 11.1 from the metaphor "cut under the microscope" has no disciplinary grounding, the tradition of language does not appear, the knowledge of the past is forgotten, knowledge that is not linked to others seems to "float", suspended in the universe of knowledge, nothing holds them back, they "fly away", they have multiple origins, nothing brings them together conceptually, there is no overview, they are fleeting, very diverse and have nothing to anchor them in terms of their identity. Yet some of them are of excellent quality.

QUESTION.– New knowledge can be generated through scientific research. If it does not have a place to settle, it gets lost in space, it simply gets lost in the universe of knowledge, even if it was financially supported by various foundations. To what body of knowledge is the new knowledge that enriches the nursing discipline, particularly within the university faculties that host it?

Multiple, but stable. This knowledge is probably hidden, at least not visible to the political authorities. And with the tendency to publish in English even in French-speaking Europe, this does not help the visibility of research at the local or regional level. It has to be discovered. This knowledge has survived over time and is at work all over the world (Figure 10.7). However, we still find a way to disperse ourselves by default to feed a hard core of knowledge for the discipline, or even to lose ourselves altogether in research. Is this a reflection of some recent academic drift from the United States, where the criteria for approval of nursing education and research programs "are now not necessarily explicit about disciplinary knowledge" [LAD 15]? Note that in Figure 11.1, some doctoral (PhD) led nursing research from a disciplinary perspective is symbolically represented by "green bubbles". Does this also mean that the visibility of the discipline (nursing science) or its purpose is not explicit for nurses and politicians alike? Let us recall the content of the Swiss Federal Law of 2016 on Health Professions in Switzerland [CON 16].

If this is the case, it is of course not to promote the development of the basic research that our discipline needs. We may also be faced with new structures that are intended to be sustainable and equitable for health systems and in which, under the term "integrated medicine"[3] (another takeover), our own discipline is disappearing. In this case, it is medicine that is meant to be "integrated" and not care. Care is simply being phagocytized by medical knowledge.

In Switzerland, when the *Hautes écoles spécialisées du domaine de la santé* (University of Applied Sciences and Arts) was founded in 2002, the schools had no budget for basic research within the disciplines taught. However, the *Hautes écoles spécialisées* (HES) differ from *écoles supérieures* (ES) in their ability to carry out scientific research to build up the knowledge that the discipline requires. As a reminder, the *Conférence suisse des hautes écoles spécialisées* stated in 2005 that "the Universities of Applied Sciences carry out basic research when this is necessary to achieve the goals set for applied research" [KFH 05]. However, as there was no funding, few school management teams aware of this message and few qualified researchers to take up the challenge, the focus remained mainly on the improvement of applied research. Applied research was funded more from a utilitarian perspective of research to respond to short-term health problems. The competence networks established in French-speaking Switzerland at the beginning of scientific research at the universities of applied sciences were generally representative of current problems in the world of health and the social field. Research themes revolved around "social and family policies", "cultural diversity and citizenship in the health and social fields", issues and new social regulations that appeared "at the frontiers of health and society", studies applied to "health, rehabilitation and reintegration practices". Research was then oriented in a general way around chronic diseases, the elderly, possible synergies between the "health and social" fields, disability, etc.), [NAD 10] and not around the perspective specific to the nursing discipline.

"It is almost impossible to obtain a comprehensive view of the knowledge accumulated in the discipline as it has evolved. While the publication of several volumes might lead us to conclude that a global overview exists, this is not the case since these volumes generally target and describe a particular theoretical level

3 "It is a personalized medicine in its four components (biomedical, educational, psychological and social), a partnership medicine that implies a relationship with the patient that is certainly asymmetrical, but equal. Thanks to the therapeutic education of the patient and the empathy of the carer, each can partly take the place of the other, while keeping his own. Finally, it is a matter of coordinated medicine between the city and the various health establishments and between the various professionals, doctors, paramedical staff and social workers, developing coherent practices, acting in a complementary way to achieve shared objectives and delivering consistent messages to patients and their families" [BEN 17].

without covering the entire body of knowledge in the discipline" [DAL 15]. In the midst of all knowledge (care theories, care processes, helping relationships, nursing diagnoses, movement of evidence, advanced practices, etc.), the fundamental knowledge specific to the discipline is almost invisible. To use a popular expression, in the face of the multitude of knowledge produced by research, "it is a real mess". How do you name and collect the green bubbles lost among the others (Figure 11.1)? As Ducharme rightly pointed out, research on the threshold of the third millennium is far from being a monolithic –entity. "It is often tinged with philosophical and methodological pluralism and the coexistence of paradigms" [DUC 02].

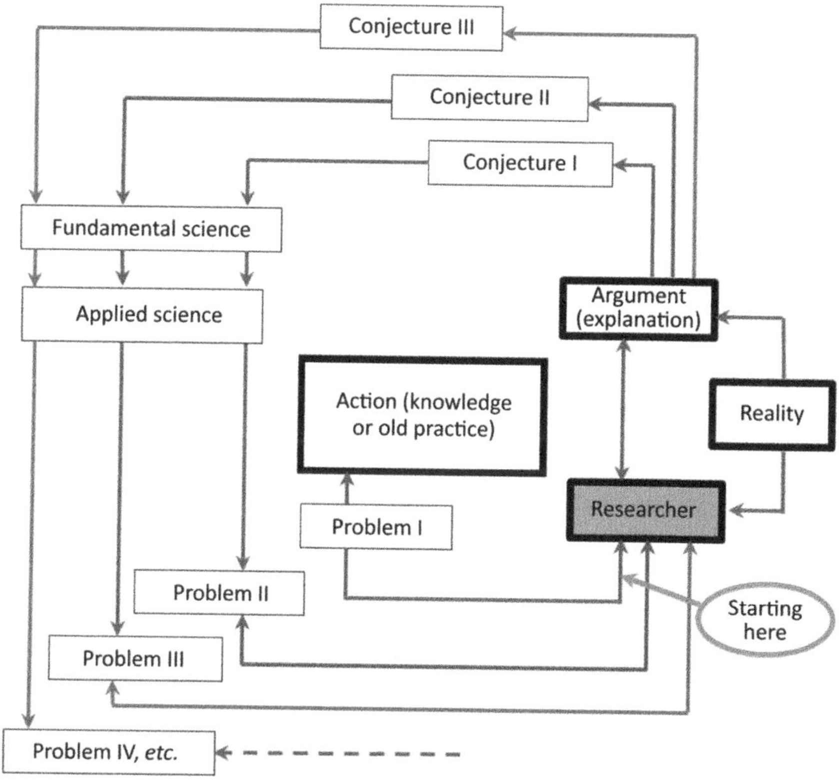

Figure 11.2. *Diagram of the construction of fundamental knowledge for a discipline. For a color version of the figure, see www.iste.co.uk/nadot/nursing.zip*

When conducting basic research to address issues arising from the questioning of fundamental knowledge from a nursing discipline perspective, there are at least three elements to consider (Figure 11.2):

– the person searching for answers, an author who provides answers to the questions he asks himself "attentively" (the researcher);

– a "reality" as an empirical context for the emergence of questioning, a space and time in which human–object interactions take place, which attract attention;

– momentarily satisfactory "explanations" (conjectures in Figure 11.2 or assumptions) based on knowledge (frame of reference) to which we conform or authoritative sources.

Among the frames of reference specific to the nursing discipline, we place the existing care theories and conceptual models in nursing.

In the absence of relevant frames of reference, we also use philosophy in basic research as a reflective science for the conceptualization of new knowledge. This activity is generally reserved for PhD holders who, as autonomous researchers, often must "advance knowledge, create new methodological approaches and create instruments to measure phenomena of interest to nursing sciences" [DUC 02].

11.1. The green knowledge theory

To address the process of building the discipline and its consolidation, we will use the notion of "green knowledge" [NAD 93]. That is, a person with the authority to conduct research, whom we call a "researcher" (Figure 11.2). Through experience and attention to what was already there (reality), the researcher extracts from an action/reflection (knowledge use or previous practice) a problem that we call "problem I". Taking hold of this problem, he seeks, through an activity of destruction and restructuring carried out by confrontation with other sources invested with authority, to formulate a conjecture, which we call "conjecture I". The explanation he finds for the perceived problem, once written and printed, produces new knowledge, a theory, which we will call fundamental science (new and starting from the existing). This theory, later applied in practice, will be tested, verified, validated, used, adopted or rejected. If it is not used, the book or article that is both the format and the vehicle of this knowledge, remains a book, a certain type of product – even if no one ever reads it. Even so, the purpose of science remains. It is to discover satisfactory explanations for everything that astonishes us and seems to need explanation. But new knowledge produces a cloud of ignorance and uncertainty, and every solution to a knowledge problem produces a new question. We will then have the appearance of a new problem that we call "problem II", which will in turn wait to be dealt with by the one who takes it up, and so on; which we can represent in Figure 11.2.

If we now symbolize the two elements that the researcher has at his disposal in a research process (real and explanatory) by colors and the mental activity of this researcher, by the work he can do on modeling clay, then we observe how, in a scientific process, knowledge that is specific to the activity of a researcher can come to take the form and color of what we will call "green knowledge"[4].

Experimentation: either two balls of modeling clay: one, blue, represents the situation as it is questioned (problem), in other words: the problem rooted in the experience and existential questioning of the researcher. The other, yellow, represents the knowledge available or sources invested with authority (explanation) in a given context or at a given time. As there can be several sources of authority within a discipline, we can also take several small yellow balls.

If you put the blue ball next to the yellow ball, nothing happens. The interrogation ignores knowledge; both balls are equal in their infinite ignorance. It takes a researcher as a dynamic element, a third element to constitute knowledge, in other words, to set the colored balls in motion. It will be an action of knowledge construction and knowledge mobilization (destruction and restructuring). This movement can only take place as a result of the researcher's activity. He can, for example, tackle (glue) and adjust the yellow knowledge on the blue situation, in order to quickly have an answer to the questions that emerge from the perceived problematic phenomena. This is either a recipe or a proliferation of applied knowledge, at best multidisciplinary.

Without the researcher's activity in empirical research and without his conceptual activity, yellow knowledge will remain yellow knowledge; it will continue to belong to the discipline that gave birth to it and will only be placed for the circumstance on the blue situation in order to mask its complexity or to alleviate the anxiety caused by the researcher's encounter with a new problem, which seemed to require a solution or even a decision quickly.

Let's take this more seriously. Let's go slower. If now the researcher, because of his cognitive–reflective activity, starts to work the modeling clay, that is, to knead it, to mix it, which requires more energy than to apply knowledge, he can progressively observe a simultaneous transformation of the yellow knowledge and the blue problem due to the specificity of his work (research practice). Provided that he continues his mixing activity, he can also observe – by progressive transformation and definitions – a homogenization of knowledge in the problematic dependent on

4 This notion was presented and argued in the presence of Marie-Françoise Collière during my thesis defense in Lyon in January 1993. The experiment that followed can be reproduced in real time.

the energy mobilized. In contact with blue and yellow, knowledge gradually becomes green.

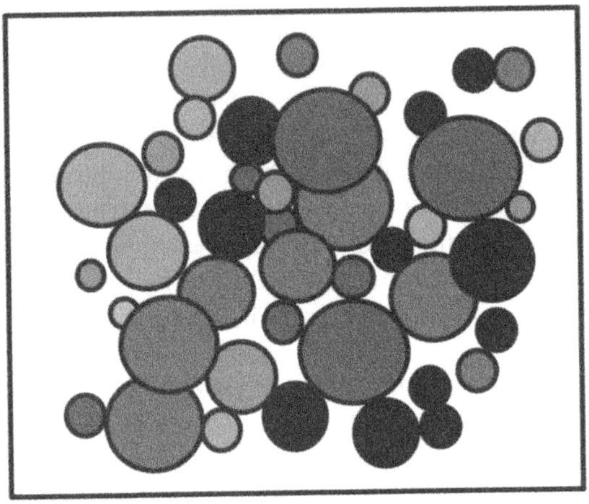

Figure 11.3. *Green knowledge. Perspectives of a discipline gradually coming together on its foundations with the development of basic research ("cut under the microscope"). For a color version of the figure, see www.iste.co.uk/nadot/nursing.zip*

This new knowledge can be communicated within the Cité Scientifique (congress, publication) in an act of authority. There is no longer just yellow knowledge associated with a blue problem; the researcher has built up green knowledge with his modeling clay balls (Figure 11.3). There is a homogenization of yellow knowledge about and with the blue problem. A little more empirical data will give dark green knowledge. A little more theoretical knowledge will give light green knowledge. All nuances are possible. But we remain in the green.

11.2. Compulsory basic knowledge

In turn, the solution to the problem or new knowledge may "give rise to new problems that in turn require solutions; the importance of the phenomenon depends on the difficulty of the initial problem as well as the boldness of the proposed solution" [POP 85]. Fundamental knowledge is growing stronger. The discipline is then constituted by the proliferation of more or less homogeneous green knowledge with all kinds of nuances. Each shade of green bears the name of the author who proposes innovative knowledge recognized by the profession (a conceptual model, for example, a green ball in Figure 11.3). The innovation, in turn, enriches the existing green knowledge (the core knowledge of the discipline) and increases the size of the ball of clay in question. Discipline-specific knowledge fundamentals develop, become closer together, attract each other and increase their reliability and visibility (Figure 11.4).

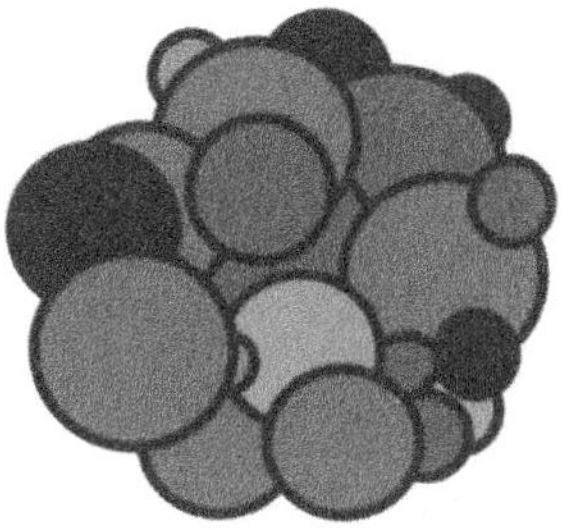

Figure 11.4. *Foundations of disciplinary knowledge carried by conceptualized language traditions over the long term (see Figure 10.7). For a color version of the figure, see www.iste.co.uk/nadot/nursing.zip*

The disciplinary basis is established. The foundations of knowledge are in place and, contrary to Figure 11.1, they are no longer suspended in any way in the history and universe of knowledge, they are held together, they are agglomerated, aggregated, they have more or less a conceptual link between them, they are much less fleeting, disparate, they can come together, they are recognized, nothing repels them (Figure 11.4).

This big green ball of modeling clay symbolizes the fundamental knowledge of the discipline with its authors. This knowledge then becomes a matrix on which several other "specialized" knowledge forms produced later then gradually come together. The accumulation of knowledge then benefits the discipline. This is no longer the case in Figure 11.1.

But we can also associate with this green knowledge, different kinds of knowledge that are grafted onto the foundations of the discipline. This knowledge produced by non-nursing research is represented by small pins of different colors that are inserted into modeling clay (Figure 11.5).

Finally, there is a format to which to attach these pins. Knowledge is no longer suspended in a vacuum. It no longer disperses. They have a disciplinary basis to hold on to. But yet, it is not fundamental knowledge. It is applied knowledge of a different nature. They add additional knowledge that focuses on the discipline. They keep their original colors and disciplinary origins.

This green basis with its little pins is part of the knowledge taught in different training institutions which in turn deliver a recognized diploma.

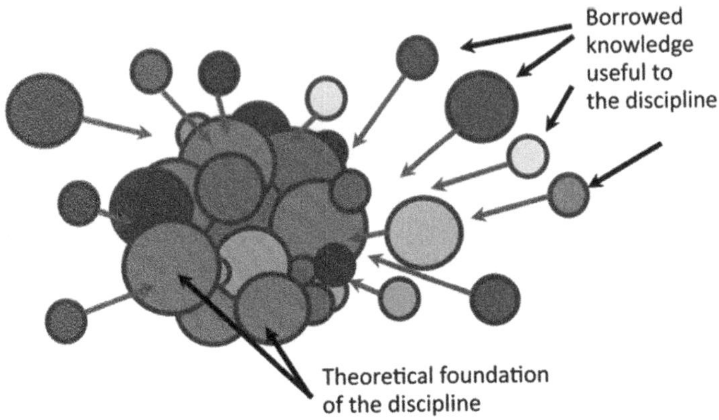

Figure 11.5. *Different long-term knowledge, more or less specialized, is gradually being inserted into the fundamental foundation of the discipline. For a color version of the figure, see www.iste.co.uk/nadot/nursing.zip*

All this knowledge, sometimes specialized according to the workplace and developed over the long term, is often the subject of training. Its presence does not prevent fundamental knowledge from continuing to develop. The green ball can continue to grow regardless of the applied knowledge of different colors. However, the knowledge brought in or borrowed, symbolized by the multi-colored head pins (Figure 11.5), is sometimes so numerous that it completely covers the surface of the fundamental base of knowledge carried by the discipline (central green core). This has the effect of making it invisible. This knowledge of colors other than green is borrowed, applied or even delegated knowledge; hence a problem of visibility and audibility of the discipline. A fair balance remains to be found! Let us note that if we continue to mix the green modeling clay, associated with other knowledge of different colors, we may well end up with brown knowledge (like the Earth), a land of knowledge that carries the transformation of the green nature of our fundamental knowledge represented by reflexive skills of the CS4 type.

We cannot, therefore, simply leave it at that: we cannot simply leave it at the level of various types of knowledge on the fundamental (green) foundation of the discipline (care theories, for example). The conceptualization work can continue. One then continues to knead the modeling clay balls in order to highlight the totality of the reflexive professional knowledge (CS4), as represented in Figure 10.4. This reflexive knowledge is that which is applied in professional situations. It is taught at school, it comes from experience in the field and it takes different forms every day. The mixing operation by continuous effort on the modeling clay is a real work (the green associated with the other colors) then giving our knowledge a brownish color. This brownish color, which has the "fundamental green nature" of the discipline as its core, can then represent the "earth" of knowledge (it is an image) as a global sum of knowledge useful for mastering professional situations (CS4). The discipline as the foundation of knowledge can then continue to develop through research. However, mixing becomes increasingly difficult, even from so-called "advanced" practices. However, it is essential to preserve the green fundamental knowledge according to the language traditions and perspective of our discipline (Figure 11.4). This green knowledge serves as an anchor for diverse knowledge from the work environment. The nurse makes permanent reflexive syntheses of it.

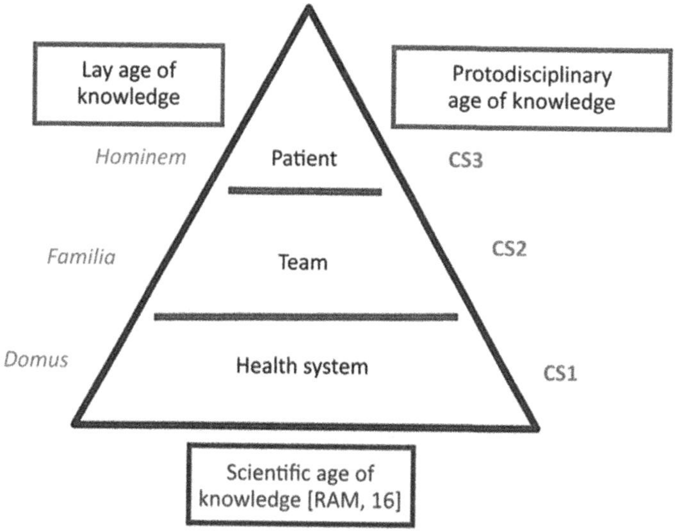

Figure 11.6. *Recipients of clinical nurse specialist (CNS) and nurse practitioner specialist (NP) services in the midst of nursing discipline language traditions. For a color version of the figure, see www.iste.co.uk/nadot/nursing.zip*

It is then deduced that the socio-constructivist and interactionist activity of the nurse (SC4) consists of using her own knowledge and language traditions to combine multiple knowledge (delegated, applied, borrowed) in interaction with the knowledge of others. It is about assuming the place that has been occupied for centuries at the heart of the healthcare system. Hence the complexity of the nursing function, which is not to be put in all hands by vocation, on the pretext that there is a lack of qualified personnel. Applied research can in turn enrich the questions raised by basic nursing research.

Surprisingly, it is still the three elements of the basic triptych of the discipline in the lay era (section 10.2.1) that appear in the diagram (in blue) of the two key professional roles and expected future scientific competencies for advanced nursing practice (ANP) (Figure 11.6), as presented by the *Institut universitaire en sciences infirmières* (IUFRS) of the University of Lausanne in 2016 [RAM 16].

In addition to the lay historical constants of nursing discipline knowledge (Figure 10.3), there are also protodisciplinary (section 10.2.2) knowledge competencies (Figure 10.4), which are divided into service to patients (CS3), service to the broader medical team (CS2) and service to the healthcare system (CS1). Figure 11.6 then accurately represents the services corresponding to the language traditions of the nursing discipline for the scientific age of its knowledge, either the service rendered to *domus–familia–hominem* or the service rendered to CS1, CS2, CS3 and their reflexive synthesis of the CS4 type of nursing activity modeling ([NAD 13] and Figure 10.4). "There are no ultimate sources of knowledge. There are no sources, no indications to eliminate, and all are open to critical review. The appropriate question for epistemology is not the question of sources. Rather, the question is whether the assertion is true, whether it is consistent with the facts" [POP 85]. Nevertheless, if we link the knowledge production approach to our sources of knowledge and those that we invest with authority through a use to which we conform (green knowledge), we can also grasp in their generalities the issues[5] that we perceive in the development of our own discipline (Figure 11.7). It is in this configuration that the knowledge of the nursing discipline is confronted with other knowledge. Thus, the increase in fundamental knowledge benefits, first of all, the strengthening of the discipline, while the increase in applied knowledge benefits the improvement of the services provided.

In this "knowledge producer" function, the knowledge produced by research then emerges. In turn, applied to a given era or culture, this leads researchers to use their own methods and techniques to achieve their goals: the aim is to produce knowledge useful both to society with a view to "orienting social life according to more enlightened choices" and to the development of our discipline in the growth of its own knowledge (Figure 11.7). Hence the question: for whom and for what do we seek and develop new knowledge (Figure 11.7)?

While the well-being of the person being cared for is always the primary focus of the profession's concerns, the development of the care discipline by theorists is also a primary focus, but it is primarily a matter of "looking to the abstract for evidence of the consistency of the concrete" [BAC 34].

---

5 "For whom", "for what" and "why" produce scientific knowledge? (see Figure 11.7).

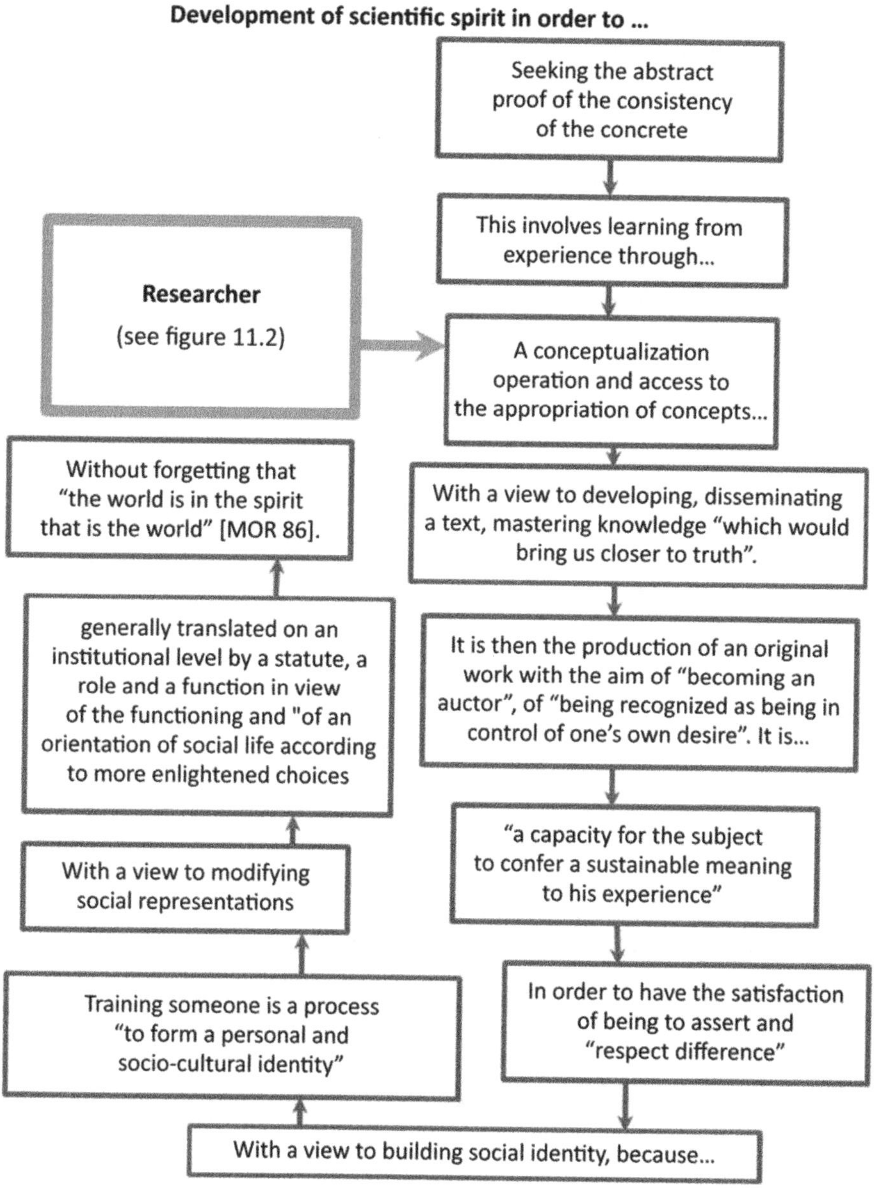

Figure 11.7. *Diagram of authoritative knowledge or the development of scientific thinking, for whom? For what? Why? For a color version of the figure, see www.iste.co.uk/nadot/nursing.zip*

For some, “basic nursing research is aimed at understanding processes related to health or care” [PÉP 17]. Not only we would say! First of all, “health” is not only a concern of the nursing discipline. At a minimum, it concerns all practicing healthcare professionals, and there are many of them. On the other hand, the processes involved in providing care, that is, the optimal functioning of the environment that used to be called “the home”, “the household”, “the hospital”, today, “the institution, the organization, the healthcare system” must also be taken into account so that the people being cared for can continue to receive the benefits to which they are entitled. However, the institutional aspect of care (the governance of care) is rarely mentioned in research within the discipline. For the neoliberal narrative, “the welfare state can no longer play its role. Only selfish management and finance are capable of stimulating progress by controlling costs” [KIE 19]. Nursing researchers must therefore seek to act on the cultural system one (SC1) to rectify the situation, but on condition that they have a good grasp of the components of the service provided to the institution and make this known. Based on the emancipatory mode of knowledge development in nursing, this consideration of the knowledge of past governments would be of great interest to the political world, that is, the world where “the language listened to and read by decision makers” [PÉP 17].

It can therefore be said that the so-called “nursing” sciences are a collection of knowledge produced by scientific research. A researcher then uses his disciplinary knowledge to grasp the problematic elements of the context by reflexivity in order to produce objective knowledge that will enrich the existing stock of knowledge. But as we have seen, in terms of language, these sciences cannot be “nursing”. So what are they? Again, this is an astonishment. Perhaps not for the nurse “lambda” in her daily practice, but certainly for researchers. Research and the production of knowledge is often a discovery of satisfactory answers to what is surprising or seems to need explanation. New knowledge may “give rise to new problems which in turn require solutions”. This is what has happened with our research, particularly with the chain of successive astonishments in the history of our knowledge. In fundamental research, knowledge progresses by eliminating the problems posed by the knowledge contained in the nursing discipline.

When we realized that Florence Nightingale was not really, as they say, “the first” to think of a training system or “the founder” of care that would be “modern” *(problem I)*, that there was already a great deal of existing knowledge about caring that was applied before the 19th Century and that is rarely mentioned *(problem II)* and that the carer often mobilized much more knowledge than was useful for caring for the sick or that health was not part of the profession’s primary knowledge *(problem III)*, we could not help but look for an additional explanation or consider a new conjecture (Figure 11.2).

Yet another astonishment: when we discover that the etymology and origin of the French term for nurse "*infirmier*" belonged exclusively to the language traditions of practical charity of the Catholic Church and that this term associated with the word science cannot only be the French translation of nursing science, we are faced with *(problem IV)*.

It was a time when, in a provocative and attention-grabbing way, we asserted that "nursing did not exist" at least in the language of lay caregivers [NAD 03a]. However, the care given by nurses existed; the same care was also sometimes given by people who did not call themselves nurses; the knowledge about care existed, but was it necessary to describe them as "nurses" for all that and by abuse of language? This discovery poses a new problem. If nursing sciences cannot, in terms of identity and language, be "nursing", what are they or what can they be in terms of their "logic"? *(problem V)*.

12

Identity and Discipline

A discipline's identity is measured by the clarity of its discourse and its authoritative sources of knowledge. These sources of knowledge define both the field of reflection and the disciplinary perspectives. The knowledge taught to nurses at the beginning of schools was often knowledge developed by other disciplines to provide insight into care practices (delegated knowledge, borrowed knowledge). However, it also reflected the representations made by the culturally dominant of the dominated, or even the dominated among themselves. The ERR chain of knowledge (see section 7.1) and the multiple borrowings from scientific referents other than those carried by language traditions resulted in an epistemological blockage around the nursing discipline. This blockage then confronted researchers who wished to develop scientific knowledge to solve the problems that the profession faced with the difficulty of choosing an identity for their own discipline. Disbelief, indifference, doubt and skepticism about a specificity of the nursing discipline, or even about its existence, were present at the end of the protodisciplinary period and at the beginning of the scientific period of knowledge until around 2010.

Scientifically, the discipline could not continue to refer to hell and demons ("*enfermière*"), nor could nursing continue to breastfeed. The nurse symbolically remains a feminine and religious emblem of a function. It is only an image. Moreover, this characteristic does not inform us at all about the "logic" of our knowledge, which often accompanies the stage of maturity of other disciplines. This problem concerns first and foremost the reflections of metatheorists, theorists and nursing researchers in the university environment. Indeed, nurses in the first field of practice (caring) are not directly concerned by this problem. They currently have other concerns. They also have a different status and salary than university researchers and work daily, facing their own problems without constantly questioning their identity. On the other hand, professors who work in nursing faculties or who participate in the development of the discipline as researchers are confronted with competition between disciplines and often have to explain to the governing or funding bodies of science why the sciences to which they belong are by nature nursing sciences (which is not obvious) and belong mainly to the humanities. As stated by Pépin *et al.* in a "reference document without equivalent in French, humanistic values are the driving force behind the authors' decision to include nursing among the human sciences" [PÉP 15]. It is not a question of creating or isolating a special group within the profession, but we know that the players in the four professional fields do not all do the same thing, do not all work in the same institutions and do not necessarily have the same reference knowledge. On the other hand, what connects these different actors is the fact that they were all once qualified as nurses and have all been confronted by experience with the knowledge conveyed by their discipline and the miseries of the human species.

Before finding its identity and its own "logic", a discipline often goes through several intermediate stages. Jean-Baptiste Lamarck was not a biologist before giving the name "biology" in 1802 to what was then called the "positive theory of the evolution of living beings", any more than Auguste Comte was a sociologist, before taking up the term "sociology" in 1839, a neologism coined by Abbé Sieyes some 50 years earlier and giving this name to "social physics". Similarly, the history of the Earth also became "geology" between 1830 and 1833, following Charles Lyell for his "principles of geology".

Nor is it a "health mediologist" who proposes before the time to give the disciplinary identity of "health mediology" to our knowledge [NAD 13]. The discipline of nursing is scientifically still "orphaned" in terms of its identity. Based on the recurrent association of the three MEDs, "*med*ium, *med*iation, cultural inter*med*iary" to qualify our practices, health mediology seems to us to be more faithful to the tradition of language to qualify our knowledge (Figures 10.4 and 12.1) than the symbolic reference "nursing science" currently used. We have mentioned the translation problems posed by these terms from French to English.

In the provision of services, it is always the recipients of our services who deliver the verbal or non-verbal information that is useful for the design and production of the service, and this, all over the world. This is a very interesting concept to study how nurses transform this information into deeds and words in the context of professional practice. This information comes from everywhere and makes the environment (medium) and the implementation of health mediations in a long occupied cultural intermediary posture in the institutional space and time of the health world, a singular space of languages specific to our knowledge (see Figure 12.1 and section 10.2.3). Let us recall the informational practice[1] already highlighted. In 2002, it represented up to 72% of a nurse's working day. Moreover, it is highly likely that, with the development of medical informatics, computerized care records and other digital innovations, such as access to data banks, informational practice will increase within coordination and management practices. Why not try to escape the symbolic representations imposed on nurses to find the logic and meaning that could scientifically structure our own knowledge?

Let us recall that it was from a somewhat hasty decision in 1977 to translate nursing as *sciences infirmières* in French without having demonstrated that the discipline was well ahead of the sciences, deserving the staff being called "*infirmières*" (nurses). What equivalence of meaning is there between nursing (breastfeeding) and *infirmière* (hell) (see Chapter 3)? An almost impossible translation that has the effect of presenting the discipline as an image or as a symbolic representation rather than from scientific representations. In terms of knowledge, "*donner le sein*" (to breastfeed) in English is not really confronting "*enfer*" in the French version. As a reminder, Nightingale never conceptualized the term nursing and it was a Canadian physician in the 1970s who proposed to Gallicize "*faculté de nursing*" by "*école des sciences infirmières*" [COH 02]. Therefore, conceptual research on the disciplinary identity of our knowledge remains to be done.

To this end, "remember that there is no consensus on the name of the discipline. Collière suggested calling it 'the care sciences' so as not to confuse the object of knowledge with the function of care. Nadot, for his part, suggests the expression health mediology, while Donaldson speaks of the science of the ecology of human personal and family health" [DAL 08a]. No univocal identity, no impossible translation between nursing and *soins infirmiers* (nursing care), no conceptualization of the symbolic terms in use, we are beginning to understand why the discipline is inaudible in the scientific sphere and in the political world.

Not only is there no consensus on the name of the discipline, but the academic world and its researchers to which the so-called "nursing" discipline belongs do not seem to be any clearer than that either. In what register of science does nursing research fit? It is sometimes found in the natural sciences, in the humanities (which seems the most logical way to take care of humans), in the life sciences, in the health

1 Combination of "information management" practices, "information gathering practices", "management and coordination practices", "professional relationship practices", "regulatory practices" (in 2002 represented between 57% and 72% of a nurse's workday) [NAD 02a, NAD 13].

sciences or in public health when it is not epidemiology or sociology. And even at a certain time (late 19th Century, early 20th Century), hospital sciences or household sciences were used as a register of attachment. How can we get out of this anomaly and the enigma conveyed by "normal science" and move on to what Kuhn called "extraordinary science" by manipulating "handling the same bundle of data as before, but placing them in a new system of relations with one another by giving them a different framework" [KUH 96]?

12.1. Why health mediology?

To deal with "Problem V" mentioned earlier (see the end of Chapter 11), we needed a new explanation of the possible identity of our disciplinary knowledge while keeping alive the link between the chosen identity and our language traditions. Indeed, we saw that the role of language traditions as a qualitative source of knowledge was important (Popper, Foucault) for the philosophy of science (see section 10.2), especially for a specific discipline such as nursing and its language traditions (see Rousseau, section 10.1).

The construction of knowledge is a long process in successive stages in which confrontation, reflection, rectification, rewriting, etc., lead the researcher to gradually approach a better understanding of the phenomena studied. It is indeed difficult to make a statement on care without first being concerned about a few definitions or objects of knowledge relating to the theoretical territories surrounding them. The task of any scientific discipline is "first to describe an empirical morphology (a corpus of empirical data) and then, once the description is complete, to provide an explanation" [NAD 93].

In the empirical morphology of knowledge in the lay period, we highlighted that hospital nurses were already establishing "acts of life mediation in a position of cultural intermediaries" (*ibid.*). We then proposed to replace the word "life" for life mediation by its Greek meaning "bios", which gave rise to the combination "biomediation" for life mediation. All that remained was to add the suffix "-logy" to refer to a science and thus to name the theory and assets resulting from life mediation (biomediatology). For a long time, our discipline has been without an identity that could constitute its "-logy". But a new semantic difficulty appeared. The act of mediation takes place well in an institutional living space (the hospital), but the term "biomediatology" was not sufficiently topical linguistically to give an indication of the action and knowledge of the caregiver as both a vector of sensitivities and a matrix of sociability. It was then that we remembered that one of the faults that altered the rest of civil society in the hospital of the 18th Century was the "lack of health" as it was represented at the time. Health was generally attributed to "salus" as a sign of preservation of life and the act of greeting to wish for health[2]. We then replaced without too many scruples "biomediatology" by "health mediology" to designate the action and the specific knowledge that accompanies it within the cultural system 3 (CS3), a cultural system that guides the reflexive practices that orient decisions (CS4) and that mobilizes caregivers in their projects [NAD 93].

The title "Health mediology" [NAD 92b] was first coined at a conference held at the January 1992 ARSI (*Association de recherche en soins infirmiers*) study days in Paris. This term, which was used in the author's doctoral thesis, is an extension of the neologism "mediology" which appeared in 1979 in his book "on intellectual power in France" in Régis Debray's *Cours de médiologie générale*, and which was the founding text of his course on general mediology. Health mediology "allows the healthcare worker to propose a set of means to avoid the appearance or excess of health problems (obstacles) or the lack of resources necessary to maintain both life and the reason for living" [NAD 93].

Definitions of course evolved. The first definition that could be given in 1992 to this science, which replaced the common meaning of "nursing science", was that health mediology could be seen as "the science that is formed from the institutional problems encountered in the practice of health mediation…" The fundamental science of the caring function, which refers to actions carried out between three value systems that are not in synergy (CS1, CS2, CS3), enables those responsible for preventing disease or restoring the health of a given population to guide their actions and explain their consequences. Health mediology is then "the science that studies the problems and theories that prevent the harmonious development of human life, despite the adverse conditions that affect humanity" [NAD 92]. It was in 2002, 10 years later, that a more substantial publication in the journal "*perspective soignante*" explained how to situate the new perspective of nursing knowledge:

> The discipline of healthcare constitutes its knowledge from the traces left by practices, both ancient and contemporary, and does not consist of prior knowledge from which it would only have to deduce its approaches. The matrix of the care discipline has the property of not being a fragmentary or residual component of dominant knowledge, nor composed of knowledge borrowed from other disciplines and applied to

2 For Collière, the salubrious term means "bearer of life" and comes from the word *salus, salutis,* which is an expression of the recognition of life [COL 82]. Saying "to your health" is still an opportunity today to toast a glass in one's hand to recognize in the other person that he or she is a "bearer of life".

> the practice in question for the circumstance (...). With the conceptual development of health mediology and its linguistic element which takes the place of so-called nursing sciences, it is also the identity of the discipline of healthcare practices and their knowledge which determines the identity of the person who refers to it and not the opposite as has been the case up to now. [NAD 02a]

While in the past, the nurse's identity was imposed by compromise on caregivers without any other form of reflection on their own knowledge, today it is their own knowledge and its combinations that determine the identity of those who refer to them. It is again through a contribution to a Canadian book in 2008 that theoretical and conceptual elements on the cultural intermediary model and its theory of "health mediology" are presented to readers [NAD 08].

To speak of health mediology for a health discipline such as nursing, a discipline, which seems to escape its own conceptualization because of the absence of basic research and references to language traditions, seems quite appropriate to the language of caring. Philosophy confirms this. For Debray, the term "mediology" is of course susceptible to extension. In this sense, the famous philosopher and writer particularly appreciates the extension health mediology to replace the old ecclesiastical term "*infirmier*" imposed on the discipline at the beginning of the 20th Century by dominant cultures. Health mediology can be used to give an account in terms of knowledge of the particularities of the position of cultural intermediary occupied in the practical field of healthcare and also to aim at a certain disciplinary autonomy.

This is precisely what the founder of the term "mediology" appreciates, as he sees no contradiction in the use and extension given to the term with his philosophy and his own reflections, especially on the language sciences. "The neologism of mediology is susceptible to extension and the title health mediology proves it with this beautiful idea of the mediation of life. An admirable name for the nursing function. Everything that concerns the transmission of knowledge and know-how belongs to the field of mediology. Michel Foucault would undoubtedly have been captivated by your words. Your fine work undeniably restores dignity to an entire profession by showing all the problems involved in the simplest gestures of hospital care"[3]. "With your research, you are opening up a new field in the history of hospital practices. I have no doubt that this will inspire further work in the future. I do not need to tell you how encouraging it is for all of us that you have chosen a

3 Letter from Régis Debray to Michel Nadot dated July 2, 1994.

mediological title"[4]. "I congratulate you on the progress you have made towards a certain degree of disciplinary autonomy"[5]. This was the disciplinary autonomy that was sought, finally recognized, at least by philosophy as a reflective science. Encouraged by Régis Debray's position of authority on the subject, it was then the moment to definitively give up replacing nursing science by "biomediatology" (study of life mediations). The term "health mediology" was then adopted. This term mediology does not lend itself so badly to health and respects the language traditions of the discipline (see Figure 12.1).

12.2. The identity of our knowledge and health mediology

In fact, being a health mediologist means applying the logistics of thought operations and using the symbolic power of languages in the health world. In health mediation, an evoked idea can indeed become a material force, allowing a patient to feel better after the interview with a nurse health mediator. And the logistics of the operations of thought concern all the nursing interlocutors and not only the patients. Health mediology (which we propose as a synonym or even as a replacement for nursing science or nursing knowledge) is naturally "in the singular since the theoretical territory examined is the one in which only the specific knowledge is found, i.e. the knowledge developed within the discipline" [DAL 08a]. Bordered, on the one hand, by the social sciences and, on the other, by the medical sciences, knowledge specific to the nursing discipline is even "at the cutting edge of the development of the human sciences in their efforts to promote a holistic vision of the human being" according to Hesook Susie Kim (1997), cited by Dallaire and Blondeau [DAL 02]. As we have seen, life, work and language, which are part of Foucault's epistemological trihedron of the social sciences and humanities [FOU 66], have been part of the daily life of the caregiver and his or her performance for generations.

A healthcare setting is an environment for transmitting and transporting messages. Meetings, symposiums, work sessions, carer–patient relationship, support, reception, relational practice, informational practice, regulatory practice, prevention messages, etc., are all part of this setting. These particular modalities of the professional relationship make it possible, through all kinds of messages, to put people in relation to each other or to objects which, without the nurse or her auxiliaries, would not have health mediology as a study of the cultural intermediary postures occupied by nurses, and the place of symbolic language in health

4 Letter from Régis Debray to Michel Nadot dated January 20, 1999.

5 Letter from Régis Debray to Michel Nadot dated August 19, 2003 [NAD 13].

institutions is therefore not exclusively concerned with a domain of objects, but with a domain of relationships. Relationship with the life and environment of the person receiving assistance in order to assume the latter; relationships through language transformed into deeds and words by the health mediologist.

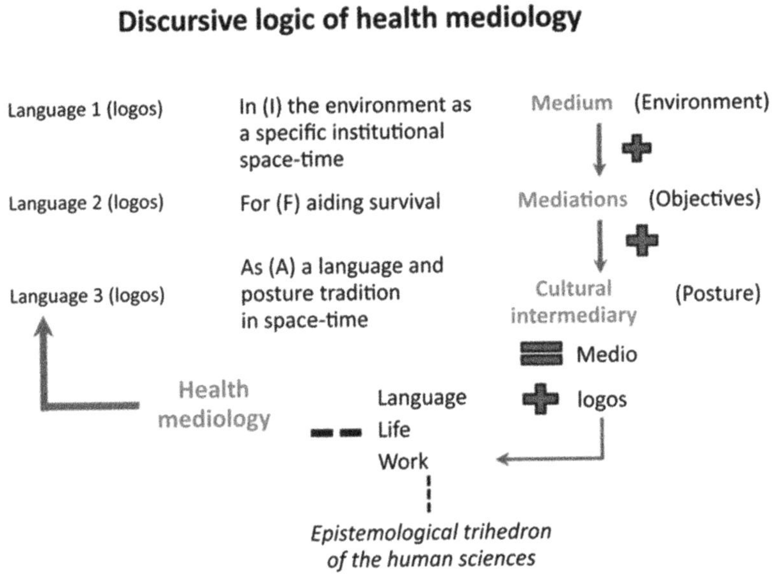

Figure 12.1. *The "3 MEDs" that determine the identity of the language of care in health mediology. For a color version of the figure, see www.iste.co.uk/nadot/nursing.zip*

The field of relations between all the languages used in the activity of institutional care since its inception seems to have become so complex that it is now diluted in a kind of language of managerial power in the health system. With information technologies, health costs that are difficult to control and the implementation of quality systems, the orders, prohibitions, rights and duties of one era are now replaced by good practice procedures and internalized principles that conform to the logic of the organization. The institution shapes practices and often invites its own actors to contribute to the improvement of their performances by the elaboration of their relational standards through quality systems. It is then for health mediology a question of restoring the place of nurses in a system which often tends to ignore them. It is a question of valuing and, making explicit, the implicit meaning of caring. Here, we value their languages, their skills, their reflexivity and the evolution of their practices. In fact, as a discipline, health mediology can study the various facets of the languages "that allow a symbol to be inscribed, transmitted, circulate and endure in human society" [DEB 93]. The words "care" and "care giving" have been part of these symbols for centuries[6].

Since language traditions also take place in a singular space and time, this space as a symbol (medium) also shows the peculiarity of language and its transformations. For example, taking care of the domain (*domus*) of the lay age, the "Household" as a place, became a gesture (one had to maintain upkeep the household, do the housework). With the arrival of the notions of hygiene, we moved on to "household sciences" which, associated with the governance of institutions, with the servants, "serving the institution", became in turn "hospital sciences". Adding knowledge in bacteriology and microbiology and we moved on to language, "hospital hygiene" and epidemiology in terms of knowledge.

In this language transformed into deeds and words, it was still a question of professional relations in a particular work environment, a space and time of speech, "The Hospital", today a medium, an institution that allows the exchange of linguistic codes. A relationship that cannot be denied between the clients of an institution, the nurse's representatives and the nurse's many interlocutors. And it is indeed through an area of relationship between life, language and work that the human sciences are constructed, in which health mediology (formerly nursing science) finds its place. "The human sciences are not an analysis of what man is by nature, but rather an analysis that extends between what man is in his positivity (living, working, speaking) and what enables this same being to know (or to seek to know) what life is, what the essence of work and its laws consist of and how he can speak about it" [FOU 66].

Acting in the "in-between" of a health institution (between oneself and others, between CS1, CS2, CS3, CS4, etc.) highlights languages, symbols on institutional assistance (technical, relational, informational) necessary to survive or to aid survival. These symbols (language acts or languages of action) are taught, transmitted and circulated from environment to environment within the health system. In the CS4 cultural intermediary position, the health mediologist nurse conveys messages from one place to another. By reflexivity, she transforms some of them into acts and gestures of care, others into information. It is a matter of carrying out a kind of techno-cultural mediation. In all cases, there are hierarchical receivers of differentiated messages. Those who connect the different worlds in which the recipients of health-related messages live and meet each other effectively and emotionally connect people who would not otherwise have done [NAD 13].

---

6 Even in the time of the hospital servants, it was known that "whoever transmitted signs meddled in serving; whoever served meddled in transmissions" [DEB 93].

This new disciplinary identity has been identified in North America since 2008. "The Swiss native Nadot, who proposes a cultural intermediary model to describe the nurse's professional activity has given, since 1992, the name of health mediology to the science or systematic study of our practices. For him, the discipline of healthcare or health mediology, refers to the study of the postures of cultural intermediaries such as nurses and the symbolic power of languages within an institution. He traces the origins of the cultural intermediary up to Nightingale and speaks of health mediations to designate the primary aspect of care, this relational and informational aspect" [PÉP 17]. Pelletier further notes that "llen (2004) reviewed several nursing research studies published between 1993 and 2003. Based on her review of recent ethnographic studies on the work of nurses, the author finds that the role of mediator in the healthcare system is now central to the nurse's contribution. As noted by several authors [NAD 01, DAL 02, NAD 03a, ALL 04], the nurse manages and negotiates multiple agendas and increasingly, she coordinates the work of others and acts as a mediator. Nadot's theoretical model compared to other approaches "is the one that best promotes awareness of the complexity of the professional role with its social, political, strategic, scientific and economic issues" [PEL 07].

With the posture of cultural intermediary, it is the third language space, the third element of the three-dimensional space specific to the caring function that appears. It combines the two previous ones (medium and mediation) by a language "in" the environment (medium) that translates the number 1 cultural system (CS1) and a language that establishes health mediations. It is now a language as a "cultural intermediary" that can be highlighted. In/for/as (IFA) is a linking principle that has long brought together the significant terms of the language of care, but it is only now that they can be highlighted (Figure 12.1). It is a bit like trying to "make mayonnaise" by analogy. You cannot remain with eggs, oil and vinegar lying side by side in terms of knowledge. We must try to homogenize this knowledge, to give a fruitful assembly to all the subsequent knowledge produced by research (see Figure 11.4). The terms in Figure 12.1 also indicate, at the same time and in order, a space (logos 1), a goal (logos 2) and a posture (logos 3). It is therefore not on health, illness and treatment that the standardization of knowledge related to institutional care explicitly begins.

It is the reception, the care of the struggling human being and the logistics required for the living and working community to function that bring together the first knowledge of care. The governesses of the past governed, they made institutions work. This is also what Florence Nightingale did in Crimea; she improved the functioning of English military hospitals. By focusing exclusively on "care" and the illnesses that require it, the profession leaves aside the skills required so that the human, the object of care, can continue to receive it properly. Today, there are fewer small papers, various notebooks, *Kardex*, etc., which are used to treat patients, than in the past. But with a world of digitized data (computerized care records, for example) created by the neo-liberal economy and not necessarily adapted to the needs of a population, the luxury of an elite is emerging [KIE 19]. Today, there is a lot of computerized, digitized data, more cost accounting of the services provided, more sound or visual perceptions coming from technology, the care environment or the economic-managerial approach at work in the health world.

To "care" yesterday as today is still to capture information, languages, decode them, question them and develop by reflexivity know-how not devoid of meaning. This knowledge enables us to manage space and time (logistical, organizational and domestic activities), to take care of the group (social activities that are not free of conflicts, fights and order) and to take care of people (in the sense of paying attention to), while providing specialized help as a "cultural intermediary" in the institutional activities of daily life. If we remove the recent knowledge about the discipline, represented by the colored pins in Figure 11.5, we soon realize that the traditions of the language of care over the centuries (green ball in Figure 11.4) have enabled the development of capacities for:

– running an organization;

– connecting with others;

– care giving;

– aiding survival;

– sympathizing with the miseries of life;

– observing what is going on, what exists;

– developing empathy, feeling, anticipating;

– moving, perceiving, acting;

– communicating;

– using intervention protocols;

– following procedures, technical or relational modalities.

The conceptual cultural intermediary model published in 2013 [NAD 13] outlines the full scope of a health mediologist's activity and introduces modern elements related to the evolution of our healthcare institutions. It gives institutional care language on practices, the *logos* it currently lacks. We know very well, following Bourdieu, that "practice is always underestimated and under-analysed, and yet understanding it requires much theoretical competence, much more, paradoxically, than understanding a theory (…) scientists are not necessarily able to invest in their descriptions of their practices the theory that would enable them to have and to give a real knowledge of these practices" [BOU 04]. The cultural intermediary model, based on original lay knowledge, follows the evolution of this knowledge and thus highlights complex, humanistic, reflexive, dynamic and innovative care knowledge, nourished at the same time by material, empirical and theoretical aspects and loaded with implicit cultural models.

While there is today an academic space in the so-called "nursing" sciences that allows the production of new knowledge and scientific journals to disseminate it, it is because there are living and committed actors who devote time to think, seek to understand, produce and write. This model integrates various care theories, from the oldest to the most recent, and values statements transmitted from generation to generation over several centuries. For Marie-Ange Coudray, former director of a training institute for health executives in France and former educational advisor to the French Ministry of Health, "the strength of the cultural intermediary model lies in its lucidity and coherence" [NAD 13, foreword].

The title "health mediology" gives the discipline a more constructed identity than the generic term "nursing science". For Coudray, "the construction around health mediology appears to be a happy future for the nursing profession. It allows us to look at all the facets of this profession, to feel its social usefulness in the diversity of its actions and the complexity of its mediations, to evaluate its impact and to continue its construction" [NAD 13, foreword]. In this conceptual model, as we have already mentioned, the nurse "health mediologist" offers services to at least three beneficiary groups, groups which do not necessarily work in synergy (the people being cared for, the medical profession and the institutional care environment). We have almost forgotten: the nurse is not "only" there for the patients as we sometimes hear! This is precisely what this new conceptual model in nursing science strongly demonstrates. Apart from knowing how to give care to patients and training their auxiliaries, what else do nurses do (at the risk of sometimes leaving their health at risk) to ensure that their activity is fully efficient and economically considered? With this questioning, we leave an interest centered almost exclusively on "caring for people" to discover the interest in focusing on the space and time of languages and the real reflexive activity of nurses demanded in order to "provide a service to all the beneficiaries of service provision" within health institutions.

13

A Return to Image: "Where Do We Go Now"?

With the title of this 13th chapter, which is also an emblematic nod to a Lebanese film by the director, screenwriter and actress Nadine Nabaki, the aim of this review is to quickly take stock of the state of thinking and perspectives around the knowledge of the discipline known as "nursing".

If we come from where we know, it is possible now to know where we are going. Despite a great deal of scientific work that proves the central role that nurses play in the functioning of health institutions, despite a high level of sympathy in civil society, it is still not clear what a nurse does and why training today must be done in nursing faculties or universities. At the beginning of the 21st Century, the foundations of the nursing discipline still seem to be a mystery. Already present in the French-speaking part of Switzerland around 1979[1], the introduction of the term "nursing sciences" in nursing curricula in France in 2009 still raises questions about the passage of nurses through the university: in which faculty? What are "the scientific foundations on which our fields of knowledge are based with regard to this entry into the academic world" [HOM 12]?

The absence of synthesis on the source of existing knowledge and an excessive timidity in the exercise of criticism of the knowledge produced does not really help to distinguish the characteristics of the nursing discipline in the midst of other disciplines. Today, many people provide care professionally without necessarily

1 Thanks to the dissemination of the reflections of Rosette Poletti, then director of the Le Bon Secours School of Nursing in Geneva [POL 79] and those of Évelyne Adam, associate professor in the Faculty of Nursing at University of Montreal [ADA 79].

being qualified as "nurses". The traditions of language and knowledge accumulated over centuries in healthcare institutions probably deserve better. The economic value of the services[2] provided by nurses will one day also have to be indicated. The cost accounting of hospitals is not yet able to account for the work done by them, and as a result, insurance companies are struggling to finance the services provided to different beneficiaries and health costs are increasing. Discursivity about implicit, tacit knowledge and the context of knowledge production are involved in the construction of the nursing discipline. Moreover, contrary to the beliefs and representations of current practices, the nurse has never had enough time to devote to the sick, and the sick have never been the sole beneficiaries of the services provided by nurses. Who then benefits from the services provided by nurses and their assistants? There is a lack of explanation on the subject!

In fact, to avoid the dispersion of knowledge, to identify it in the long term, to give a certain homogeneity to this knowledge, it consists of conceptualizing at the same time, the traditional feminine household sciences (which nurses do not/no longer want to hear about!), the hospital sciences derived in hospital hygiene knowledge, the sciences of organizations (often hidden in care theories!), the human sciences including within them nursing sciences (not truly integrated yet!) and biomedical sciences (often overvalued!).

13.1. An intergenerational continuity of knowledge

However, it can be shown that the languages carried by the nursing discipline are transmitted from generation to generation, pass through time and social events and often undergo cultural domination in the long term. This intergenerational transmission merits attention to the institutional environment in which the first care words were born. The hospital is changing, but professional knowledge continues to be transmitted horizontally between peers, even when there are schools. The lack of basic research in nursing faculties also explains why the nursing discipline has been slow to position itself in the university environment. It was hard to see women positioning themselves in the scientific field to talk about their discipline in the 18th Century. Their status, especially for the underprivileged classes, the working classes and the servants, did not allow it. What is also important to note is that the practical languages of the nursing discipline identified in the diagram in Figure 13.1 are transmitted from generation to generation in space and pass through time without great difficulty with the events of society. This language does not necessarily belong to

2 The nursing profession in the economic world today is certainly in the tertiary sector, that of services.

a single country. It can cover several continents in an almost identical way with a few temporal variables, particularly in the French-speaking world[3]. And it is only when this knowledge passes through the door of the university that it is called upon to become a discipline.

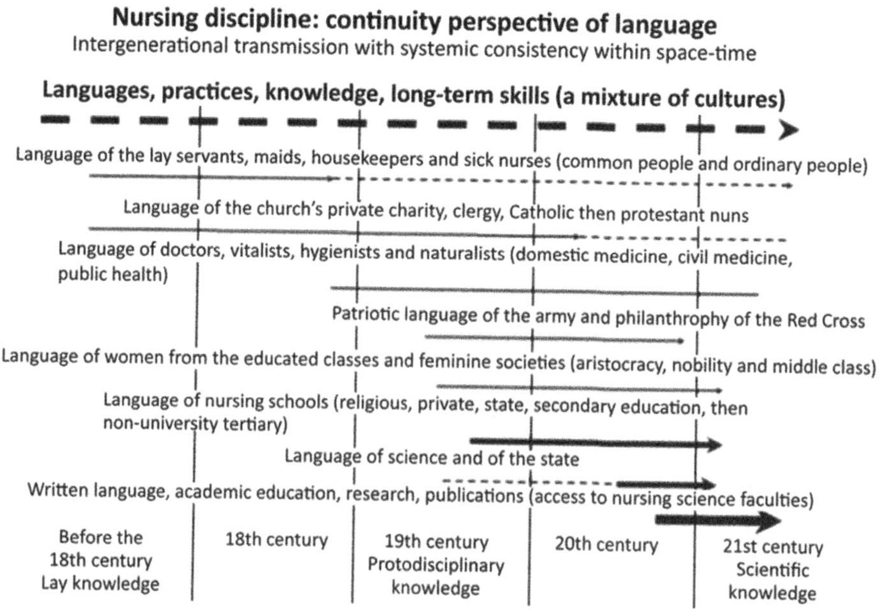

Figure 13.1. *Continuity of caregiver language over the long term [NAD 12a]*

These languages and those that have them often suffer long-term cultural domination. Think, for example, of the cultural domination by the Church at the end of the 18th Century (language of practical charity), by the Army around 1864 (patriotic and philanthropic language of the Red Cross) and by medicine (biomedical scientific language from the birth of the clinic). Then, the educated classes also sought to

3 Even in an era when the "Internet" did not yet exist, languages, ideas and types of care organization were slowly moving from one country to another, including from old Europe to North America. In the 19th Century, the elite of the nursing profession was aware of what was happening around the first schools of care simultaneously in France (Anna Hamilton), Switzerland (Valérie de Gasparin), Great Britain (Florence Nightingale), the United States (Elisabeth Blackwell) and Germany (Pastor Fliedner and the deaconesses of Kaiserswerth on the Rhine).

impose themselves in public health (the language of the aristocracy and/or the bourgeoisie), and finally, the state also came to impose itself, first in the field of health, then in the field of funding and recognition of higher education in nursing and research in the academic environment (see Figure 13.1).

Thus, in his report to the Ministry of Health and that of the Ministry of Higher Education, Research and Innovation in France, Le Bouler, responsible for an interministerial project that occupied the French government in 2018, states that "the development of advanced practices is in any case certainly an important aspect of the university integration of paramedical training" [LEB 2018]. Why especially "advanced practices" when there is not yet a consensus within the discipline on ordinary practices and the political or economic world does not know what they are made of? Between nursing circles reluctant to take on practices that do not belong to them and medical circles resistant to assigning new roles to nurses, it is not surprising to see controversies emerging around advanced practices. We could begin to verify whether the totality of ordinary practices carried by the discipline is currently taken into account in their complexity instead of only satisfying the political demand to fill medical deserts.

13.2. Ordinary practices before advanced practices

NOTE.– The Le Bouler report clearly shows the concern of the French government, but at the same time the ambiguity of the nursing profession in France (and sometimes in Quebec and French-speaking Switzerland) which is trying to promote "advanced practices" while the nursing profession is still struggling today to find a consensus to describe and explain scientifically at the global level, the foundations of "ordinary practice". What is the scientific name of the discipline and the specificity of its own university faculties? In which academic world does the care discipline find its place? To what science does the academic knowledge of institutional care belong? Here are some more questions that the profession must try to answer.

In Green Knowledge Theory (section 11.1), we can see how fundamental knowledge is constructed according to the nursing discipline's own orientations. It is the foundation of the fundamental knowledge specific to the discipline of nursing before the Nightingale era that had to be rediscovered. How, from yellow fundamental knowledge in nursing science and the energy mobilized by a doctor of nursing to carry out blue research, can green knowledge be manufactured? How can we avoid the dispersal of knowledge once research results have been published and how can we bring together and agglomerate the different productions of green knowledge? Behind multiple paradigms, different schools of thought find their place. A matrix basis needs to be created. The knowledge is there! It is on this (green) basis, instead of going nowhere, that the new green care theories come to be established (Figure 11.4). It is on this basis that the different types of knowledge produced by basic scientific research from the perspective of nursing are established. Who is motivated or interested today in funding basic research and the development of nursing knowledge and therefore the size of this green ball? In addition, we might ask how was basic research funded in comparison, in the 19th and the 20th Centuries for other academic disciplines in place long before the nursing discipline?

NOTE.– Not having been there at the right time (19th Century?) and in the right place (university?) is perhaps a chronic female intellectual disadvantage with which the nursing discipline must learn to live and overcome.

It was necessary to find historically what could make sense in our language traditions in order to create this place that would make it possible to give meaning to the different layers of our knowledge by bringing them together (Figure 10.7). New knowledge often builds on previous knowledge. The green modeling clay ball (Figure 11.4) can thus receive new knowledge. It can also continue to grow in size. Some basic knowledge probably needs to be refined, becoming more compact, more explicit and less volatile. If they are in line with the green logic, that of the growth of scientific knowledge, they can be integrated without further questioning into the care discipline, that is, the existing green ball. On the other hand, if they are of different colors, which is often the case in applied research, they focus on green knowledge without necessarily becoming homogeneous, without changing into green knowledge. This then remains useful knowledge for care practices, but it does not necessarily enrich the discipline. The knowledge produced falls short of disciplinary orientations and language traditions. It may be knowledge from another discipline (borrowed knowledge, delegated knowledge) and placed for the circumstance on the nursing discipline. Be careful, with borrowed knowledge and delegated knowledge, not to mask the fundamental knowledge of the nursing discipline so that it remains visible. It is still on this basis that so-called "advanced" practices of the CS2 type can be grafted on, provided that they respect the principles of the disciplinary perspective which, by its very essence, belongs to the human sciences. It was necessary to find a place, a soil, a fertile ground on which to grow the knowledge specific to the discipline of healthcare while remaining faithful to its traditions of green language (Figures 11.4 and 11.5). Knowledge can no longer be scattered only in the multiple documents produced by the profession and contained in publications. It can no longer float freely in the world of knowledge (Figure 11.1). It can and must attach itself to a hard core that has been built up over many centuries (Figures 10.7, 11.4 and 11.5). The growth of the green colored ball of clay (this is a picture) is indicative of the volume of knowledge in the discipline (Figure 11.4).

A faculty of nursing or health mediology[4] can then accommodate future researchers in the field.

While the dominant ideology in our healthcare systems today seems to place the patient at the center of the concerns of healthcare institutions (that is what they say!), the close observation of a nurse's working day nevertheless makes us doubt the assertion. What if this fine speech simply served to gain acceptance for a measure of hospital productivity based on industrial models through quality systems? It is clear that the word "quality" does not mean the same thing to everyone. Let us not forget that "quality is part of a rhetorical strategy, which we use to legitimize our own interests and positions. When insurers talk about quality, they are talking about cost containment, while doctors, families and nurses also take into account the living environment of their patients" [ABR 12]. No less than 42 Swiss associations were concerned about the quality of care in 2018 without the nursing discipline being mentioned in the documents. Isn't the medical narrative which "sometimes served to create a myth of omnipotence, a discourse aimed at reassuring people or exploiting their naivety" [KIE 19] just as present behind "omnipresent marketing and the emergence of gigantic digital powers" at the service of quality systems? This book then shows that the knowledge used by nurses over the long term enables them to offer quality of service, with a view to respecting the integrity of the people being cared for, ensuring the quality of the service provided to the medical profession and preventing organizational chaos within institutions. On what knowledge are the different practices based and how much are they charged to the different beneficiaries of the service provision? While we talk every year about the increasing health costs and the overload of nurses at work, no one knows!

A minority within the profession, nursing researchers and their research findings are often unknown to politicians, the insurance industry, publishers, the media[5] or the healthcare community. Not only do the research results do not reach the average politician, but they are also often not well known to the public or the manager of a health insurance fund, but the very fact that there may be a discipline specific to healthcare simply escapes any perception or argument that would allow us to escape the existing "big do-it-yourself" approach to the reimbursement of healthcare. Who trains the various people responsible for the governance of health systems on the discipline of nursing? It seems that only medicine is financed. The meaning of the

4 "In mediology, mediology does not mean media or medium but mediations, that is to say, the dynamic set of procedures and intermediate bodies that are interposed between a production of signs and a production of events" [DEB 94].

5 Note, for example, that nursing sections in bookstores or with some health science publishers are generally difficult to find. One finds the "medicine" or "medical sciences" section, sometimes even the "paramedical" category, at best "nursing" or "health sciences".

word "care" differs according to whether it is used by male or female parliamentarians and according to whether the parliamentarian is a member of the party in power or of a political grouping more to the left on the chessboard. As a scientific study conducted by the Research and Development Unit of the Haute école spécialisée La Source à Lausanne on the revision of the Swiss Health Insurance Act (2008) shows, "efforts to reconceptualize healthcare are in any case hampered by a number of culturally embedded ideas" [GAI 09].

Politicians do not really have time to waste trying to verify their perception of nurses. Everyone knows what a nurse looks like and what she does! It is true, within society, nurses have a strong potential for sympathy (what a wonderful vocation that can be exploited to the fullest!). Students are attracted to university studies in nursing. But at the same time, they often leave the profession after only a few years of practice! This also means that there is little return on investment in terms of training (new schools, status of professors and researchers, publications). Lack of recognition? Low salary, perhaps? Not only that. On the other hand, the dilution of tasks in an amalgam of knowledge that is difficult for politicians and leaders of health-related institutions to grasp seems to be a problem that might be worth studying. We see terms being used to show that nurses can exercise their power (nursing power, nursing leadership), but this is more an injunction to implement decisions made at the health system level than to participate themselves in decisions affecting both the population's need for care and the profession's need to develop its own discipline. We cannot be concerned only with the needs of the population, and we are not alone in this concern, if at the same time we are prevented, inhibited or powerless to produce knowledge useful to the services provided. Hart (2004), quoted by Dallaire, even states that nurses are more compelled to implement decisions made by the Department of Finance "in response to multiple national and international economic pressures" [DAL 13] than to be attentive to the needs of the people who benefit from their services and to promote the knowledge developed by their own discipline.

It is not surprising, therefore, that the workload of nurses poses problems in terms of recognition and optimal staffing. The great do-it-yourself approach to care reimbursement is much more dependent on images, prejudices and symbolic and social representations of nurses than on the knowledge they actually apply within the care discipline. The role of nurses in supervising their nursing auxiliaries, trainee students and volunteers in action is rarely taken into account at the economic level. Yet, they are the ones who train all these people. The structure of the discipline (CS3), the service provided to the medical profession (CS2) and to health institutions (CS1) remain at a level implicit in the function. "Care is imbued with implicit meanings and can therefore be used to mean different things. It is difficult to engage in discussion or to involve representatives of care in policy discussions when there are so many implicit meanings" [DAL 13]. These implicit meanings have accumulated over the long term, especially in the political world, and represent a body of knowledge that has never really been taken into account. It is precisely this implicit knowledge contained in reflexive knowledge that inhabits the three stages of knowledge according to our five layers of knowledge schematized in Figure 10.7.

Subject to struggles for influence and power, the nursing discipline, which includes approximately 1,055,982 healthcare professionals in part of the French-speaking world (Quebec, France, Belgium, Switzerland, Lebanon) and more than 3.5 million in the United States, is struggling to mark its place in the world of knowledge. And yet, it is indeed within the university that the notion of discipline was born. Not everyone has access to the academic world. The three periods of knowledge that structure the nursing discipline in a complex (heterogeneous and multicultural) way over the long term have slowly and progressively developed without everyone's knowledge because they are intertwined around multiple images and symbolic representations that continue to dominate the role of women, the role of hospitals and the power of medicine in society between the 18th and 21st Centuries.

Conclusion

The object of struggles for influence and power that allow a discipline to make its place in the world of knowledge, nursing today seems to be in a position identical to that of physicians in the period immediately preceding the birth of the clinic. Indeed, in order for the medical discipline to be recognized as scientific, particularly in the United States throughout the 19th Century, power games, tensions and struggles for influence allowed graduate doctors of medicine (regulars) to establish themselves and gain the upper hand over the crowd of competing unqualified empirical practitioners, traditional healers, midwives and other practitioners "who had dominated the medical scene in the United States throughout the 19th century" and "ensured the true medical profession a lasting monopoly of the medical arts" [EHR 15]. These "regular" physicians were "almost always more expensive than their competitors without credentials". Regular doctors "almost exclusively treated members of the middle and upper classes who could afford the prestige of being treated by a 'gentleman' of their own class" [EHR 15]. Their formal studies meant little, even by European standards at the time. "The regulars, because of their close links with the ruling class, were able to influence legislation" [EHR 15]. This is probably still the weak point of the nursing profession today! Indeed, when reading the legislation on the nursing profession in several countries, it is difficult to perceive the cost and scientific anchoring of the discipline's own knowledge. Add to this religious, lay, domestic and feminine components and we will have all the dimensions necessary to understand the difficulty of the emergence of care as a body of knowledge in an institutional framework. But this body of knowledge, which exists in a fragmentary way, also probably lacks homogeneity (it is not yet "homemade mayonnaise"!).

Nurses' access to university did not, however, mark the beginning of basic scientific research within their own discipline. When the first academic nurses referred to science, it was above all a reference to knowledge borrowed from hygiene, biomedical science or the human and social sciences. Penetrating new spaces of knowledge (unity) and normative language (science) exposed the first Academic nurses to use the symbolic language they heard around them. University nursing in North America is a "discourse on" care, but not yet a sign of an existing core discipline. Rather, it is a matter of training good care directors and managers or good teachers, as is the case in Europe with the creation of executive schools. It is also implicitly about trying to become sociologically a profession first before thinking about defining the discipline or nursing science. Epistemology in nursing was not one of the issues on the agenda at the birth of the discipline and hardly finds its place in the first university nursing programs. Care theories, first from the United States (1960) and then the creation of various nursing faculties, reinforced the idea of the advent of nursing. A structure of higher education at the university level was put in place. We agree that nursing is a disciplinary field in which new knowledge is developed. The *ministère français de l'Enseignement Supérieur, de la Recherche et de l'Innovation* (French Ministry of Higher Education, Research and Innovation) was not mistaken. On October 30, 2019, the Council of Ministers adopted a decree that paves the way for the creation of three qualification sections of the *Conseil national des universités en sciences infirmières* (National Council of Universities in nursing sciences) (CNU 92), in maieutics (CNU 90), and in re-education and rehabilitation sciences (CNU 91). This allows nursing sciences to leave the "paramedical" and to take an important step towards their attractiveness and recognition[1]. But much remains to be done and it is not a foregone conclusion! Even with this 92nd scientific section, future research professors will not spare the effort to explain why nursing is a discipline in the humanities in its own right in the health sciences (we take care of humans by helping them to survive, don't we?). They will have to explain its origin, nature and scope. What is this disciplinary field in which knowledge is produced and what knowledge is produced? At the university level, the disciplines will be in competition. Nursing will have to be careful to distinguish itself from other health disciplines in order to avoid confusion and amalgamation of knowledge, and to protect itself from the desires and aims of other disciplines and related disciplines. This means not only raising the status of training, but also subsequently enriching the discipline specifically, instituting forums for reflection and producing and disseminating scientific knowledge so that it is recognized.

1 Among the texts published in the *Journal officiel de la République Française* on November 30, Decree No. 2019-1107 of October 30, 2019, which amends Decree No. 87-31 of January 20, 1987, has the strongest symbolic significance as it replaces the "*Conseil national des universités pour les disciplines médicales, odontologiques et pharmaceutiques*" with the "*Conseil national des universités pour les disciplines de santé*". The three new university sections (CNU 90, CNU 91 and CNU 92) will be hosted there.

With the development of research, including the beginnings of basic research in Europe towards the 2000s, it is also the production and dissemination of scientific knowledge and its recognition[2] within the Cité Scientifique that is taking center stage. As the study conducted for SIDIIEF in 2015 notes, based on humanistic values, the knowledge produced by the nursing discipline "is consistent with that of the human, social and health sciences" [PÉP 15]. The nursing discipline is therefore not in the order of nature, as some researchers sometimes implicitly claim. Rather, it is the social sciences and humanities that should be looked at.

Moreover, as the Swiss Academy of Medical Sciences rightly points out, "the way nurses see it is more focused on the condition related to the disease rather than on the disease itself and is oriented towards assistance that will enable the daily control of impairments resulting from health disturbances" [ACA 07]. In other words, and to put it simply... Medicine deals with the illnesses of man and nursing science (health mediology) deals with man in his illnesses. In Switzerland, for example, a bachelor's degree in nursing is not a degree dependent on a bachelor's degree in medicine! One is in the natural sciences (medicine), the other in the humanities and social sciences (nursing science or health mediology). Hence, there is complementarity and non-interchangeability or subordination of the nursing role to the medical role. Nurses are not there to make up for the medical shortage either. They are already facing their own shortage and the development of the next generation. To position oneself well scientifically is also to find the right words to explain what one is doing. It also helps researchers to clarify the type of knowledge concerned by their research and makes it possible to make progress in strengthening the disciplinary identity that is still lacking today.

Despite the development of academic faculties of nursing or graduate schools of nursing, doctoral schools of nursing, scientific research aimed at producing new knowledge, despite the involvement of nurses in health promotion both in institutional settings and in private practice, the nature of the nursing discipline still seems to be an enigma. There is knowledge. But the polymorphism that consists of bringing together hybrid entities with knowledge from different disciplines around a common object represents nursing as a fragmented discipline [HOM 12]. The knowledge mobilized by a nurse, including tacit knowledge, is so varied that these varieties make it complex, and it is difficult to stick to the only dominant representations in order to account for the skills deployed on a daily basis. Often, when we realize the cost of nursing services, good souls, under various pretexts, take it upon themselves to set up hybrid training courses that are less expensive and, above all, lead to a diploma or a less remunerated qualification. We would so much like to have at our

2 Notably through funding and the allocation of research grants to the researcher.

disposal an "interchangeable pawn", who is nevertheless a learned one, capable of managing the uncertainty of care organizations on a daily basis and of meeting all the challenges encountered by the system. In 2018, for example, the Swiss regional press offered a post of "billing nurse" with an ES or HES diploma or a title deemed equivalent to "ensure that billing rules are applied" in a hospital in the canton of Vaud[3]. It should be remembered that in terms of knowledge as well as science, a discipline cannot be HES or ES (university or community colleges). In terms of knowledge and science, it is simply developed and taught at the highest level of the education system.

For more than 30 years, a group of professors, researchers and scientists in various nursing faculties, some with scientific skills identical to those of researchers in other disciplines, have been demonstrating that nursing practice is a complex practice of information management, a high-risk practice, a service provision essential to the functioning of the healthcare system. In spite of this, why are representations, work structures and available means not necessarily reviewed and adapted to the requirements of the service provided? More than that: the economic burden of highly qualified personnel is generally reduced by trying to lower the qualification level, especially if they have a university education[4]. In the political system, such highly trained personnel find nothing to complain about when they are qualified for the occasion as "skilled labor". Is the physician also part of the skilled workforce? Here, we see the weight of representations. Health is certainly expensive! But for years, we have also been denouncing the risks of errors, overloads, malfunctions, blockage of institutions, demotivation of nurses to work in the conditions that are theirs. Don't naïve representations of the nursing discipline also come at a certain cost?

Both in the training of students and within the dominant social representations, nursing knowledge is rarely situated as a dynamic and development of a specific culture. Nursing professors, political leaders, managers of health insurance funds or scientists in other disciplines continue to perceive nursing knowledge as synonymous with symbolic representations in which women are certainly useful, kind and caring, but must also retain the place once attributed by society at the end of the 18th or the beginning of the 19th Century. In particular, that of servants and nuns, auxiliaries involved in the care of the sick or in the greatness of hygiene and medicine. Representations not yet completely erased from collective representations. The

---

3 Journal *La Liberté* from September 24, 2018.

4 In French-speaking Switzerland, the basic diploma, Bachelor of Science in Nursing, is obtained at a university of applied sciences and is the first level of the international academic division of higher education, i.e. Bachelor, Master and Doctorate in Nursing (see Figure 10.1).

discipline is still looking for its place. It is not surprising that in France, for example, in terms of representations, "nursing thought is confiscated by medical thought" in the context of the university development of the training of Advanced Practice Nurses (IPA) as "new" medical auxiliaries [5] with semi-professional status [DEL 19b].

IMPORTANT.– What if, in the end, the nursing discipline was something quite different from what is scientifically talked about it in the 21st Century? In order to remain faithful to the language traditions that form the basis of the nursing discipline and to the critical analyses that make it possible to collectively construct new knowledge, is it not necessary to present a new arrangement of the knowledge in question?

In terms of a perspective for talking about the nature of the nursing discipline, should we not consider a subtle philosophical combination of knowledge related to historical representations of the ordinary social status of women[6], those who knew how to care for both a household and an estate. For the old hospital was often a large estate. In general, this work of hospital care is obscured and could explain in part the difficulty in identifying the characteristics of the knowledge required and the lack of analysis of the epistemological status of this knowledge. It includes a maternal role[7], a domestic role, a housewife role, with household functions[8], domestic functions and governance functions. As for the relationship with illness, it was, at the beginning of the institutionalization of care, that of a housewife with her family and guests, who, if necessary, often followed a doctor's recommendations with the help of "her servants". But with the development of hospitals, medicine and health systems towards the end of the 18th Century, these already complex traditional female functions of course continued to grow (to what extent?) in terms of values, knowledge, ideologies and skills.

But beware of the temptation to draw conclusions too quickly from this in order to say that, basically, the nursing discipline in the lay age only covered an ordinary

5 To avoid the use of "health care auxiliary" as a euphemism.

6 By status, we mean all the texts (laws, regulations, etc.) that define a person's situation or group in a given society, with the aim of communicating around oneself a social identity that is as precise or recognizable as possible.

7 The role is the dynamic aspect of the status. It is influenced by the actor's culture and personality.

8 In general terms, function is what a person must accomplish in order to play his or her role in a social group. In the hospital setting, there are often job descriptions for nurses.

function as a servant, a mother, a domestic helper[9] or a housekeeper. There was a risk of developing guilt at being just that! So, nothing very professional. Should the scientific period of knowledge be seen as a so-called advanced practice built on a new delegation of medical knowledge? Today's knowledge is neither one nor the other, quite the contrary, as we have just explained in this book! Even today, women's ordinary household and maternal work (care and cleanliness) and voluntary work, and the skills deployed to accomplish it, are unpaid and the volume of invisible service goods produced at this time escapes any modeling

At a time when there was a serious shortage of staff in healthcare institutions in 2018 and a time when university nursing education is filling up with students, we must still ask ourselves what place does nursing and its expert knowledge occupy in political and economic decisions in the health sector? We do not have to fill the medical shortage; it is not in the orientations of the discipline and its history. How are the complexities and demands of nursing care perceived? Faced with the economic demands of healthcare that often do not take into account the characteristics of the discipline (only medicine, cost accounting, medical informatics, etc.), there is a risk that nursing students will turn away from the greatness displayed by their profession. Nurses on duty risk becoming disillusioned with their daily reality, with the values they learned during their training and which do not correspond to the values and constraints operated blindly, particularly under pressure from health insurers who are completely unaware of the orientations of the nursing discipline within health institutions.

The nursing profession can no longer think only of care and the sick. It must also think about the environmental, structural, political, economic and scientific conditions for the production of knowledge and its use within the healthcare system. All the more so since "the economic-managerial approach to which politics has entrusted the answers to medicine does not offer any human and humanizing narrative" [KIE 19]. This may be the time for nurses to position themselves with their humanistic values and to make this known. Let us not forget that "the key position occupied by nurses within the organization, between doctors and patients, at the crossroads of technical and relational lines, designates them socially and practically as interfaces between the demands of the organization, those of therapy and those of the patients" [GRO 99]. This is not a revelation, but it seems that only nurses know this! Forced, but willing, to live with and for humans, the nurse is often faced with the uncertainty of their reactions, behaviors, motivations for living or dying, or desires. The traditional cultural intermediary role may be a politically and

9 It is not surprising that "nurses first appeared in Canadian statistics in the 1911 census and were identified as home helps" [COH 00].

economically sensible one to take into account if we want to avoid, for example, excessive waiting times in emergency departments and serious dysfunctions in healthcare institutions. In such cases, it is necessary to act in a coordinated manner on the environmental conditions that make care activities what they are, with all their risks. Today, as in the past, the nurse has many interlocutors. She has always had only the patients as clients. Several professions and human groups depend on the quality services provided by nurses.

At the heart of the healthcare system for a long time, the nurse supports the human object of care and attention in an environment that oppresses or overwhelms them. The profession is, of course, affected by economic turbulence and changes in direction or new issues in the health system. Despite this, through an increase in humanism, reflexivity, skills and adaptive competencies, they nonetheless pursue their mission properly. But at what cost and for how much longer? Scientific research and its imperatives in an academic environment are a requirement like any other for future nursing professors. They also have an obligation to produce new knowledge and to develop the knowledge carried by the nursing discipline and the health sciences in both basic and applied research, to innovate, disseminate and promote this knowledge (publications, conferences). Being well positioned scientifically also helps researchers to emancipate themselves from previous cultural dominations and avoids the collective professional imagination from projecting itself through advanced nursing practice into the conquest of new medical knowledge while clarifying the type of knowledge concerned by their research. The discipline known as “nursing” has its place in the university, but it must be capable of homogenizing the theories and the different schools of thought that are specific to it. It would then be possible, without necessarily seeking to relieve the medical profession of its responsibilities, but by assuming our own, to make progress in the emergence and strengthening of our knowledge and of a disciplinary identity which is still lacking today.

References

[ABR 12] ABRAHAM A., "Rhétorique de la qualité en médecine", *Horizons, le magazine suisse de la recherche scientifique*, no. 93, p. 25, 2012.

[ACA 94] ACADÉMIE FRANÇAISE, *Dictionnaire de l'Académie Française*, Chez la Veuve de Jean-Baptiste Coignard imprimeur ordinaire du Roy et de l'Académie Française avec Privilège du Roy, Paris, 1694.

[ACA 62] ACADÉMIE FRANÇAISE, *Dictionnaire de l'Académie Française*, 4th ed., Chez la Veuve B. Brunet, Paris, 1762.

[ACA 07] ACADÉMIE SUISSE DES SCIENCES MÉDICALES, "Les futurs profils professionnels des médecins et des infirmiers dans la pratique ambulatoire et clinique", *Bulletin des médecins suisses*, vol. 88, no. 46, pp. 1942–1952, 2007.

[ACT 80] ACTA NURSOLOGICA 3, "Première conférence francophone sur les théories de soins infirmiers", Geneva, Switzerland, 7–9 February 1980.

[ADA 79] ADAM E., *Être infirmière*, HRW Ltée, Montreal, 1979.

[ADA 83] ADAM E., *Être infirmière*, 2nd ed., HRW Ltée, Montreal, 1983.

[AUB 13] AUBIN J.-P., "Indisciplinés de toutes les disciplines, dispersez-vous !", *Hermès 67, la revue, Interdisciplinarité : entre disciplines et indiscipline*, 2013.

[AUF 96] AUFFRAY J.-P., *L'espace-temps*, Flammarion, Paris, 1996.

[AVA 91] AVANZINI G., *L'école d'hier à demain, des illusions d'une politique à la politique des illusions*, Érès, Toulouse, 1991.

[BAC 83] BACHELARD G., *La formation de l'esprit scientifique*, Librairie philosophique J. Vrin, Paris, 1983.

[BAC 84] BACHELARD G., *Le nouvel esprit scientifique*, 16th ed., Presses universitaires de France, Paris, 1984.

[BAL 93] BALY M., *Florence Nightingale à travers ses écrits*, InterEditions, Paris, 1993.

[BAN 99] BANCEL-CHARENSOL L., DELAUNAY J.-C., JOUGLEUX M., "Une société de services, comment gérer des biens invisibles ?", *Sciences humaines*, no. 91, pp. 36–39, February 1999.

[BAR 99] BARTES Y., "Commentaires", *Cahiers de la sécurité intérieure : une approche réflexive du partage entre savoir expert et savoir profane, " Risque et démocratie "*, no. 38, pp. 219–220, 1999.

[BAT 05] BATES C., DODD D., ROUSSEAU N. (eds), "Introduction", in *Sans frontières, quatre siècles de soins infirmiers canadiens*, Presses de l'université, Ottawa, 2005.

[BEN 91] BENDER P., "La genèse et le contenu de la Convention du 20 mai 1976", in VALSANGIACOMO E. (ed.), *La Croix et la carrière, la Croix-Rouge suisse et l'histoire des infirmières*, Schwabe & Co AG, Bâle, 1991.

[BEN 17] BENDAOUD M.L., CALLENS S., *New Health Systems: Integrated Care and Health Inequalities Reduction*, ISTE Ltd, London and Elsevier Ltd, Oxford, 2017.

[BER 04] BERTHELOT J.-M., *Les vertus de l'incertitude*, Quadrige/Presses universitaires de France, Paris, 2004.

[BLO 75] BLOCH O., WARTBURG W., *Dictionnaire étymologique de la langue française*, 6th ed., Presses universitaires de France, Paris, 1975.

[BOK 18] BOKOBZA M., *Madame la comtesse de Gasparin, protestantisme radical, genre et pèlerinage au XIXe siècle*, L'Harmattan, Paris, 2018.

[BOT 84] BOTTÉRO J., "La magie et la médecine règnent à Babylone", in LE GOFF J., SOURNIA J.-C. (eds), *Les maladies ont une histoire*, L'histoire/Le Seuil, Paris, 1984.

[BOT 87] BOTTÉRO J., *Mésopotamie, l'écriture, la raison et les dieux*, Gallimard, Paris, 1987.

[BOU 70] BOURDIEU P., PASSERON J.C., *La reproduction, éléments pour une théorie du système d'enseignement*, Les Éditions de Minuit, Paris, 1970.

[BOU 82] BOURDIEU P., *Ce que parler veut dire, l'économie des échanges linguistiques*, Fayard, Paris, 1982.

[BOU 84] BOURDIEU P., *Questions de sociologie*, Les Éditions de Minuit, Paris, 1984.

[BOU 04] BOURDIEU P., NICE R., *Science of Science and Reflexivity*, University of Chicago Press, Chicago, 2004.

[BRA 10] BRAUNSCHWEIG S., FRANCILLON D., *Cultiver les valeurs professionnelles, 1910-2010, 100 ans de l'ASI*, Médecine & Hygiène, Geneva, 2010.

[BRO 98] BROCARD N., "Soins, secours et exclusion. Établissements hospitaliers et assistance dans le diocèse de Besançon XIVe et XVe siècles", *Annales littéraires de l'université de Franche-Comté*, Besançon, 1998.

[BRU 02] BRUNHES H., "L'enseignement ménager en Suisse et particulièrement dans le canton de Fribourg", *La revue municipale de Paris*, pp. 3499–3504, January 1902.

[BUG 04] BUGNON-MORDANT M., "Cet endoctrinement qui passe par PISA", *La Liberté*, 16 December 2004.

[CAB 89] CABANIS P.J.G., *Du degré de certitude de la médecine*, Éditions de la Cité des Sciences et de l'Industrie, Paris, 1989.

[CAH 85] CAHIER-BUCCELLI G., "L'hôpital général de Genève à une époque charnière (1676-1712)", in LESCAZE B. (ed.), *Sauver l'âme, nourrir le corps, de l'hôpital général à l'hospice général de Genève, 1535-1985*, Hospice général et Bernard Lescaze, Geneva, 1985.

[CAR 86] CARRÈRE J.-B., *Manuel pour le service des malades ou précis de connaissances nécessaires aux personnes chargées du soin des malades, femmes en couche, enfans nouveaux-nés, & cc*, Lamy Libraire, Paris, 1786.

[CHA 79] CHARLES G., *L'infirmière en France d'hier à aujourd'hui*, Le Centurion, Paris, 1979.

[COH 00] COHEN Y., *Profession infirmière, une histoire des soins dans les hôpitaux du Québec*, Presses de l'Université, Montreal, 2000.

[COH 02] COHEN Y., PÉPIN J., LA MONTAGNE E. *et al.*, *Les sciences infirmières, genèse d'une discipline*, Presses de l'Université, Montreal, 2002.

[COL 82] COLLIÈRE M.-F., *Promouvoir la vie. De la pratique des femmes soignantes aux soins infirmiers*, InterÉditions, Paris, 1982.

[COL 88] COLLIÈRE M.-F., "Une histoire usurpée… L'histoire des femmes soignantes ", *Cahier de l'AMIEC – Pour une histoire des soins et des professions soignantes*, no. 10, pp. 23–45, 1988.

[COL 92] COLLIÈRE M.-F., "Difficultés rencontrées pour désentraver l'histoire des femmes soignantes", in WALTER F. (ed.), *Peu lire, beaucoup voir, beaucoup faire. Pour une histoire des soins infirmiers au XIXe siècle*, Zoé, Geneva, 1992.

[COL 94] COLLIÈRE M.-F., *Virginia Henderson, la nature des soins infirmiers*, Éditions du renouveau pédagogique, Saint-Laurent, 1994.

[COL 96] COLLIÈRE M.-F., *Soigner… Le premier art de la vie*, InterÉditions, Paris, 1996.

[CON 16] CONFÉDÉRATION SUISSE, Loi fédérale sur les professions de la santé (LPSan) du 30 septembre 2016, Law, Assemblée fédérale de la Confédération suisse, 30 September 2016.

[CRO 42] CROIX-ROUGE SUISSE, *Bulletin des gardes-malades*, no. 4, pp. 62–80, 15 April 1942.

[CRO 59] CROIX-ROUGE SUISSE, *Revue suisse des Infirmières*, no. 4, pp. 101–136, April 1959.

[CRO 60] CROIX-ROUGE SUISSE, *Revue suisse des Infirmières*, no. 10, pp. 305–340, October 1960.

[CSS 10] CSST, Recherche dans les hautes écoles spécialisées de Suisse, Coups de projecteur sur son état de développement, Recommendations, Conseil suisse de la science et de la technologie, February 2010.

[CUS 86] CUSENIER R., "L'hôpital de Montbéliard vers l'an 1500", *Bulletin de la Société d'Émulation de Montbéliard*, no. 109, 1986.

[DAL 02] DALLAIRE C., BLONDEAU D., "Le savoir infirmier : une problématique", in GOULET O., DALLAIRE C. (eds), *Les soins infirmiers, vers de nouvelles perspectives*, Gaëtan Morin Éditeur, Boucherville, 2002.

[DAL 08a] DALLAIRE C., AUBIN K., "Les soins infirmiers, les sciences infirmières ou la science infirmière", in DALLAIRE C. (ed.), *Le savoir infirmier, au coeur de la discipline et de la profession*, Gaëtan Morin, Montreal, 2008.

[DAL 08b] DALLAIRE C. (ed.), "Le savoir profane dans le savoir infirmier", in *Le savoir infirmier : au cœur de la discipline et de la profession*, Gaëtan Morin, Montreal, 2008.

[DAL 13] DALLAIRE C., "Entre sens politique des infirmières et réceptivité de la société, quelles voies sont à envisager ?", in CHAGNON V., DALLAIRE C., D'ESPINASSE C. *et al.* (eds), *Prendre soin : savoirs, pratiques, nouvelles perspectives*, Presses de l'université Laval, Quebec, 2013.

[DAL 15] DALLAIRE C., "La difficile relation des soins infirmiers avec le savoir", *Recherche en soins infirmiers*, no. 121, pp. 18–27, June 2015.

[DEB 79] DEBRAY R., *Le pouvoir intellectuel en France*, Ramsay, Paris, 1979.

[DEB 93] DEBRAY R., *L'État séducteur*, Gallimard, Paris, 1993.

[DEB 94] DEBRAY R., *Manifestes médiologiques*, Gallimard, Paris, 1994.

[DEB 00] DEBRAY R., *Introduction à la médiologie*, Presses universitaires de France, Paris, 2000.

[DEB 08] DEBOUT C., "Théories de soins infirmiers, un retour sur l'histoire", *Soins, la revue de référence infirmière*, no. 724, pp. 28–31, April 2008.

[DEB 10] DEBOUT C., EYMARD C., ROTHAN-TONDEUR M., "Une formation doctorale dans la filière infirmière : plus-value et orientations dans le contexte français", *Recherche en soins infirmiers*, no. 100, pp. 134–144, March 2010.

[DEG 37] DE GASPARIN A., *Rapport au Roi sur les Hôpitaux, les hospices et les services de bienfaisance*, Imprimerie royale, Paris, April 1837.

[DEG 54] DE GASPARIN V., *Des corporations monastiques au sein du protestantisme*, vol. 1, Librairie Meyrueis, Paris, 1854.

[DEG 55] DE GASPARIN V., *Des corporations monastiques au sein du protestantisme*, vol. 2, Librairie Meyrueis, Paris, 1855.

[DEG 60a] DE GASPARIN A., *École normale de gardes-malades à Lausanne. Premier compte-rendu*, Imprimerie Georges Bridel, Lausanne, 1860.

[DEG 60b] DE GASPARIN A., *Les perspectives du temps présent. Quatrième série de discours prononcés à Genève*, Ch. Meyrueis et Cie, Paris, 1860.

[DEG 78] DE GASPARIN V., *Voyage au Levant par l'auteur des horizons prochains, tome 1, La Grèce, l'Égypte et la Nubie*, 4th ed., Calmann Lévy éditeur, Paris, 1878.

[DEG 86] DE GASPARIN A., *Questions diverses*, 3rd ed., Calmann Lévy éditeur, Paris, 1886.

[DEL 87] DELAUNAY J.-C., GADREY J., *Les enjeux de la société de service*, Presses de la fondation nationale des sciences politiques, Paris, 1987.

[DEL 19a] DELMAS P., "Pratique avancée infirmière : les occasions ratées de la profession", *Santé mentale*, no. 234, pp. 6–7, January 2019.

[DEL 19b] DELMAS P., "La notion d'IPA ne se limite pas à l'exercice d'une pratique médicale !", infirmiers.com (accessed 13 April 2019), available at: https://www.infirmiers.com/profession-infirmiere/presentation/la-notion-d-ipa-ne-se-limite-pas-a-l-exercice-d-une-pratique-medicale.html, 2019.

[DEM 99] DE MUNCK J., *L'institution sociale de l'esprit*, Presse universitaires de France, Paris, 1999.

[DES 19] DESCHAMPS J., *Mediation: A Concept for Information and Communication Sciences*, ISTE Ltd, London and Wiley, New York, 2019.

[DIÉ 87] DIÉBOLT E., "Les savoirs infirmiers", *Revue de l'infirmière*, no. 2, pp. 43–46, January 1987.

[DIÉ 88] DIÉBOLT E., COLLIÈRE M.-F., "Présentation", *Cahier de l'AMIEC – Pour une histoire des soins et des professions soignantes*, no. 10, pp. 18–21, 1988.

[DIÉ 90] DIÉBOLT E., *La maison de santé protestante de Bordeaux, (1863-1934), vers une conception novatrice des soins et de l'hôpital*, Érès, Toulouse, 1990.

[DON 03] DONZÉ P.-Y., *Bâtir, gérer, soigner. Histoire des établissements hospitaliers de Suisse romande*, Georg éditeur/Médecine et Hygiène, Geneva, 2003.

[DRO 92] DROUX J., "Personnel soignant et médicalisation de l'hôpital : les liaisons fiévreuses", in WALTER F. (ed.), *Peu lire, beaucoup voir, beaucoup faire, pour une histoire des soins infirmiers au XIXe siècle*, Zoé, Geneva, 1992.

[DUB 88] DUBY G., *Seigneurs et paysans. Hommes et structures du Moyen Âge*, Flammarion, Paris, 1988.

[DUB 05] DUBAR C., TRIPIER P., *Sociologie des professions*, 2nd ed., Armand Colin, Paris, 2005.

[DUC 02] DUCHARME F., "Les soins infirmiers et la recherche : perspectives au seuil du troisième millénaire", in GOULET O., DALLAIRE C. (eds), *Les soins infirmiers, vers de nouvelles perspectives*, Gaëtan Morin, Boucherville, 2002.

[EHR 15] EHRENREICH B., ENGLISH D., *Sorcières, sages-femmes & infirmières*, Cambourakis, Paris, 2015.

[FAB 13] FABIANI J.-L., "Vers la fin du modèle disciplinaire ?", *Hermès 67, la revue, Interdisciplinarité : entre disciplines et indiscipline*, 2013.

[FIN 89] FINGER M., "Apprentissage expérientiel ou formation par les expériences de vie ?", *Éducation permanente*, nos 100–101, pp. 38–46, 1989.

[FON 40-96] FONDS DE L'HÔPITAL DES BOURGEOIS, Livre des sentences, Urteil Buch, Serment du médecin à l'hôpital 1790, Document, Archives de l'État de Fribourg, pp. 180–181, 12 August 1740–10 October 1796.

[FON 44] FONDS DE L'HÔPITAL NOTRE-DAME, Règlement pour la direction de l'hôpital général de Genève, Document, Archives de l'État de Fribourg (AEF), 1744.

[FON 59-62] FONDS DE L'HÔPITAL NOTRE-DAME, Manuel de la Chambre de l'hôpital, Archives de l'État de Fribourg, 17 May 1759–31 May 1762.

[FON 61-74] FONDS DE L'HÔPITAL NOTRE-DAME, Manuel de la Chambre de l'Hôpital, Archives de l'État de Fribourg, 12 July 1761–23 June 1774.

[FON 71-82] FONDS DE L'HÔPITAL NOTRE-DAME, Manuel de la Chambre de l'Hôpital, Archives de l'État de Fribourg, 4 August 1771–14 April 1782.

[FON 84] FONDS DE L'HÔPITAL NOTRE- DAME, Règles des Religieuses hospitalières sous le titre de Notre-Dame de sept douleurs pour le Grand Hôpital de Fribourg en Suisse, Document, Archives de l'État de Fribourg, 1784.

[FOU 66] FOUCAULT M., *Les mots et les choses*, Gallimard, Paris, 1966.

[FOU 69] FOUCAULT M., *L'archéologie du savoir*, Gallimard, Paris, 1969.

[FOU 72] FOUCAULT M., *L'histoire de la folie à l'âge classique*, Gallimard, Paris, 1972.

[FOU 88] FOUCAULT M., *Naissance de la clinique*, Presses universitaires de France, Paris, 1988.

[FRA 94] FRANCILLON D. (ed.), *Valérie de Gasparin, une conservatrice révolutionnaire*, École La Source/Ouverture, Lausanne/Le Mont-sur-Lausanne, 1994.

[FRA 09] FRANCILLON D., *150 ans d'histoire 1859/2009. La Source en images*, La Source, Lausanne, 2009.

[GAI 09] GAINCHARD B., Remboursement partiel des soins : quel statut politique pour les soins dans l'assurance maladie ?, Research report, Research and Development Unit, Haute école de santé La Source, 2009.

[GÉL 88] GÉLIS J., "Préface", *Cahier de l'AMIEC – Pour une histoire des soins et des professions soignantes*, no. 10, pp. 13–16, 1988.

[GHA 99] GHANEM-NADOT N., Les supports écrits dans la formation du personnel soignant, extraction, réduction et reproduction des écrits : un processus de domination culturelle en trois actes, Undergraduate thesis, Université de Genève, 1999.

[GOD 84] GODEFROY F., *Dictionnaire de l'ancienne langue française et de tous ses dialectes du IXe au XVe siècle*, vols III and IX, Vieweg F. éd., Paris, 1884.

[GRO 99] GROSJEAN M., LACOSTE M., *Communication et intelligence collective, le travail à l'hôpital*, Presses universitaires de France, Paris, 1999.

[HOM 12] HOMERIN M.-P., *La discipline infirmière dans le champ scientifique. Visibilité et lisibilité d'un savoir professionnel*, De Boeck/Estem, Paris, 2012.

[IMB 47] IMBERT J., *Les hôpitaux en droit canonique*, Librairie philosophique Vrin, Paris, 1947.

[JOB 85] JOBERT G., "Processus de professionnalisation et production du savoir", *Éducation permanente*, no. 80, pp. 125–145, September1985.

[KED 05] KEDDY B., DODD D., "Les infirmières en service privé et les infirmières de l'Ordre de Victoria (1900-1950)", in BATES C., DODD D., ROUSSEAU N. (eds), *Sans frontières, quatre siècles de soins infirmiers canadiens*, Presses de l'Université, Ottawa, 2005.

[KFH 05] KFH, Recherche et Développement dans les hautes écoles spécialisées, Document de référence, Conférence suisse des hautes écoles spécialisées (HES – KFH), 21 September 2005.

[KIE 19] KIEFER B., "La crise du discours médical", *Revue médicale suisse*, no. 640, p. 516, February 2019.

[KLE 13] KLEINPETTER E., "Taxonomie critique de l'interdisciplinarité", *Hermès 67, la revue, Interdisciplinarité : entre disciplines et indiscipline*, 2013.

[KNI 83] KNIBIEHLER Y., FOUQUET C., *La femme et les médecins*, Hachette, Paris, 1983.

[KNI 84] KNIBIEHLER Y., *Cornettes et blouses blanches, les infirmières dans la société française 1880-1980*, Hachette, Paris, 1984.

[KRA 95] KRAFFT C., La Source, École normale de gardes-malades de Lausanne, Rapports du directeur et du trésorier sur l'année 1894, Imprimerie L. Vincent, Lausanne, 1895.

[KRA 00] KRAFFT C., La Source, École normale de garde-malades de Lausanne, Rapports du directeur et du trésorier sur l'année 1899, Imprimerie L. Vincent, Lausanne, 1900.

[KRA 01] KRAFFT C., La source, École normale de garde-malades de Lausanne, Rapports du directeur et du trésorier sur l'année 1900, Imprimerie L. Vincent, Lausanne, 1901.

[KRA 07] KRAFFT C., *Thérapeutique à l'usage de la garde malade*, Imprimerie Georges Bridel, Lausanne, 1907.

[KRE 32] KREBS-JAPY Y., *Florence Nightingale, sa vie et son œuvre*, Poinat éditeur, Paris, 1932.

[KUH 96] KUHN T.S., *The Structure of Scientific Revolutions*, University of Chicago Press, Chicago, 1996.

[LAC 01] LACOSTE M., "Peut-on travailler sans communiquer ?", in BORZEIX A., FRAENKEL B. (eds), *Langage et travail, communication, cognition, action*, CNRS, Paris, 2001.

[LAN 84] LANGLOIS C., *Le catholicisme au féminin, les congrégations françaises à supérieure générale au XIXe siècle*, Les éditions du Cerf, Paris, 1984.

[LAR 91] LARCHET J.-C., *Théologie de la maladie*, Les éditions du Cerf, Paris, 1991.

[LEB 18] LE BOULER S., Mission Universitarisation des formations paramédicales et de maïeutique, bilan intermédiaire de la concertation et propositions d'orientation, Rapport à Madame la ministre des Solidarités et de la Santé et à Madame la ministre de l'Enseignement supérieur, de la Recherche et de l'Innovation, Paris, 2018.

[LER 92] LEROUX-HUGON V., "Quelles infirmières pour l'Assistance Publique ? Les ambiguïtés d'un projet politique à travers le Progrès médical (1873-1914)", in WALTER F. (ed.), *Peu lire, beaucoup voir, beaucoup faire, pour une histoire des soins infirmiers au XIXe siècle*, Zoé, Geneva, 1992.

[LES 85] LESCAZE B., "Pouvoirs publics, charités privées. L'hôpital dans la cité au XVIe siècle", in LESCAZE B. (ed.), *Sauver l'âme, nourrir le corps, de l'hôpital général à l'hospice général de Genève, 1535-1985*, Hospice général et Bernard Lescaze, Geneva, 1985.

[LÉV 13] LÉVY-LEBLOND J.-M., "Éloge de la discipline", *Hermès 67, la revue, Interdisciplinarité : entre disciplines et indiscipline*, 2013.

[LOI 07] LOISELLE C.-G., PROFETTO-MCGRATH J., POLIT D.F. *et al.*, *Méthodes de recherche en sciences infirmières, approches quantitatives et qualitatives*, Éditions du Renouveau pédagogique, Saint-Laurent, 2007.

[LOU 83] LOUX F., *Traditions et soins d'aujourd'hui*, InterÉditions, Paris, 1983.

[LOU 85] LOUIS-COURVOISIER M., "L'Hôpital général et ses assistés (1585-1555), L'Hôpital, ses responsables et ses pensionnaires", in LESCAZE B. (ed.), *Sauver l'âme, nourrir le corps, de l'hôpital général à l'hospice général de Genève, 1535-1985*, Hospice général et Bernard Lescaze, Geneva, 1985.

[LOU 00] LOUIS-COURVOISIER M., *Soigner et consoler, la vie quotidienne dans un hôpital à la fin de l'Ancien Régime, Genève 1750-1820*, Georg éditeur/Médecine et Hygiène, Geneva, 2000.

[MAG 88a] MAGNON R., "Propos sur la bibliographie des manuels, livres ou traités destinés à l'enseignement des soins donnés aux malades", *Cahier de l'AMIEC – Pour une histoire des soins et des professions soignantes*, no. 10, pp. 257–264, 1988.

[MAG 88b] MAGNON R., "Entre le sabre, le Goupillon et la Faculté", *Cahier de l'AMIEC – Pour une histoire des soins et des professions soignantes*, no. 10, pp. 49–60, 1988.

[MAR 54] MARROU H.-I., *De la connaissance historique*, Le Seuil, Paris, 1954.

[MAT 96] MATHY P., Les choix épistémologiques, les idéologies et les valeurs dans les manuels de biologie : production d'instruments d'analyse pour la formation des enseignants, PhD thesis, Université de Genève, 1996.

[MCP 05] MCPHERSON K., "L'influence de Florence Nightingale dans l'essor de l'hôpital moderne", in BATES C., DODD D., ROUSSEAU N. (eds), *Sans frontières, quatre siècles de soins infirmiers canadiens*, Presses de l'Université, Ottawa, 2005.

[MOR 34] MORIN J., *Manuel théorique et pratique des gardes-malades, et des personnes qui veulent se soigner elles-mêmes, ou l'ami de la santé*, Roret Libraire, Paris, 1834.

[MOR 86] MORIN E., *La méthode 3, la connaissance de la connaissance*, Le Seuil, Paris, 1986.

[MOR 91] MOREAU C., "L'infirmière, d'abord une hospitalière", *Revue de l'infirmière*, no. 2, pp. 21–23, 1991.

[MOR 92] MOREL P., Les diaconesses vaudoises dans la tourmente, les attaques de la Comtesse Valérie de Gasparin contre les diaconesses vaudoises, Undergraduate thesis, Université de Lausanne, 1992.

[MOR 14] MOREILLON S., "Valérie de Gasparin : une chrétienne contestataire", *Le temps*, 15 July 2014.

[MOS 05] MOSER M.-H., "L'hôpital Notre-Dame de Lausanne", in JOMINI M., MOSER M.-H., ROD Y. (eds), *Les hôpitaux vaudois au Moyen Âge, Lausanne, Lutry, Yverdon, Cahiers lausannois d'histoire médiévale*, Faculté des lettres de l'Université, Lausanne, 2005.

[MÜT 94] MÜTZENBERG G., "Portrait et destinée", in FRANCILLON D. (ed.), *Valérie de Gasparin, une conservatrice révolutionnaire*, École La Source/ Ouverture, Lausanne/Le Mont-sur-Lausanne, 1994.

[NAD 83] NADOT M., De moniteur à enseignant, Diploma thesis, Université Lyon II, 1983.

[NAD 90] NADOT M., "En quoi les soins infirmiers sont-ils infirmiers ?", *Krankenpflege/Soins infirmiers*, no. 10, pp. 15–19, 1990.

[NAD 92] NADOT M., "Une médiologie de la santé comme science", *Recherche en soins infirmiers*, no. 30, pp. 27–36, September 1992.

[NAD 93] NADOT M., Des médiologues de santé à Fribourg, Histoire et épistémologie d'une science soignante non médicale, PhD thesis, Université Lyon II, 1993.

[NAD 02a] NADOT M., "Médiologie de la santé, de la tradition soignante à l'identité de la discipline", *Perspective soignante*, no. 13, April 2002.

[NAD 02b] NADOT M. *et al.*, Rapport de recherche au Fonds national Suisse de la recherche scientifique (FNS), project N° DO-RE 01008 and CTI 5545 FHS, Mesure des prestations soignantes dans le système de santé, Report, Unité de recherche et de développement – Haute école de santé de Fribourg, 2002.

[NAD 03a] NADOT M., "Les soins infirmiers, ça n'existe pas !", *La revue de l'encadrement et de la formation, Soins Cadres*, no. 46, pp. 59–62, May 2003.

[NAD 03b] NADOT M., "Mesure des prestations soignantes dans le système de santé", *Recherche en soins infirmiers*, no. 73, pp. 116–122, June 2003.

[NAD 07] NADOT M., "Leviers et obstacles à l'activité du chercheur en sciences infirmières", *La revue de référence infirmière, Soins*, no. 717, pp. 37–40, July-August 2007.

[NAD 08] NADOT M., "La fin d'une mythologie et le modèle d'intermédiaire culturel", in DALLAIRE C. (ed.), *Le savoir infirmier, au coeur de la discipline et de la profession*, Gaëtan Morin, Montreal, 2008.

[NAD 10] NADOT M., La recherche en Suisse", *Recherche en soins infirmiers*, no. 100, pp. 94–100, March 2010.

[NAD 12a] NADOT M., "La recherche fondamentale en science infirmière, La recherche historique sur les fondements de la discipline", *Recherche en soins infirmiers*, no. 109, pp. 57–68, June 2012.

[NAD 12b] NADOT M., *Le mythe infirmier ou le pavé dans la mare !*, L'Harmattan, Paris, 2012.

[NAD 13] NADOT M., BUSSET F., GROSS J., *L'activité infirmière, le modèle d'intermédiaire culturel, une réalité incontournable*, De Boeck/Estem, Paris, 2013.

[NAD 14] NADOT M., "L'enseignement des sciences infirmières : une discipline inaudible à géométrie variable", *Recherche en soins infirmiers*, no. 119, pp. 75–84, December 2014.

[NIQ 21] NIQUILLE J., L'Hôpital Notre-Dame à Fribourg, PhD thesis, Université de Fribourg, 1921.

[NOI 18] NOIRIEL G., *Une histoire populaire de la France de la guerre de Cent Ans à nos jours*, Agone, Marseille, 2018.

[PEL 07] PELLETIER F., L'activité infirmière dans deux groupes de médecine de famille (GMF) de la région de Québec, Master's thesis, Faculté des sciences infirmières de l'université Laval, 2007.

[PÉP 08] PÉPIN J., "L'évolution du savoir infirmier au Québec", in DALLAIRE C. (ed.), *Le savoir infirmier, au cœur de la discipline et de la profession*, Gaëtan Morin, Montreal, 2008.

[PÉP 10] PÉPIN J., DUCHARME F., KÉROUAC S., *La pensée infirmière*, 3rd ed., Chenelière éducation, Montreal, 2010.

[PÉP 15] PÉPIN J., LARUE C., ALLARD E. *et al.*, *La discipline infirmière, une contribution décisive aux enjeux de santé*, Centre d'innovation en formation infirmière de la faculté des sciences infirmières de l'université de Montréal et SIDIIEF, Montreal, 2015.

[PÉP 17] PÉPIN J., DUCHARME F., KÉROUAC S., *La pensée infirmière*, 4th ed., Chenelière éducation, Montreal, 2017.

[POI 12] POISSON M., "Infirmières, enseignantes et pionnières : le personnel infirmier dirigeant et enseignant permanent à l'ouverture de l'École internationale d'enseignement infirmier supérieur de Lyon en 1965", *Recherche en soins infirmiers*, no. 109, pp. 69–92, June 2012.

[POL 78] POLETTI R., *Les soins infirmiers, théories et concepts*, Le Centurion, Paris, 1978.

[POP 85] POPPER K., *Conjectures and Refutations: The Growth of Scientific Knowledge*, Payot, Paris, 1985.

[POP 94] POPPER K., *Objective Knowledge: An Evolutionary Approach*, Oxford University Press, Oxford, 1994.

[PRO 02] PROVENCHER H., FAWCETT J., "Les sciences infirmières : une structure épistémologique", in GOULET O., DALLAIRE C. (eds), *Les soins infirmiers, vers de nouvelles perspectives*, Gaëtan Morin, Boucherville, 2002.

[RAM 16] RAMELET A.-S., Rapport d'activité, Institut universitaire de formation et de recherche en soins (IUFRS), Report, Université de Lausanne – Faculty of biology and medecine, 2016.

[REY 92] REY A., *Dictionnaire historique de la langue française*, Dictionnaire Le Robert, Paris, 1992.

[RIC 61] RICHELET, *Dictionnaire portatif de la langue françoise. Extrait du grand dictionnaire de Richelet*, Bruyset Imprimeur Libraire, Lyon, 1761.

[RIC 86] RICŒUR P., *Du texte à l'action, essais d'herméneutique, II*, Le Seuil, Paris, 1986.

[RIC 88] RICŒUR P., *Philosophie de la volonté, vol 1, Le volontaire et l'involontaire ; vol 2, Finitude et culpabilité*, Aubier, Paris, 1988.

[ROC 68] ROCHER G., *Introduction à la sociologie*, vol. I, HMH Ltée, Paris, 1968.

[ROD 05] ROD Y., "L'hôpital d'Yverdon", in JOMINI M., MOSER M.-H., ROD Y. (eds), *Les hôpitaux vaudois au Moyen Âge, Lausanne, Lutry, Yverdon, Cahiers lausannois d'histoire médiévale*, Faculté des lettres de l'Université, Lausanne, 2005.

[ROU 97] ROUSSEAU N., "De la vocation à la discipline", *Infirmière canadienne*, pp. 39–44, May 1997.

[ROU 08] ROUSSEAU N., "Sacrifier l'autonomie pour obtenir la profession : les choix des élites infirmières à travers l'histoire et leurs conséquences", in DALLAIRE C. (ed.), *Le savoir infirmier, au cœur de la discipline et de la profession*, Gaëtan Morin, Montreal, 2008.

[SAI 56] SAINTE PALAYE J.B.C., *Dictionnaire historique de l'Ancien langage François depuis son origine jusqu'au siècle de Louis XIV*, vol. 5, L. Favre, Niort, 1756.

[SAI 85] SAINSAULIEU R., *L'identité au travail*, Presses de la Fondation nationale des sciences politiques, Paris, 1985.

[SEY 33] SEYMER L.R., *L'infirmière à travers les âges*, Éditions de l'œuvre nationale de l'enfance, Brussels, 1933.

[SID 11] SIDIIEF, La formation universitaire des infirmières et infirmiers, une réponse aux défis des systèmes de santé, Document, SIDIIEF, 2011.

[SIN 08] SINOUÉ G., *La Dame à la lampe, une vie de Florence Nightingale*, Gallimard, Paris, 2008.

[SMI 92] SMITH A., "Madame Agénor de Gasparin ou les délices de la chaire", *Romantisme, Les femmes et le bonheur d'écrire*, no. 77, pp. 47–54, 1992.

[TAI 18] TAILLENS F., Interview avec Gilles Lugrin, Directeur de l'IUFRS, le système de santé suisse a besoin de nouveaux rôles", *Krankenpflege, Soins infirmiers, Cure infermieristiche*, pp. 58–59, September 2018.

[TAN 15] TANNER J., LAMBERCY L., *Mes yeux n'étaient pas assez grands pour voir, voyage au Levant, 1747-1748*, Éditions d'en bas, Lausanne, 2015.

[TEY 93] TEYSSEIRE D., "Présentation", in S. TISSOT (ed.), *Avis au Peuple sur sa santé*, Edima, Paris, 1993.

[THO 83] THOM R., *Paraboles et catastrophes, entretiens sur les mathématiques, la science et la philosophie*, Flammarion, Paris, 1983.

[TUR 89] TURIN Y., *Femmes et religieuses au XIXe siècle*, Nouvelle Cité, Paris, 1989.

[VAL 91] VALSANGIACOMO E., *La Croix et la carrière, la Croix-Rouge suisse et l'histoire des infirmières*, Schwabe & Co AG, Basel, 1991.

[VIL 33] Ville de Romont, Revue des règlements souverains servant de règle, d'économie, de police et de subordination pour la Noble ville de Romont (Original des statuts), Document, Archives de la ville de Romont, 1733.

[VIN 42] VINCENT J., *Aux écoutes de la souffrance. Histoire de l'Institution des diaconesses de Saint-Loup 1842-1942*, La Concorde, Lausanne, 1942.

[VIN 95] VINCK D., *Sociologie des sciences*, Armand Colin, Paris, 1995.

[VIN 00] VINCK D., *Pratiques de l'interdisciplinarité, mutations des sciences, de l'industrie et de l'enseignement*, Presses universitaires de Grenoble, Grenoble, 2000.

[VIO 05] VIOLETTE B., "Guérir le corps et sauver l'âme : les religieuses hospitalières et les premiers hôpitaux catholiques au Québec (1639-1880)", in BATES C., DODD D., ROUSSEAU N. (eds), *Sans frontières, quatre siècles de soins infirmiers canadiens*, Presses de l'Université, Ottawa, 2005.

[WAL 94] WALTER F., *La Suisse urbaine 1750-1950*, Zoé, Geneva, 1994.

[WYN 99] WYNNE B., "Une approche réflexive du partage entre savoir expert et savoir profane", *Les cahiers de la sécurité intérieure*, no. 38, pp. 219–236, 1999.

[YOU 05] YOUNG J., ROUSSEAU N., "Le nursing laïc de l'époque de la Nouvelle-France à la fin du XIXe siècle (1608-1891)", in BATES C., DODD D., ROUSSEAU N. (eds), *Sans frontières, quatre siècles de soins infirmiers canadiens*, Presses de l'université, Ottawa, 2005.

[ZIN 14] ZINN H., *Une histoire populaire des États-Unis, de 1492 à nos jours*, Agone, Marseille, 2014.

[ZUM 85] ZUMKELLER D., "Les domaines ruraux de l'Hôpital général de Genève au 18e siècle", in LESCAZE B. (ed.), *Sauver l'Âme et nourrir le corps, de l'Hôpital Général à l'Hospice Général de Genève, 1535-1985*, Hospice Général, Geneva, 1985.

Index

H, I, J

K, L, M

N, O, P, R

Other titles from

iSTE

in

Health Engineering and Society

2020

BARBET Jacques, FOUCQUIER Adrien, THOMAS Yves
Therapeutic Progress in Oncology: Towards a Revolution in Cancer Therapy?
(Health and Patients Set – Volume 2)

PAILLIART Isabelle
New Territories in Health
(Health Information Set – Volume 3)

2019

CLAVIER Viviane, DE OLIVEIRA Jean-Philippe
Food and Health: Actor Strategies in Information and Communication
(Health Information Set – Volume 2)

PIZON Frank
Health Education and Prevention
(Health and Patients Set – Volume 1)

2018

HUARD Pierre
The Management of Chronic Diseases: Organizational Innovation and Efficiency

PAGANELLI Céline
Confidence and Legitimacy in Health Information and Communication (Health Information Set – Volume 1)

2017

PICARD Robert
Co-design in Living Labs for Healthcare and Independent Living: Concepts, Methods and Tools

2015

BÉRANGER Jérôme
Medical Information Systems Ethics

Printed and bound by CPI Group (UK) Ltd, Croydon, CR0 4YY
16/09/2026
14963077-0005